Early
Language
Intervention

An Introduction

Linda McCormick
University of Hawaii

and

Richard L. Schiefelbusch
University of Kansas

Charles E. Merrill Publishing Company
A Bell & Howell Company
Columbus Toronto London Sydney

Published by
Charles E. Merrill Publishing Co.
A Bell & Howell Company
Columbus, Ohio 43216

This book was set in Korinna.
Cover Designer: Tony Faiola.
Production Editor: Jeffrey Putnam.

Cover photograph by Austin Wolff.

Library of Congress Catalog Card Number: 83–42997
International Standard Book Number: 0–675–20091–1

Printed in the United States of America

2 3 4 5 6 7 8 9 10—88 87 86 85

To Kelli, Mark, and Cami McCormick

Contents

Preface

I n planning the contents of this book, we have aimed at a synthesis of
theoretical and applied information. Our purpose is two-fold: to introduce prospective teachers and communication specialists to normal
and deficient or delayed language and communication development
and to present a sampling of the programs, materials, and procedures
available for teaching language. We focus primarily on the language and
communication deficits and programming needs of children functioning
within the developmental range from birth to mental age four for two reasons. The first reason arises from our functional training bias: an understanding of basic skill development is critical for students preparing to
work with severely and profoundly handicapped students, high-risk infants, and preschool populations. The second reason is conceptual: there
is a rich array of factual information relevant to this developmental range
that has not been brought together in a form that teachers and clinicians
can use.

This book is designed to be an introductory text: it assumes no specific prior knowledge about language and communication concepts. An
effort has been made to give readers some sense of the depth and breadth
of basic research in such fields as linguistics, psycholinguistics, sociolinguistics, psychology, speech/language/pathology, special education, and
anthropology, but our main purpose is to familiarize preservice professionals with the language/communication assessment and intervention procedures these disciplines have generated in the past decades. It is important for future practitioners to be aware that the production of valuable
training-relevant information is not limited to a single discipline. Each of
the above fields has contributed enormous volumes of empirical data. The
problem has been locating and synthesizing these data. Because each
discipline reports its findings in separate, and often very technical journals,
teachers and language communication specialists are either unable to locate the data or they lack the theoretical background and vocabulary to
understand and translate potentially valuable theoretical data into practice
(or both). We have tried to avoid this interpretation/translation problem by
keeping technical terminology at a minimum and defining essential terms
and constructs. Further, to avoid confusing beginning students we have
narrowed the content to areas where there seems to be general consensus

rather than controversy. We have deliberately tried to present clear and concise intervention/relevant information in a scholarly manner.

It is our sincere hope that all students will share our excitement and sense of wonder about the most miraculous of accomplishments—learning language—when they finish reading this text. We want this book to stimulate so much interest and curiosity that readers will rush to their bookstores and libraries for more theoretical and comprehensive volumes. More importantly, we hope students will seek out infants and young children to observe and listen to, in every possible context. Ultimately, they are our best teachers: children themselves are the only real and valid source of information about child language learning.

Even though each chapter in this text can stand alone and be read and understood without reference to other chapters there is a definite logical and procedural sequence to the content and a continuity between chapters. Overall the flow is from past to present to future. The intent of the first chapter is to provide some theoretical background, familiarity with the terminology and historical perspectives. The basic assumptions and implications of the interactionist perspective are introduced in this chapter. This viewpoint, which holds that nature-nurture, adult-child, and environment-organism interactions are the key contributors and facilitators of language learning, provides the book's unifying theme. The second chapter provides an overview of normal language learning from birth to age four with special attention to the environmental variables which contribute to normal language learning. Chapter Three provides some data regarding the language and communication characteristics of subgroups of children within the larger population of atypical learners and language users. Further, it proposes an alternative, program-relevant classification system derived from the interactionist perspective. Chapters Four through Six are the core of the book. They lead readers through the problem-solving and decision-making aspects of assessment, planning service delivery and evaluation. Chapters Seven through Nine are provided to complement and broaden the reader's perspective of the *application* of procedures presented in the three previous chapters. Each presents an exemplary program model for a different child population. Chapter Ten provides an overview of augmentative communication systems and the decisions pursuant to introduction of alternative communication strategies. Chapter Eleven deals with support interactions—the professional-professional and professional-parent networks so critical to successful intervention in any area. The book culminates with an overview of the "state-of-the-art" and suggestions for bridging the gap between "real" and "ideal."

Numerous colleagues and students assisted and supported our writing efforts. Chief among these were Joy McGehee, Luanna Voeltz, and Rick Hoogs at the University of Hawaii. The first author is especially grateful to Faye Yamamoto for her patience in locating, listing, and checking references, and to Gayle Tsukada for typing of early drafts. In addition, many graduate students in the Special Education Department of the University of Hawaii provided valuable feedback, suggestions, and encouragement.

The authors would like also to thank Ms. Marianne Taflinger of Charles Merrill for her efficient guidance and encouragement. The contributions of Ms. Marilyn Fischer have been varied and critical to the project at all stages. Together with Mr. Robert Hoyt, Ms. Mary Beth Johnston and Ms. Thelma Dillon, also of the Bureau of Child Research, University of Kansas, she has contributed generously to the final manuscript.

We thank our reviewers, whose comments helped us write more clearly and effectively: Robert L. Carpenter of the University of Washington; Gerald Mahoney of the University of Michigan; George Karlan of Purdue University; and Barbara Culatta of the University of Kentucky. We especially thank Ann Rogers Warren of Vanderbilt University and Katherine Butler of Syracuse University, who read the entire manuscript.

The planning and the execution of this book has been lengthy but exhilarating. We hope that its readers will share in the excitement we experienced in attempting to capture, not only the most pertinent and useful information currently available, but also in possible future designs for assisting handicapped children to develop functional language.

CHAPTER ONE

AN INTRODUCTION TO LANGUAGE INTERVENTION

Linda McCormick and Richard L. Schiefelbusch

You have an excellent command of the English language. You have no problem selecting the precise words and sentences that signal the meanings you wish to express, and you are skilled in using language for appropriate and effective interactions. Because language seems automatic, you probably have little idea of how you learned it or of the extent of the knowledge underlying your competence. You do not consider speaking and understanding as particularly complex or mysterious because as Chomsky (1972) points out, "We lose sight of the need for explanation when phenomena are too familiar and 'obvious'" (p. 25).

Although you may take your own language competence for granted, you recognize how important it is to your social life and your professional career. Language is the skill your parents were most concerned for you to acquire because they recognized that, in addition to its central role in the transmission of knowledge, language has a profound effect on social, academic and vocational opportunities. Language may be the most distinctive attribute of human beings; its acquisition is an integral part of human development. It is not surprising that how language is learned and taught are major issues in education and other human service fields.

In confronting these issues, we must acknowledge that language is complex and enigmatic. Consider the fact that even though computers can be programmed to play chess, to fly airplanes, and to analyze huge banks of statistical data, we have not been able to program them to simulate the generative nature of human language. This gives you some idea of why the challenges of language assessment and intervention are so formidable. Most teachers and communication specialists will readily corroborate this perception, as well as the urgent need for research results that they can translate into curriculum. Front line personnel working with severely and profoundly mentally retarded children indicate that communication skills is the curriculum area where information is most desperately needed (Lynch, Shoemaker, & White, 1976; Maurer, Wehman & Reichle,

1977). It may also be the area where relevant information is most obscure to the practitioner.

Informed decisions are, by definition, data-based decisions (Miller, 1978). Regardless of whether you hold to developmental biases, a basic understanding of the nature of language and normal language acquisition is critical to informed decision making in the area of language intervention. Both developmental and applied published research assume that readers have substantial background knowledge about language. Without it, this important literature is almost impregnable.

Informed decisions require a basic understanding of what language is, and how it is acquired.

A certain amount of theoretical background and familiarity with the terminology is necessary to understand and integrate the research literature. Every discipline studying language (linguistics, psycholinguistics, sociolinguistics, psychology, special education, speech/language pathology) has its own traditions, terms, methods, priorities, and biases related to language and language intervention. Their books and journals reflect this diversity. The unfortunate consequence for teachers and language specialists is greater than usual difficulty in translating language and communication theories and research results into curriculum content, materials, and procedures.

The goal of this book is to bridge the research-application span, to disseminate and translate language constructs, terms and practical techniques for assessment and remediation. Specifically, the book focuses on the language problems of children who are functioning below the 4-year normative level. This population includes most children served by infant programs, early childhood handicapped services, and classes for the severely and profoundly handicapped. A single volume could not address all issues related to language training for these youngsters, but one book can provide enough background to introduce you to this exciting field and suggest sources for additional study.

This book focuses on language and communication skills normally acquired by age 4.

This chapter explains key terms and constructs and provides some historical background and perspectives on language development. Views about the products and processes of language acquisition have changed over the past two decades, and they may change even more in this decade. A full account of this evolution would require considerably more space than we are willing to commit to historical chronology; only a brief overview of five major theoretical perspectives on language acquisition, with some advantages and limitations of each, is presented. The fifth and most recent—the interactionist position—reflects our own theoretical orientation, which is further expanded in subsequent chapters.

IMPORTANT TERMS AND CONSTRUCTS

You may have encountered and used many of the following terms. However, the way they are used in the language development and intervention literature may be confusing unless you understand the literal definitions. The constructs presented in this section are a small subset of those you will encounter in the relevant literature. Other terms are defined in context throughout the book.

Language is defined by Bloom and Lahey (1978) as "knowledge of a code for representing ideas about the world through a conventional system of arbitrary signals for communication" (p. 4). The term **signal** in this definition can refer to movements (as in manual communication), as well as to words. Speech and communication are not synonyms for language. Each of the three terms has a different and distinct meaning, and there are practical, as well as theoretical reasons, for maintaining a precise distinction among these terms.

The terms *speech, language,* and *communication* are not synonymous.

Language is only one of a number of ways to communicate. It is a code, an abstract system with rules governing the sequencing of its basic units (sounds or signs and words) and rules governing meaning and use. These rules underlie both understanding (decoding) and production (encoding) but they are usually "known" only in the sense that they are applied. Children give evidence of "knowing" many of these rules at a very early age. One of the important questions in the study of child language is precisely how this important rule learning occurs.

The most important points to remember about language rules are: (a) they are socially acquired, (b) they are basically covert (not directly observable), and (c) they specify how to arrange symbols to express ideas. The rules of language are of great importance, but they are only a part of the picture. By the time you finish reading this chapter and the next one, you will realize that viewing language only in terms of its rules (structural characteristics) is comparable to describing the anatomy or physiology of the human body without reference to how the various parts function and relate to one another.

Speech is one of many possible vehicles for language. Other vehicles include manual signing, gesturing, written symbols, pictures, diagrams, and even body postures and facial expressions. Speech is an overt, observable motor behavior which is heavily dependent upon physiological and neuromuscular coordination. Compared to other ways of conveying ideas and intentions, speech is probably the most difficult. Speech production requires precise coordination of **respiration** (the act of breathing), **phonation** (the production of sound by the larynx and vocal folds), **resonance** (the vibratory response which controls the quality of the sound wave), and **articulation** (the use of the lips, tongue, teeth, and hard and soft palates to form speech sounds).

Communication is the interchange of ideas or information. More general than the other two terms, it includes the encoding of a message to stimulate meaning in the mind of another, and the accurate decoding of the intended meanings of others. The defining characteristic of communication is that it entails an exchange of ideas and intentions.

Some scholars (e.g., Goffman, 1969) have suggested that an individual's ability to communicate and his ability to function in society are closely related. Being a competent communicator entails substantially more than producing and understanding language (Hymes, 1971). It involves knowledge of social and cultural conventions such as conversational turn-taking, forms of address, standard verbal routines, and sufficient motivation to apply this knowledge. Some form of communication takes place at all levels of the phylogenetic scale, from the amoeba to man. There is some evidence that, not only can members of the same species communicate with each other, they can communicate with other species as well (Menzel, 1969). Animal communications do not employ language, but animals generally achieve desired results. Few people misinterpret a dog's intentions when it growls at the postman, whines and scratches at the door, or barks and leaps about when it sees a favorite person.

Linguistics is the scientific study of language. Formal linguists attempt to take language apart in much the same way as a mechanic takes an engine apart. Unlike mechanics, however, who are then concerned with reassembling the engine, linguists are most concerned with describing the parts of language and how they work. Linguists also study language as an area of anthropology or cultural history.

Linguistics, psycholinguistics and sociolinguistics are separate knowledge domains.

Psycholinguistics is the study of language acquisition, general language behavior, and underlying psychological mechanisms. Psycholinguists study language differences and the relationships between language and thinking. In particular, they are concerned with how language influences, and is influenced by, memory, attention, and perception.

Sociolinguistics is the study of how language varies in relation to social situations and cultures. Sociolinguists are concerned with describing the knowledge that underlies socially appropriate verbal behavior and the way language is acquired and used in social contexts. The recent research on pragmatic functions (how language is used) has come from these professionals who study children's experiences in different social contexts.

Grammars are theories—systems of rules—that attempt to describe how language works. A grammar represents a hypothesis about the organization of language in the mind of speakers of that language. It is essentially a guess about the mental plan (underlying knowledge about language) people use when they produce and understand sentences. No one has yet succeeded in writing a grammar capable of describing the English language (or any other language), though many have tried. If a grammar is ever formulated, it will have to account for at least five sets of operations: semantic, syntactic, morphological, phonological and pragmatic processes. (Each of these operations is described below.)

There are two uses of the term *grammar.*

Use of the term grammar as an explicit description of the tacit knowledge underlying language differs from the more common, but restricted, use of the term to refer to linguistic etiquette. When someone says, "He doesn't use good grammar," the person is usually judging a speaker's utterances in a morphological and/or syntactic sense. Used in this narrower sense, the term means language usage rather than the mental plan and internal operating principles.

Semantics is the study of language meaning and how it is acquired. The semantic component of language includes meanings as well as rules for linking meaning with words and word sequences (phrases and sentences). Speakers create and understand language by applying semantic rules in some complex way that is not clearly understood. (The discussion of language content in this chapter will explain more about semantics and semantic development.)

Semantics is particularly concerned with the relationships between language and knowledge of the real world of objects and events. Until fairly recently it was considered the domain of philosophers rather than linguists.

The most important point to remember about language meaning is that words do not represent things per se; they represent ideas about things. Words and combinations of words represent what people know about the world they live in. They have no meaning in themselves. Words and sentences are elements of a code in some ways similar to a picture, map, or graph, but more abstract. Words are arbitrary because they do not reproduce (except in the case of onomatopoetic words), but instead represent objects, events, and relationships.

Semantic knowledge is a subset of cognitive knowledge.

The difference between semantic knowledge and cognitive knowledge is subtle, but very important. Semantic knowledge can be thought of as a subset of cognitive knowledge. The structure we give to our experiences as we organize them into perceptually and/or functionally equivalent categories and somehow relate these concepts to each other, is cognitive knowledge (Wells, 1974). Cognitive knowledge cannot properly be labeled semantic knowledge until the concepts become linked to language (Bowerman, 1976). When a concept about the world (nonlinguistic knowledge formed through experiences with objects, actions and relationships) is properly linked to a word or sequence of words, it has semantic meaning. For example, when a child says "doggie" for all four-legged animals, we can say she has a concept for animals (though it does not resemble that of an adult), but she does not have a semantic concept for dogs. The cognitive knowledge is not yet linked properly to language.

The organization of conceptual and linguistic classifications (cognitive and language categories), and precisely how they become linked to each other in semantic memory so that they can be retrieved for speaking and understanding, is an area of some controversy. Two views of how this occurs will be discussed as part of the definition of lexicon. You can understand why semantic knowledge is more difficult to study than, for example, phonology or syntax, which have overt features to observe and quantify. Particularly with children we have to infer semantic knowledge from the way they use words and sentences. Children cannot define and clarify what they "mean" by a word or multiword construction, so we must guess about how they arrive at word meanings, their underlying organization of meanings and words, and the rules they have worked out for these linkages.

Syntax refers to the principles for combining words to form grammatical sentences.

Syntax is sentence structure. The syntactic component of language has to do with word order, inflections, and relationships between words. Syntax is one level of grammar—an aspect necessary for the explicit description of a language. Syntactic rules specify which strings of words are acceptable and which are not. Without syntactic organization, language would be an incoherent jumble of words.

As a speaker of English, you demonstrate knowledge of syntax (you can differentiate acceptable from unacceptable word strings) even though you may not be able to explain this knowledge or diagram sentences properly. Look at these sentences. Which is acceptable?

1. The waitress poured the coffee.
2. The poured coffee the waitress.

Because the words of the second sentence are out of order, it makes little sense. If you recognize this you have what is called **linguistic competence** —intuitive knowledge about what is correct in your native language. Every time you form a sentence you demonstrate this intuitive knowledge.

Describing a sentence in terms of its structural or syntactic aspects could include describing parts of speech (verbs, nouns, etc.), constituent parts (noun phrases, verb phrases, etc.), or sentence type (negative, passive, interrogative, imperative, etc.). Sentences have two levels of syntax, or structure—a surface or syntax structure level and a deep or meaning structure level (Chomsky, 1957, 1972). **Transformations** are operations that relate surface structures to their corresponding deep structure. Consider the following sentences that have different surface structures (one is active and the other passive), but share the same deep structure:

Sentences have surface structure and deep structure.

1. The girl hit the baseball.
2. The baseball was hit by the girl.

Among other operating principles, the transformational-generative grammar, proposed by Chomsky, has what are called "rewrite rules" which specify and explain how the above sentences are derived from the same deep structure, or core meaning. Rewrite rules also specify how different underlying structures can generate the same surface structure. Consider this sentence, for example:

The shooting of the hunters was terrible.

You realize immediately that this could mean that (a) the hunters were not good marksmen, or (b) they were shot. The sentence has two deep structures (plausible meanings) and one surface structure.

Syntactic descriptions of language attempt to describe the intuitive rules that speakers use in generating and understanding sentences. Among the mysteries associated with language acquisition is precisely how children master these rules. The fact that they master most rules of syntax by age 4 or 5 is no less than miraculous. There is even some question about exactly when syntactic rule learning begins. Children literally send "mixed messages": some investigators interpret certain early utterances as evidence of syntactic knowledge, while others view the same messages as lacking syntactic knowledge.

8

Morphology is the study of words and their meaningful parts.

Morphology is concerned with the internal structure of words, how they are built up from roots, prefixes, suffixes, etc.—the morphemes of language. To be a morpheme, a sound unit must be a word or a part of a word with stable meaning; it must be indivisible (not separable into smaller parts without violating the meaning or leaving meaningless remainders). Words like "red," "straw," "berry" consist of one morpheme each. Each can stand alone, or be combined with another morpheme, to form a different word (redhead, strawberry). This type of morpheme is a **free morpheme.** Other morphemes such as -ing, -ful, un-, -ed cannot stand alone. These meaningful prefixes and suffixes are called **bound morphemes.**

Phonology is the study of speech sounds.

Phonology is the study of the system of speech sounds employed by native speakers of a language. English has approximately 43 sounds; other languages have different numbers of sounds (Spanish, for example, uses about 24) as well as some different sounds. Phonology should not be confused with **phonetics,** which studies the properties of human soundmaking—the ways people form, transmit, and hear sounds.

A **phoneme** is the smallest sound unit in language that signals a meaningful difference. Say the words "bat" and "pat" to yourself. The only difference between the way they sound is the initial sound. Since this initial sound difference produces two different words, the difference is a meaningful one. Therefore, /b/ and /p/ are, by definition, two different phonemes. The reason for defining a phoneme so precisely, instead of just saying sounds are different if they sound different, has to do with differences in sound systems across languages.

Phonemes are discriminated by their acoustic properties (the sound waves involved) and their articulatory properties (where and how they are articulated). They are divided generally into consonants and vowels. Consonants are further classified according to place and manner of articulation, i.e., stop or fricative sounds. Vowels are more open sounds that are classified according to the shape of the tongue during phonation.

Lexicon is the term for a speaker's mental dictionary. Actually a lexicon is more like an encyclopedia than a dictionary because it includes not only words, but also general and specific information about each lexical item. In addition to information about the meaning of words, a lexicon includes information about the pronunciation, and the linkages between words and words, words and concepts, and concepts and concepts.

There are two basic hypotheses about how early lexical meanings are acquired.

There are two distinct views regarding lexical development: the semantic features hypothesis and the functional core hypothesis. Clark (1973) contends that the meaning of a referential word (a word that refers to an object or objects) can be broken down into a set of constituent elements called **features.** These features, or meaning elements, account for what the child knows and has stored about the meaning of the word. For example, "four-legged," "barks," "animate," etc., might be attached to the word "dog." Accordingly, "dog" would be used for any object possessing these features. This view, the **semantic features hypothesis,** suggests that children derive meaning features by attending to the perceptual attributes of objects. Over time, features are added to this collection (from more general to specific) with the result that the child's meaning for a word gradually becomes highly specific. Eventually the child's concept will resemble the adult meaning.

The alternative view of lexical development, called the **functional core hypothesis,** is put forth by Nelson (1974, 1978). According to this view, the child derives her word meanings from functional, rather than from perceptual, experiences. The basic premise is that, instead of attending to how things look and sound and categorizing according to perceptual similarities, children attend to functional variables (how, where, and when things are used) and base their categorizations on this knowledge. They experience a ball as *rollable, bounceable, throwable;* these properties define the core meaning of the concept *ball.* Nelson argues that the child begins concept formation with this functional core meaning. After a functional core has become *attached* to the word, the peripheral perceptual information necessary for future identification of similar balls (e.g., *roundness*) is added.

These two theories share at least two assumptions (Rice, 1980): both view the child's development of word meanings as heavily dependent on nonlinguistic experience, and both view concepts as composed of elements which share common attributes (things that look alike, sound alike, or are acted on in the same way, etc.). In the final analysis, both will probably be found to be correct. The point to remember is that children use functional and perceptual information to arrive at their early lexical meanings.

Suprasegmental phenomena are the tonal/rhythmic characteristics of language such as intonation contour (where stress is placed in a word, phrase, or sentence), pitch, and rhythm or pause time. These characteristics are extremely important in interpreting sentences. When they are used to signal word and sentence differences, they are called **prosodic features.** When suprasegmentals are used to signal emotional and attitudinal aspects of communication, they are often called **paralanguage** (meaning "beside language") features. The term paralanguage includes nonlanguage sounds such as laughing, crying, sighing, and whining.

> Suprasegmental features play an important role in communication.

A change in any one or several suprasegmental features can change the meaning and the effect of a message. For example, by changing the intonation contour of a sentence from rising to falling one can change a sentence from a question to a statement. Adults are capable of communicating irony entirely through suprasegmental features.

Mean length of utterance (MLU) is a relatively simple measurement method for quantifying language development. It is obtained by counting the total number of morphemes in 50 (or 100) consecutive utterances from a spontaneous speech sample and then dividing by 50 (or 100). Because it does not reflect all qualitative language changes, MLU must be considered a gross index. Still, it is quite useful.

> A child's MLU can provide a useful index of language development.

Many of the problems inherent in matching delayed and normal children for research purposes on the basis of mental age or chronological age can be avoided by matching according to MLU. Until the child's utterances exceed four morphemes, MLU is a reliable index of linguistic competence because early linguistic attainments result in increased length. After that, it is not particularly useful because increased sentence length does not necessarily mean increased language ability.

When two children's MLUs are about the same, essentially parallel development in content, form, and use can be expected. If there are significant differences in the types of words and structures used and the meanings expressed, the difference may be an indication of a problem. At least, it is reason for additional observation and more precise evaluation of the less competent child.

Brown (1973) used MLU as the index for defining five stages of language development based on his analyses of speech samples from many children (see Table 1-1). One reason his descriptions of attainments in each stage are so useful for assessment and intervention is that the stages are not tied to chronological ages. Stages I and II are referred to most often in subsequent chapters.

The terms discussed in this section are basic to the study of language and introduce germane background information. However, definitions alone cannot provide a sufficient groundwork for understanding language development and use. This requires some historical context and awareness of the numerous perspectives which have contributed to our present conceptualizations. We strongly urge you to supplement this brief introduction to the history, assumptions, limitations, and contributions of these theories about language with additional readings.

FIVE PERSPECTIVES ON LANGUAGE ACQUISITION

PSYCHOLINGUISTIC PERSPECTIVE

HYPOTHESIS: Children have an innate predisposition to apply linguistic rules (Chomsky, 1957).

HISTORY

Psycholinguistic views on language development.

In the late fifties and early sixties, psycholinguistics was concerned with structuralism and mental processes. Linguistic structuralism took the form of hypothesizing about the mental plan speakers use in understanding and generating sentences, and Noam Chomsky, professor of linguistics at MIT, was the dominant theorist. Chomsky (1957, 1965) formulated a complex and formal theoretical model (transformational grammar) to describe the abstract internalized knowledge that each of us, as a native speaker of our language, uses in deriving sentences. This theory also had strong implications for how that knowledge is acquired.

Chomsky was, in his own words, interested in "studying language as an instrument or tool, attempting to describe its structure with no explicit reference to the way in which it is put to use" (1957, p. 103). His theoretical model provides many tenets that remain basic to psycholinguistics.

TABLE 1-1 Brown's Stages, MLUs, and Major Attainments

Stage	MLU	Attainments
I	1.75	Basic semantic roles and syntactic relations within simple sentences
II	2.25	Appropriate use of some inflections such as *-ing, -s* (for plural), and *-ed* and previously omitted prepositions, conjunctions
III	2.75	Uses questions, imperatives, and negatives
IV	3.50	Uses embedded sentences and other complex constructions
V	4.00	Gains control over more complex relations between simple sentences

The competence-performance distinction is one example of a significant contribution. Chomsky differentiates between what a person knows about language (competence) and the psychological capacities such as memory, perception, and attention implicated in realizing that knowledge (performance). In some contexts this distinction is useful.

Chomsky's model is structural and heavily dependent upon syntactic explanations. He describes the relationships between sentence elements (e.g., noun phrase, verb phrase) and formally defines such grammatical concepts as subject and object of a sentence relative to noun phrases, verb phrases, and sentences. Chomsky formulates explanations for different sentence types (e.g., declarative, passive, negative, and imperative) and specifies rules for generating these different sentence types, which he called "transformations." (Transformations are syntactic operations that change the form or structure of a sentence without changing the meaning.) He describes language as a set of simple "kernal" sentences, plus transformational rules for changing the kernals into a variety of complex sentences.

ASSUMPTIONS

The basic assumptions of Chomsky's theory relative to language acquisition are nativistic. In theory, the origins of language are explained by reference to an inborn capacity—an innate linguistic mechanism. This innate mechanism (called *Language Acquisition Device* [LAD]) is characterized as a set of rules or underlying principles for forming sentences, and procedures for discovering how these principles apply to the particular language to which the child is exposed. In other words, according to Chomsky's theory, the infant is "prewired" for language acquisition. Presumably, LAD automatically "activates" when the child is exposed to linguistic input. The assumption is that a child uses the advance knowledge in his language acquisition device to process the linguistic environment and generate hypotheses about how things should be said. How else could children learn rules for forming sentences? Rules are never explained (at least until a child is some years into his schooling), and they are neither explicit nor obvious in the language addressed to a young child.

From Chomsky's perspective, the child's task is one of narrowing the range of possibilities through a hypothesis-testing process until he eventually arrives at an accurate conceptualization of the syntactic rules of his language culture. Chomsky considers this preprogramming-activation hypothesis the only way to explain the "miraculous" ability of even very young children to produce an infinite number of novel, but grammatical, utterances. At the time, Chomsky's theory seemed a more adequate explanation for language acquisition than the principles of association, reinforcement, and generalization which behaviorists of that day were espousing because it seemed to explain the tacit knowledge young children demonstrate about how things can be expressed. However, there were, and still are, many outspoken critics of Chomsky's nativist proposals.

LIMITATIONS

Chomsky's innateness hypothesis makes certain assumptions about cognitive development and linguistic input which were strongly attacked in the seventies. As Schlesinger (1977) has pointed out, the nativists actually treated language learning as if it occurred independently of cognitive development. The respective roles of syntax and semantics became hopelessly confused in vague explanations of how a child "knows" what to do with linguistic input. Precisely what children are born "knowing" versus what they come to know about the objects, events, and relations in the physical world was unclear. Also difficult to ascertain in nativist proposals was precisely how and when the understanding children come equipped with, and the understanding they acquire are linked to words and phrases.

Because Chomsky's position on the role of linguistic input is more explicit than his conceptualizations of LAD, researchers have found it easier to criticize. Chomsky considers linguistic input to be important for activation of LAD, but too fragmented, confusing, and unsystematic to serve an instructional function. He describes the speech addressed to young children as basically ungrammatical, replete with false starts, hesitations, and slips of the tongue, and totally unsuited to facilitate the child's acquisition of grammar. As we discuss in Chapter Two, this premise has since been contradicted by many investigators (e.g., Brown, 1973; Nelson, 1973; Newport, 1976; Phillips, 1973; Snow, 1972). The importance of parents' speech to children for teaching the forms and structures of language seems indisputable.

In summary, it is not difficult to see why the early structural and nativistic perspectives have been so adamantly contested by psycholinguists and researchers in related fields. Semanticists (e.g., Fillmore, 1968) argue that language acquisition depends heavily on underlying semantic, rather than syntactic, representations. Cognitive theorists (Sinclair-de Zwart, 1973), citing Piaget's writing, argue that language acquisition does not so much reflect innate knowledge of syntax as innate cognitive propensities; and psycholinguists (e.g., Broen, 1972; Phillips, 1973) challenge the view that language acquisition is not directly dependent on linguistic input.

CONTRIBUTIONS

Although it proved inadequate to explain or describe language acquisition, Chomsky's model stimulated important research. Researchers began to look for parallels among children learning language in widely different language communities (linguistic universals). More importantly, they began to realize the value of naturalistic observations. A range of studies of normal and disordered language users was inspired by Chomsky's formulations (Miller, 1962; Menyuk, 1964; Morehead & Ingram, 1973). One outgrowth of this perspective, pivot grammar conceptualizations, is still very evident in the literature.

While analyzing child language transcripts for evidence of grammatical rule knowledge, Braine (1963) noted an interesting pattern in the spontaneous productions of three children who had just begun forming two-word utterances. Certain words are heavily used, and they are always used in a particular position. A second, larger set of words is not so popular, but considerably more varied; these words also are used in a specific way, that is, in the second position in two-word utterances. Braine calls the first set of heavily used words "pivots," and those belonging to the larger set "open." He noted that the children seemed to be consistently producing "pivot-open" constructions: they almost always combined a word from a small set of heavily used initial words (e.g., "here" or "there") with one from the large open class of nouns, verbs, and adjectives. Sometimes the children would produce "open-open" constructions, and occasionally "open-pivot" constructions, but never "pivot-pivot" combinations. Based on these observations, Braine and others (Miller and Ervin, 1964) characterize children's language knowledge at this two-word stage as a pivot-open grammar. Two-word combinations are described as usually "pivot-open" (e.g., "more milk," "more cookie," "more book"), sometimes "open-pivot" (e.g., "Mommy come," "baby come," "doggie come"), and occasionally "open-open" (e.g., "milk cup"). Here is the theory: In early language acquisition, children expand their vocabulary mostly by adding new members to the open class and only occasionally by adding new pivot words. This grammar, reduced to a single rule, is that an utterance consists of either an open word or a pivot word, followed by an open word.

> Pivot grammar states that utterances include either an open word or a pivot word followed by an open word.

Pivot grammar was eventually found to be inadequate to account for language learning—even at the earliest stages. Pivot grammar descriptions ignore the content of the utterances altogether. Bloom (1970) contends that it provides little more than a superficial description of child language, not an explanation for how language is learned. Further dissatisfaction arose when it became evident that the multiword utterances of some children simply do not fit, and cannot be explained by, pivot grammar rules.

At about the same time Braine was considering pivot grammar as a means of characterizing children's utterances, Brown and Fraser (1963) suggested the term "telegraphic" to describe early sentences. They noted that first sentences resemble telegrams: nouns and verbs are over-

> Telegraphic utterances resemble adult telegrams.

represented, and prepositions, conjunctions, articles, and auxiliary verbs are omitted or only rarely included. The telegraphic characterization was strengthened by a subsequent report by Brown and Bellugi (1964) describing the early sentences of two children in a longitudinal study. The imitations, in addition to spontaneous sentences, produced by these children showed what the telegraphic characterization predicted. Contentives (nouns, verbs, and adjectives making concrete reference to persons, objects, actions, and qualities) and word order were retained, and functors (e.g., pronouns, prepositions, articles, and the like) were largely omitted.

Unfortunately, the telegraphic account of early sentences is only slightly more valid than pivot grammar. There is clearly an element of truth in both pivot-open and telegraphic grammar accounts of two-word utterances, but neither account provides anything approaching a satisfactory representation of the child's underlying knowledge of language. Neither considers the intended meanings or purposes of the utterances. In general, the psycholinguistic perspective is not particularly useful to teachers and clinicians concerned with language training. The most that can be gleaned from theoretical research of the sixties is a hierarchical description of the structural complexity of sentences. Although these data conceivably could influence the selection of training goals if a child is producing sentences, they are virtually useless for the pre-syntactic child.

BEHAVIORIST PERSPECTIVE

Behavioral views on language development.

HYPOTHESIS: Children learn language because their verbal behavior is selectively rewarded by significant others in their environment (Skinner, 1957).

HISTORY

The behaviorist position, first presented by B.F. Skinner (1957) in *Verbal Behavior,* views language learning as dependent upon imitation, practice, and selective reinforcement. Taking exception to the idea of an innate "language acquisition device," behaviorists have described language as the gradual accumulation of vocal symbols and sequences of symbols and emphasized the role of parents in modeling and reinforcing increasingly more grammatical utterances. Many of the behavioral (operant) principles presented by Skinner are derived directly from animal studies, but the functional analyses he advocates parallel those emphasized in the pragmatic approach of Dore (1975), Halliday (1975), and Bates (1976). Conceptually, behavioral functions and pragmatic functions are similar. Both refer to defining behaviors (or acts) in terms of their effects. (See the later section on pragmatic perspectives.)

Staats (1963), an early proponent of the behavioral perspective, contends that language acquisition can be explained by reference to stimulus-response principles. Strongly objecting to the lack of specification of either past or present learning conditions in psycholinguistic conceptualizations, Staats argues for (a) consideration of the functions served by different types of utterances; and (b) manipulative and cause and effect-type research, rather than total reliance on descriptive methodology.

ASSUMPTIONS

The behaviorist position assumes that environmental variables play an important role in language acquisition. Verbal responses are assumed to be directly related to, and subsequently controlled by, contingent events (reinforcement and punishment). Parents model appropriate utterances and then gradually shape the young child's vocalizations until they are acceptable.

LIMITATIONS

Arguments against total reliance on operant conditioning principles to *explain* language acquisition have come from many sources. First, consider the rate of language acquisition. Beyond the earliest stages of word acquisition, the child's verbal repertoire increases too rapidly to depend on conditioning mechanisms alone. Furthermore, contrary to Skinner's assumption, parents do not provide either positive or negative reinforcement for correct syntax; they do not correct or punish grammatical errors (Brown & Hanlon, 1970). Parents generally respond to the truth value of their child's utterances. They correct semantic inaccuracies, *not* syntax. The child who says, "Me eated ice cream," when she actually ate jello, will be corrected ("No, you had jello"). However, if she had, in fact, eaten ice cream, her parents would probably not have corrected her verbalization.

There continues to be a great deal of controversy about the precise role of imitation in language acquisition. However, most now reject the notion that it is *solely* responsible for language learning (Bloom & Lahey, 1978). Children would not say the things they do. Such productions as "I goed," "mouses," and "allgone cookie" are evidence against exclusive reliance on imitation for language learning. Finally, the abstractness and complexity of the meanings and structures normal children acquire in a remarkably short time are additional evidence that more than conditioning mechanisms are involved. In summary, while operant techniques utilizing imitation, modeling, and selective reinforcement have been proven effective in helping some children acquire basic language forms and structures, they do not *seem to explain* all language learning.

CONTRIBUTIONS

Behaviorists have contributed enormously to our understanding of what language *is,* as well as what it is *not.* Their contributions have led to the delineation of systematic training designs and important demonstrations of their application with nonspeaking individuals (Schiefelbusch, 1978; Schiefelbusch & Hollis, 1979; Schiefelbusch & Bricker, 1981).

Primate research has been particularly fruitful in highlighting functional criteria and alternative language modes for nonspeakers (Schiefelbusch & Hollis, 1979). With the chimpanzee as a "model" for language re-

Primate research has generated meaningful and useful constructs.

search, Premack (1970) and others set out to analyze and functionally define language and the language learning process. Premack began by asking the fundamental question *what is language?* What behaviors must Sarah, his chimp, demonstrate before she could be said to have language? Sarah eventually learned to respond to and produce more than 130 "words" using plastic pieces as basic word units. She demonstrated knowledge of interrogatives, metalinguistics (the use of language to teach language, as in the case *X is the name of Y*), class concepts, simple and complex sentence structures, pluralization, quantifiers, the logical connective (*if-then*), and the conjunctive *(and)*.

Washoe, a chimp under the tutelage of the Gardners (1969), and four young chimps trained by Fouts (1973) learned to understand and transmit sign language signals. The key observation about their signing vocabularies is that they are not limited to names or labels, but also use a range of verbs and adjectives in appropriate social contexts. Another chimpanzee, Lana, has been taught to use a computer instrumentation system (Rumbaugh, 1977). Lana communicates her desires and controls her experimental environment by pressing the appropriate sequence of keys connected to a computer. She can obtain M&Ms, music, different play activities with her trainers, and other treats by producing the correct sentence. The symbols in Lana's system (called "Yerkish") were formed by combining simple geometric elements into more complex figures fastened to a wall panel that functioned as a computer keyboard. She learned, apparently without direct instruction, to tell her trainers about machine malfunctions and the trainers' own mistakes. She invented new "sentences" when the ones she had been taught proved inadequate.

The achievements and capabilities of Sarah, Lana, Washoe, and other "talking" chimpanzees are impressive; they are also extremely informative to language interventionists. Is language "innate" and the province of humans alone? Are chimps similar enough to humans to warrant theoretical generalizations from apes to children? Do the nonspeech productions of chimpanzees qualify as "real" language? These are questions we cannot yet answer. However, primate research has had a profound impact on practical programming issues (Schiefelbusch & Hollis, 1979). These investigations have highlighted:

1. new and potentially promising analysis, planning, design, and implementation strategies for intervention.
2. the value of substituting nonspeech symbol forms and alternative response modes where conventional auditory-vocal communication is not attainable.
3. important constructs about the nature of the functional relationships between cognitive, social, and communication processes.

Another valuable contribution of the behaviorist tradition is to provide a format for asking and answering instructionally relevant questions (see Chapter Five). Regardless of the type of linguistic or nonlinguistic responses being sought, applied behavior analysis provides techniques to guide selection and empirical validation of the training arrangements. Though often criticized for concentrating too heavily on short-term gains, behaviorists have added significantly to our knowledge of language learning by addressing such issues as modeling, shaping, chaining, prompting, response class development, generalization, and training designs. All of these constructs are discussed in detail in subsequent chapters.

SEMANTIC-COGNITIVE PERSPECTIVE

HYPOTHESIS: Children learn language to talk about sensorimotor experiences (Nelson, 1973).

Semantic-cognitive views on language development.

HISTORY

A combination of events in the late sixties and early seventies was responsible for what came to be known as the semantic revolution. Many linguists and psycholinguists were already beginning to question Chomsky's formulations when a significant study by Lois Bloom (1970) sparked the revolution. Bloom's published research began with the intention of applying syntactic analysis techniques, in the tradition of transformational grammar. Her plan was to analyze and describe the language development of three young children by writing a set of rules that could generate the sentences they were producing. Writing such a grammar entailed identification of forms and structure regularities, such as the frequency of occurrence of different forms, and of word order sequences.

Suspecting that specification of the meanings the children intended with their multiword utterances would aid her in assigning different words to grammatical categories (nouns, verbs, etc.), she approached the task somewhat differently from others who had attempted the same type of analysis (Braine, 1963; Miller & Ervin, 1964). She carefully recorded the context of all the children's utterances. She also noted where the child was at the time, where she had been immediately before producing the utterance, what she was doing, what others were doing and saying, and to whom she was talking. The important products of Bloom's observational data were a classification system and a description of children's meanings when they are beginning to combine two or three words in short sentences. Her hypotheses about their semantic intentions provided far more information about their knowledge of language than did details about structure (e.g., the number of noun-verb constructions produced) which are generated by syntactic analysis techniques. Bloom's conclusion was that the emergence of language probably depends as much, if not more, on prior cognitive knowledge than on knowledge of syntax.

The first cannon of the semantic revolution had sounded. Almost simultaneously, three other psycholinguists (Brown, 1973; Schlesinger, 1971; Slobin, 1970) arrived at essentially the same conclusions as Bloom, using different data. All four came up with sets of semantic categories assumed to reflect the meanings children express when they first begin to produce two-word utterances. The fact that the lists were amazingly similar strengthened the semantic-cognitive position. The conclusion was that children seem to possess a range of semantic intentions (also called semantic relations and semantic functions) and express these meanings long before they know anything about syntax (Brown, 1973).

ASSUMPTIONS

Based on analysis of vast amounts of data he and his colleagues had collected, Brown notes that the meanings children express around the age of 2 are precisely what one would expect children to understand, considering their cognitive development during the sensorimotor period. "Representation starts with just those meanings that are most available to it, propositions about action schemas involving agents and objects, assertions of nonexistence, recurrence, location and so on" (p. 200). This maxim of the semantic revolution, that language is predicated upon, and can best be explained by reference to general cognitive development, is called the "cognitive hypothesis" (Cromer, 1974) or "cognitive determinism" (Schlesinger, 1977). It states simply and logically that children talk when they have something to talk about, and they talk about what they understand.

The reasoning that language has a cognitive base and that language learning cannot proceed without certain cognitive attainments revived interest in the writings of Piaget (1952, 1954, 1962). Sinclair-de Zwart (1973), the major interpreter of Piaget's sensorimotor tenets, hypothesized direct linkages between specific sensorimotor concepts and early linguistic constructions. A general consensus emerged that, at the very least, attainment of the concept of object permanence must precede expression of words with stable meanings (Bloom, 1973; Brown, 1973; Clark, 1973, 1977; Nelson, 1974, 1977).

Reminiscent of some of Chomsky's notions, the cognitive hypothesis suggests an innate "seed" and assigns relatively less importance to linguistic input. However, the inherited mechanism Piaget describes is not a linguistic device like LAD but more like a "cognitive acquisition device." Piaget suggests that the child has a propensity to develop cognitively in certain ways, and also outlines what appear to be universal sensorimotor adaptations and "knowing" activities.

LIMITATIONS

The cognitive hypothesis did not survive the seventies unscathed. Although many investigators still persist in their arguments for a direct relationship between mastery of certain sensorimotor concepts (usually object permanence) and particular features of early language (e.g., Bloom, 1973), definitive data have not appeared. The problems associated with relying on cognitive development alone to account for language development have been enumerated by Bowerman (1978). First, the cognitive hypothesis reduces to little more than conjecture when it comes to explaining how the linkages between specific cognitive attainments and the emergence of particular language capacities occur. While it may serve as a general description of what happens in the language acquisition process, the important question of how children figure out precisely which linguistic devices (words, word order, intonation) express which meanings and, subsequently, form the appropriate associations is unanswered. A second unanswered question is why children's language repertoires increase. The cognition-determines-language hypothesis provides no clues as to why, after mastering one device to express a particular meaning, children go on to learn increasingly more complex forms and structures to encode the same intention.

A third conspicuous inadequacy of the cognitive hypothesis is the neglect of linguistic input. As Schlesinger (1977) and others have pointed out, some aspects of language knowledge and competence simply cannot be explained without reference to linguistic input. There are important language concepts that children would not learn were it not for exposure to language. Such words as "why" and "how" which have no perceptible referents appear to require both cognitive and linguistic inputs (Blank, 1974, 1975). Production may precede understanding for some, as yet unspecified, set of words and phrases. The fourth reason for suggesting that the cognitive hypothesis may not be sufficient to explain language acquisition comes from research with nonverbal children. That there are some children who, in spite of seemingly normal cognitive attainments, do not learn to talk suggests that abilities other than purely conceptual knowledge are implicated in the language learning process (Cromer, 1974).

CONTRIBUTIONS

In summary, it seems unlikely that cognitive development alone can account for the complexity of language in all its manifestations. We cannot ignore its contributions, but we cannot ignore the roles of linguistic input and social interactions either. The regularities observed in the social and language environments of language-learning children must be at least as important as the universal aspects of their cognitive development. Like the linguistic and behaviorist approaches, the semantic-cognitive approach has serious limitations. The literature does not yet offer a unified basis for teacher and clinician decisions in language intervention. Although cognitive development is undoubtedly a powerful force, we have come to realize that some knowledge and some skills necessary for communicative competence are not traceable to manipulations of the physical world.

PRAGMATIC PERSPECTIVE

HYPOTHESIS: Children learn language in order to socialize and direct the behavior of others (Bruner, 1974).

Pragmatic views on language development.

HISTORY

The conceptual origins of pragmatics, or speech acts theory, can be traced to Morris (1938). He characterized language as having three dimensions—syntax, semantics, and pragmatics—and elaborated on the relation of signs in each dimension. Some years later the philosophical writings of Austin (1962) and Wittgenstein (1953) extended the speech act theory. Current work draws from a number of disciplines, including sociology, psychology, linguistics, and speech pathology, but most researchers in this area identify themselves as sociolinguists.

Pragmatics has been defined as: (a) the study of speech acts and the context in which they are performed, and (b) the rules governing how language is used in context (Bates, 1976). This perspective has contributed enormously to the study of child language acquisition during the past few years. Garvey (1977) describes the speech act (basic unit of analysis in pragmatics) as "an intentional, verbally encoded social gesture directed by one person to another" (p. 41). The following major categories of speech acts are proposed by Searle (1975): (a) representations (statements that can be classed as true or false), (b) directives (statements with which the speaker attempts to get the listener to do something), (c) commissives (statements committing the speaker to a course of action), (d) expressives (expressions of a psychological state), and (e) declaratives (statements of presumed facts).

Function is central to the pragmatic approach as *critical effect* is central to the behavioral approach. As noted in that section, they are almost identical constructs. As used in speech acts theory, function refers to intent which is the purpose or desired effect of an utterance. To understand the function of an utterance, we must understand why the speaker said what she did. The central question is *What act is the utterance intended to perform?*

ASSUMPTIONS

Pragmatics makes a basic distinction between the meaning, the form (words), and the structure (syntax) of an utterance and its function (e.g., demand, request, indicate). Researchers in this area emphasize that describing language and accounting for language acquisition entails substantially more than explaining how children construct meanings and learn to decode and encode linguistic forms and structures (Bruner, 1975, 1978; Bates, 1976; Ryan, 1974; Halliday, 1975). There is a difference, for example, in knowing what milk is, simply saying the word "milk," and the child using the word in context to request that the glass be refilled. The first has to do with conceptual knowledge; the second, saying the word, involves linguistic knowledge; and the third, requesting, depends on pragmatic knowledge. Though the interdependence of the three dimensions is readily acknowledged, Dore (1979) and others insist on the importance of differentiating between conceptual, linguistic, and pragmatic knowledge in explaining the nature of language and language development. They contend that even at the single-word utterance stage, children are using words to realize "primitive speech acts," such as "request," "protest," "calling," and "greeting."

The pragmatic orientation views language acquisition as one aspect of social development. Strategies for acquiring syntactic knowledge and the development of semantic categories are described as dependent on social interactions and on an awareness of social relationships (Clark, 1973; Nelson, 1974; Ryan, 1974; Lock, 1978). Caregiver-child interactions are considered "the originating force as well as the conditions for language learning" (Rees, 1978, p. 238). In fact, socialization is considered basic, and cognitive development secondary. Sociolinguists argue that an innate predisposition may account for the fact that children learn language and that cats do not, but it does not explain how this is accomplished (Newport, Gleitman, and Gleitman, 1977). Regarding innate or biological origins, Richards (1974, 1976) points to established infant preferences for human faces and human speech-like sounds. He argues that the infant's biological structure provides for selectivity in perceptual processes and that the infant is predisposed to attend to the social features of her environment. The infant's selective attention to certain aspects of her environment, namely, adults and adult communication modes, enables communications between infant and caregiver and predicts how language acquisition occurs. Research demonstrating that infants and their caregivers communicate almost from the moment of their first contact certainly lends credence to this hypothesis (e.g., Richards, 1976). (Research in this area is discussed in the next chapter.)

LIMITATIONS

Ultimately only very detailed conceptual and empirical work will tell us if pragmatic measures are more fruitful than cognitive and linguistic measures to investigate and explain language acquisition. First we need reliable and valid methods of working with the data. Speech acts have been investigated by analyzing spontaneous speech and by structuring tasks designed to elicit certain functions (Snyder, 1978). At least three separate classification systems have been proposed for categorizing children's speech acts (Dore, 1975; Halliday, 1975; Bates, 1976). The problem is twofold: (a) all three systems are based on data from a small number of children, and (b) there are, as yet, no reliable and valid criteria for assigning utterances to appropriate categories. Because there have been no definitive statements about what to consider evidence for attribution of a given function to a child, interpretations are made rather subjectively (Rees, 1972). This is a methodological limitation which undoubtedly will be solved in the near future. A theoretical limitation that the pragmatic perspective shares with the other approaches is that it does not answer the question of how children learn the structures (syntax) of their language.

CONTRIBUTIONS

The significance of the pragmatic perspective is that it provides many of the missing clues in the complex mystery of language acquisition. It has asked, and is beginning to answer, many of the questions raised by other perspectives: the role of linguistic input; the continuity between gestures and words; and the ways children learn the complex social devices through which people make their intentions known.

Pragmatics puts communication in the center stage. Shared understanding is considered to pre-date the emergence of language both ontogenetically and phylogenetically (Lock, 1978; Newson, 1978). (This brief discussion is restricted to individual development. The reader is referred to Lock [1978] for elucidation of the evolutionary argument). The contention is that because caregivers impute intentions to their infant's actions, these behaviors eventually achieve an intentional status as far as the child is concerned. Caregivers are so anxious to establish shared understanding with their baby that from birth they treat her as an intentional communicator. By treating their infant's actions as if they are intentional, parents establish and maintain a variety of communicative gestures—many as subtle as a trembling lower lip or a grimace.

A basic aim of research stimulated by pragmatics is to discover the conditions and contexts in which communicative competence develops. Bruner (1975) and Bates (1976) suggest that children begin learning the how, when, and where of communication in joint action routines such as peekaboo and build-and-knock-down play. In the context of these joint action "dialogues," the infant learns that she can influence the behavior of others in verbal and nonverbal ways.

Bates (1976) proposes a three-stage sequence in the earliest development of communicative functions, identifying three types of speech acts in the sensorimotor period as precursors to intentional communication. In the first, the perlocutionary stage, the child's signals such as crying, smiling, cooing, etc. are interpreted and differentially responded to as if intentional communications. At around 8 months, the infant enters the illocutionary stage. She begins using more conventional signals (extending her arms to be picked up, handing a mechanical toy to an adult to be activated) and uses them intentionally to affect the behavior of others. By the last half of the second year, children are using locutionary acts—conventional verbalizations—to get things done. A child will say "more milk," for example, to request that her glass be refilled. She may or may not produce the words in combinations with a gesture (displaying her glass) in the locutionary stage.

Greenfield and Smith (1976) claim that the specific words young children select to produce in their early attempts to communicate are determined by pragmatic factors. They select those words that are needed and most useful in promoting accurate adult interpretation of their intentions. At the one-word stage, the child would, for example, say "cookie" rather than "want" to request a cookie, with the understanding that the former has a higher probability (if she is limited to one word productions) of conveying her request.

INTERACTIONIST PERSPECTIVE

Interactionist views on language development.

HYPOTHESIS: Infants are born prepared to learn to talk and the environment teaches them about talking.

HISTORY

The interactionist approach provides arguments for linkages and interactions, rather for a dichotomous than for an either/or position. Piagetian theory is a prime example of this tradition. Fundamentally an interactionist, Piaget conceived of cognitive development as determined by internally guided activity (i.e., adaptation) that interacts with the environment and gradually becomes modified as a function of the interaction process.

Another variant of interactionism is illustrated by Schlesinger's (1977) well-reasoned case against viewing the cognitive determinism hypothesis and the linguistic input hypothesis as conceptually incompatible. He presents four interaction hypotheses to support his position. First, cognitive development may be responsible for the emergence of some language attainments (possibly the child's earlier productions), and linguistic experiences may account for others. Second, there is the possibility that language acquisition varies across children. Some children may rely more on sensorimotor learning strategies (as claimed by the cognitive determinism hypothesis), while others rely more on linguistic experiences. A third possibility is that both may operate, but not concurrently, within a single child acquiring a particular discrimination. Cognitive development and linguistic experiences could interact and facilitate each other at different points in the acquisition process. A final possibility would be that the processes are mutually supportive and essentially simultaneous; they function as equal working partners all along the way in the language acquisition process.

ASSUMPTIONS

Finding a contemporary theorist, teacher, or clinician at this time who dogmatically espouses the extreme form of any of the four previously discussed perspectives on language acquisition would be most unusual. Most would place themselves at some point on an interactionist continuum. They would acknowledge, with a variety of qualifications, the validity of interactionist arguments and agree to some role for internal factors. However, there would be little agreement about the propensities or acquisition strategies children bring to language learning. (These strategies probably resemble a collection of perceptual, organizational, and problem-solving plans, but this is only speculation.) What is most important is that we are approaching a consensus that the child does not arrive empty-handed (or empty-headed). She is neither a blank slate nor a passive recipient, but an adapting, communicating organism from birth.

Comparison of the various perspectives on language acquisition leads to the conclusion that it is not their views on the relative influence of innate versus environmental forces that distinguishes them so much as differences in the way they conceptualize the early products of the language acquisition process. Differences are most apparent in descriptions of what emerges as a child learns to talk and understand, not the of acquisition processes themselves. Is it syntax? Is it meaning? Is it a form of social interaction? Or is there, as Bloom and Lahey (1978) and others have maintained, evidence of all three dimensions in early language?

CONTRIBUTIONS

The interactionist model presented by Bloom and Lahey depicts language as a three dimensional system—content-form-use. The interactions of semantic-cognitive, structural-linguistic, and pragmatic-functional knowledge domains are described. More important, however, from the perspective of teachers and clinicians, the Bloom and Lahey model provides a scaffold and frame of reference for assessment and intervention. As an interactionist perspective, the content-form-use model provides a framework for consideration of the nature of language and normal language acquisition. From the standpoint of assessment and intervention, it is a way of describing the expressive capabilities of handicapped children. The excellent volume, *Language Development and Language Disorders,* by Bloom and Lahey (1978) has greatly influenced our treatment of the three dimensions and organization of the next few chapters.

> The content-form-use model provides a framework for assessment and intervention.

Content, or semantics, is the *what* of language. Think of content as a mental dictionary with complex vertical and horizontal linkages between linguistic and nonlinguistic information. There are two ways of categorizing content. Language content or meaning can be conceived of as having a general (and universal) knowledge level and a specific (idiosyncratic) knowledge level. At the general level there are three types of knowledge, each with subcategories; at the specific level are the particular concepts or topics the child actually talks about. Table 1-2 presents the general content categories and subcategories, and examples of topics at the specific level.

> Content has a general level and a specific level.

The content-topic distinction makes it easy to see how all children (and adults too) can share common knowledge categories and yet talk about different topics. Regardless of culture or context they will all learn about and talk about objects, relationships among objects, and relationships within and between events. What will vary across different children and cultures is the specific topics—the particular objects, events, and relations understood and talked about. Where there are large differences in the particular objects, events and relation in the environment (such as we see across cultures), there will be large differences in children's vocabularies. They will still talk about objects, events, and relations but very different topics. As interests shift and experiences accumulate, topics obviously change. Two-year-olds talk about juice, six-year-olds talk about Cokes or sodas, and adults talk about coffee or wine.

> Form can be viewed in terms of sounds, words, or sentences.

Form is the *how* of language, its shape or surface structure and the all-important linkages with meaning. Form may be described in a number of different ways. As discussed earlier, sounds can be described phonetically, in terms of where and how they are articulated, and/or in terms of distinctive articulatory features. Words can be described grammatically, whether they are nouns, verbs, adverbs, adjectives, prepositions, etc. Sen-

TABLE 1-2 General and Specific Levels of Content

General Level	Specific Level (particular topics)
1. Knowledge about objects	
a. classes of objects	"dogs"
b. particular objects	"Spot"
2. Knowledge about object relations	
a. existence, nonexistence, recurrence (how objects relate to themselves or other objects in the same class)	"all gone"
b. color, size, etc. (properties and attributes that distinguish one object from another in the same class)	"big," "red"
c. location, action, possession (how an object or objects in one class relate to object(s) in another class)	"my sweater" "book on chair"
3. Knowledge about event relations	
a. time, causality (how different events relate to each other)	"before lunch" "if . . . then"
b. time the event occurs, mood of speakers, speakers' ideas about the event (relations within an event)	"eat now" "I want to swim"

tences can be described according to type, whether declarative, negative, yes/no question, *wh-* question, or imperative. The clauses and phrases within a sentence can also be classified. However, describing form in this way provides little information about content connections (linkages with meaning).

An important property of form is its linking function. Form is the means for linking sounds (or, in the case of manual languages, signs) to meaning. Descriptions of language based only on syntactic and grammatical analysis often fail to take this linkage property into account. One classification that does take meaning connections into account is the substantive-relational dichotomy. Words are classified and described according to whether they represent object knowledge (substantive words) or relation knowledge (relational words). Relational words are verbs, prepositions, adverbs, and adjectives. "Milk," "baby," and "Daddy" are substantive words while "more," "gone," and "red" are relational words.

Another way to classify form and take meaning into account, when combinations of words are involved, is to consider the semantic-syntactic relations between words. This method requires information about the context and purpose of the utterance. It allows classification of an utterance by whether it represents an action relation (e.g., "the girl ate the cookie"), a locative relation (e.g., "the baby is in the bed"), or a state relation encoding possession or attribution (e.g., "my new doll," or "the red ball"). A third method of describing form which also takes account of meaning is to delineate the use of morphological inflections. Grammatical morphemes attached to nouns, verbs, and adjectives add to or change the meanings of sentences. For example, -s, when added to count nouns, indicates plurality; when added to animate nouns it can indicate possession; when added to a verb, such as "eat" or "hit," -s indicates present or habitual action.

Language comprehension assumes a mental representation of sound sequences (words) so that they can be recognized when heard. Words must also be retrievable for production. Understanding and production both assume linkages between mental representations of sound sequences (language knowledge) and mental representations of experiences of the world (cognitive knowledge). There are many different ways of "knowing" words which children begin to learn at around 1 year. At another level, knowing language form also entails knowing how to understand and say sentences. Sentence elements must be interrelated according to rules of grammar that specify word order and meaning relations between words. Regardless of how language form is described, whether by reference to vocabulary words, sentence types, or one of the other methods noted above, the function it serves as a connector, linking sounds (or signs) and meaning, is as important as the code and the structure.

Use is the *why, when,* and *where* of language, the communication or social interaction aspect. Language use assumes a concern for the listener, a reason for speaking, the ability to use contextual knowledge to choose among alternative forms of different messages, and understanding of the dynamics of discourse. Data a speaker uses in choosing among alternative forms of a message include information about the listener and the context. Generally speaking, the more accurate a speaker's ability to "read" her listener and the context, and the more sophisticated her grasp of the rules and devices for expressing intentions, the more appropriate and effective the communication. This third dimension of language—the communication component—is also discussed in the subsections on communication and pragmatic perspectives.

There are basically three types of related pragmatic knowledge-skill domains: *performatives, presuppositions,* and *conversational postulates* (Bates, 1976). The first major category of language use rules has to do with performatives (or speech acts). A performative or speech act is the intention or goal of a sentence. Some performatives are specific in the sense that they are constrained to certain forms and contexts. Introductions, greetings, and pledging allegiance to the flag are examples of this type of limited, highly ritualistic speech act. Other performatives that promise, request, warn, prohibit, apologize, etc. are more varied with respect to the forms with which they can be expressed and the context in which they can be used. Consider, for example, the differences between greeting (performatives of the first type) and requests (performatives of the second type). There are only a limited number of greetings (e.g., "Hi," "Hello," "How are you?"), and there are limitations as to when and where they are used (always upon first meeting or encountering someone). Acts of re-

There are three related categories of language use rules.

questing, on the other hand, can take many forms depending on the context. "I'm hungry" would serve as a request in some contexts. But any number of other forms, including "Let's get dinner," "I'd like some nachos," and "Please cut me a piece," also could be requests in different contexts. The request form selected will depend on the speaker, the listener, the relationship between the two, and the context.

The second major category of language use rules is concerned with listener and context variables. Presuppositions are judgments about the capacities and needs of listeners in different social contexts. Competent communicators decide which of the many possible forms for a message will best serve the desired function, considering the participants and the context of the particular exchange. The speaker must know how to take into account information about what the listener already knows and does not know about the particular topic of the exchange, as well as information about the context. This information then guides the selection of words and sentence forms. For example, when a potential speaker is about to address someone, the person's age, occupation, rank, marital status, and sex, as well as situational variables (e.g., if it's church, whisper) will be considered. The form of the utterance will be influenced also by whether the topics of the message are present in the situation in which the utterance occurs. A listener applies similar rules to decoding the speaker's intentions (Gordon and Lakoff, 1975). This is tacit knowledge in that it is rare for a speaker or listener to be able to delineate these presuppositions. Nevertheless, appropriate and effective communication is heavily dependent on this knowledge-skill domain.

A third knowledge-skill domain in language use has to do with conversational rules—rules of dialogue. These mechanics of discourse include rules for (a) entering and initiating conversations, (b) leaving or terminating conversations, (c) taking turns, (d) shifting topics, (e) handling digressions, (f) asking questions, and (g) temporal spacing of pauses. These relationship devices are important for setting up and maintaining all types of exchanges.

By the end of their second year, children give evidence of specific knowledge and skills in the three language use domains. Evidence from analyses of their early utterances and conversations indicates that they know how to infer what their listeners already know versus what they need to know and to take this information into account in deciding what forms to use in their messages (e.g., Bates, 1976; Cazden, 1970; Garvey, 1975). There is also evidence of the ability to participate appropriately as partners in conversation (Bloom, Rocissano, and Hood, 1976). Appropriate language use is the culmination of a learning process which begins shortly after birth, when infants begin to learn that their behavior can influence the behavior of others and then begin to behave with the intention of maintaining that influence.

Content, form and use necessarily intersect in language understanding and production. The three components also interact in language development. Language acquisition is the gradual construction of a plan and operations for content, form, and use integration and subsequent realization. In the next chapter, the basic hypothesis of the interactionist perspective and some of the data supporting this hypothesis will be discussed as they relate to normal language acquisition.

In summary, we restate the inadequacy of such a brief overview of these rich perspectives. Our intent is not to perpetuate the dichotomies which have plagued the field for two decades. Later chapters will moderate much of the variance among these positions and emphasize the points of reconciliation. You will come to realize that, in many instances, the major differences have more to do with terminology than conceptual underpinnings.

SUMMARY

1. The theoretical and applied literature related to language learning is almost as complex as language itself, but understanding and interpreting this literature is critical to *informed* decision making.

2. Language is an abstract code with rules governing its construction, use, and understanding.

3. Speech, because it is a precise motor behavior that depends on physiological and neuromuscular coordination, is probably the most difficult language mode.

4. Communication is substantially more than producing and understanding language; it is the *exchange* of ideas and intentions.

5. Psycholinguistics, sociolinguistics, and linguistics are related but separate areas of study.

6. Grammars are attempts to describe the organization of language in the mind of the language user.

7. Semantics, the study of language meaning, is particularly concerned with the relation between language and cognitive knowledge.

8. The syntactic component of language has to do with word order, inflections, and relationships between words.

9. A morpheme is a word, or part of a word, that has a stable meaning; it cannot be divided into smaller units without violating the meaning or leaving meaningless remainders.

10. Phonemes are the smallest sound units which signal a *meaningful* difference and they are discriminated by reference to their respective acoustic and articulatory properties.

11. A speaker's lexicon includes information about the meaning of words, how they are pronounced, and linkages between words and words, words and concepts, and concepts and concepts.

12. When suprasegmental features are used to signal word and sentence differences they are called prosodic features; when used to signal affect they are paralanguage features.

13. MLU is a gross but useful index of language development prior to the time a child's utterances exceed four morphemes.

14. The basic assumptions of Chomsky's psycholinguistic perspective are that language can be explained by reference to an innate linguistic mechanism (LAD) and that language is basically a set of simple sentences plus transformational rules.

15. The basic assumption of the strict behaviorist perspective is that language learning depends on imitation, practice, and selective reinforcement.

16. The basic assumption of the semantic-cognitive perspective is that language acquisition depends on mastery of certain sensorimotor concepts.

17. The basic assumption of the pragmatic perspective is that language acquisition is one aspect of social development. Early caregiver—child interactions are the force behind, as well as the conditions for, language learning.

18. The basic assumption of the interactionist perspective is twofold: (a) infants are born with a general propensity to perceive, organize and interact in certain ways, and (b) the number and variety of experiences provided to the infant significantly affect learning.

19. The interactionist perspective points to nature-nurture, adult-child, and environment-organism *interactions* as the key contributors and facilitators of language acquisition.

REFERENCES

AUSTIN, J.L. *How to do things with words.* Cambridge, Mass.: Harvard University Press, 1962.

BATES, E. *Language and context: The acquisition of pragmatics.* New York: Academic Press, 1976.

BLANK, M. Cognitive functions of language in the preschool years. *Developmental Psychology,* 1974, *10,* 229–245.

BLANK, M. Mastering the intangible through language. In D. Aaronson & R. Rieber (Eds.), *Developmental psycholinguistics and communication disorders. Annals of the New York Academy of Sciences,* 1975, *263,* 44–58.

BLOOM, L. *Language development: Form and function in emerging grammars.* Cambridge, Mass.: The MIT Press, 1970.

BLOOM, L. *One word at a time: The use of single-word utterances before syntax.* The Hague: Mouton, 1973.

BLOOM, L., & LAHEY, M. *Language development and language disorders.* New York: John Wiley & Sons, 1978.

BLOOM, L., ROCISSANO, L., & HOOD, L. Adult-child discourse: Developmental interaction between information processing and linguistic knowledge. *Cognitive Psychology,* 1976, *8,* 521–552.

BOWERMAN, M. Semantic factors in the acquisition of rules for word use and sentence construction. In D. Morehead & A. Morehead (Eds.), *Directions in normal and deficient child language.* Baltimore: University Park Press, 1976.

BOWERMAN, M. Words and sentences: Uniformity, individual variation and shifts over time in patterns of acquisition. In F.D. Minifie & L.L. Lloyd (Eds.), *Communicative and cognitive abilities—Early behavioral assessment.* Baltimore: University Park Press, 1978.

BRAINE, M. The ontogeny of English phrase structure: The first phase. *Language,* 1963, *39,* 1–13.

BROEN, P. The verbal environment of the language learning child. *ASHA Monographs,* Number 17. Washington, D.C.: American Speech and Hearing Association, 1972.

BROWN, R. *A first language, the early stages.* Cambridge, Mass.: Harvard University Press, 1973.

BROWN, R., & BELLUGI, U. Three processes in the child's acquisition of syntax. *Harvard Education Review,* 1964, *34,* 133–151.

BROWN, R., & FRASER, C. The acquisition of syntax. In C.N. Cofer & B. Musgrave (Eds.), *Verbal behavior and verbal learning: Problems and processes.* New York: McGraw Hill, 1963.

BROWN, R., & HANLON, C. Derivational complexity and order of acquisition in child speech. In J. Hayes (Ed.), *Cognition and the development of language.* New York: John Wiley & Sons, 1970.

BRUNER, J. The organization of early skilled action. In M.P.M. Richards (Ed.), *The integration of a child into a social world.* London: Cambridge University Press, 1974.

BRUNER, J. The ontogenesis of speech acts. *Journal of Child Language,* 1975, *2,* 1–19.

BRUNER, J. On prelinguistic prerequisites of speech. In R.N. Campbell & P.T. Smith (Eds.), *Recent advances in the psychology of language* (Vol. 4a). New York: Plenum Press, 1978.

CAZDEN, C. The neglected situation in child language research and education. In F. Williams (Ed.), *Language and poverty, perspectives on a theme.* Chicago: Markham, 1970.

CHOMSKY, N. *Syntactic Structures.* The Hague: Mouton, 1957.

CHOMSKY, N. *Aspects of the theory of syntax.* Cambridge, Mass.: MIT Press, 1965.

CHOMSKY, N. *Language and mind.* New York: Harcourt Brace Jovanovich, 1972.

CLARK, E. Non-linguistic strategies and the acquisition of word meanings. *Cognition,* 1973, *2,* 161–182.

CLARK, E. Strategies and the mapping problem in first language acquisition. In J. Macnamara (Ed.), *Language learning and thought.* New York: Academic Press, 1977.

CROMER, R. The development of language and cognition. The cognitive hypothesis. In B. Foss (Ed.), *New perspectives in child development.* New York: Penguin Education, 1974.

CROMER, R. An experimental investigation of a putative linguistic universal: Marking and the indirect object. *Journal of Experimental Child Psychology,* 1975, *20,* 73–80.

DORE, J. Holophrases, speech acts, and language universals. *Journal of Child Language,* 1975, *2,* 21–40.

DORE, J. What's so conceptual about the acquisition of linguistic structures? *Journal of Child Language,* 1979, *6,* 129–138.

FILLMORE, C. The case for case. In E. Bach & R.T. Harms (Eds.), *Universals in linguistic theory.* New York: Holt, Rinehart & Winston, 1968.

FOUTS, R.S. Acquisition and testing of gestural signs in four young chimpanzees. *Science,* 1973, *180,* 978–980.

GARDNER, R.S., & GARDNER, B.T. Teaching sign language to a chimpanzee. *Science,* 1969, *165,* 664–672.

GARVEY, C. Requests and responses in children's speech. *Journal of Child Language,* 1975, *2,* 41–63.

GARVEY, C. The contingent query: A dependent act in conversation. In M. Lewis & L. Rosenblum (Eds.), *Interaction, conversation and the development of language.* New York: Wiley, 1977.

GOFFMAN, E. *Strategic interaction.* Philadelphia: University of Pennsylvania Press, 1969.

GORDON, D., & LAKOFF, G. Conversational postulates. In P. Cole & J.L. Morgan (Eds.), *Syntax and semantics, Vol. 3: Speech acts.* New York: Academic Press, 1975.

GREENFIELD, P.M., & SMITH, J.H. *Communication and the beginnings of language: The development of semantic structures in one-word speech and beyond.* New York: Academic Press, 1976.

HALLIDAY, M.A.K. Learning how to mean. In E. Lenneberg & E. Lenneberg (Eds.), *Foundations of language development* (Vol. 1). New York: Academic Press, 1975.

HYMES, D. Competence and performance in linguistic theory. In R. Huxley & E. Ingram (Eds.), *Language acquisition: Models and methods.* New York: Academic Press, 1971.

LECOURS, A.R. Methods for the description of aphasic transformations of language. In E.H. Lenneberg & E. Lenneberg (Eds.), *Foundations of language development: A multidisciplinary approach* (Vol. 2). New York, Academic Press, 1975.

LENNEBERG, E.H. Aphasiology. In E.H. Lenneberg & E. Lenneberg (Eds.), *Foundations of language development: A multidisciplinary approach* (Vol. 2). New York: Academic Press, 1975.

LOCK, A. (Ed.) *Action, gesture and symbol: The emergence of language.* London: Academic Press, 1978.

LYNCH, V., SHOEMAKER, S., & WHITE, O. Training needs survey. *AAESPH Review,* 1976, *1,* 1–16.

MAURER, S., WEHMAN, P., & REICHLE, J. *Inservicing teachers of severely and profoundly handicapped children: The IOWA model.* Unpublished manuscript, Iowa Department of Public Instruction, 1977.

MENYUK, P. Alternation of rules in children's grammar. *Journal of Verbal Learning and Verbal Behavior,* 1964, *3,* 480–488.

MENZEL, E.W. Naturalistic and experimental approaches to primate behavior. In E. Willems and H. Raush (Eds.), *Naturalistic viewpoints in psychological research.* New York: Holt, Rinehart & Winston, 1969.

MILLER, G.A. *Psychology: The science of mental life.* New York: Harper & Row, 1962.

MILLER, J.F. Assessing children's language behavior: A developmental process approach. In R.L. Schiefelbusch (Ed.), *Bases of language intervention.* Baltimore: University Park Press, 1978.

MILLER, W., & ERVIN, S. The development of grammar in child language. In U. Bellugi & R. Brown (Eds.), The acquisition of language. *Monographs of the Society for Research in Child Development, 1964, 29,* (Serial No. 92).

MOREHEAD, D., & INGRAM, D. The development of base syntax in normal and deviant children. *Journal of Speech and Hearing Research. 1973, 16,* 330–352.

MORRIS, C.W. Foundations of the theory of signs. In O. Neurath, R. Carnap, & C.W. Morris (Eds.), *International encyclopedia of unified science* (Vol. 1, no. 2). Chicago: University of Chicago Press, 1938.

NELSON, K. Structure and strategy in learning to talk. *Monographs of the Society for Research in Child Development, 1973, 38,* 149.

NELSON, K. Concept, word and sentence: Interrelations in the acquisition and development. *Psychological Review, 1974, 81,* 267–285.

NELSON, K. The conceptual basis for naming. In J. Macnamara (Ed.), *Language learning and thought.* New York: Academic Press, 1977.

NELSON, K. Semantic development and the development of semantic memory. In K.E. Nelson (Ed.), *Children's language* (Vol. 1). New York: Gardner Press, 1978.

NEWPORT, E. Motherese: The speech of mothers to young children. In N. Castellan, D. Pisoni & G. Potts (Eds.), *Cognitive theory* (Vol. 2). Hillsdale, N.J.: Lawrence Erlbaum Associates, 1976.

NEWPORT, E., GLEITMAN, H., & GLEITMAN, L.R. Mother, I'd rather do it myself: Some effects and non-effects of maternal speech style. In C.E. Snow & C.A. Ferguson (Eds.), *Talking to children: Language input and acquisition.* London: Cambridge University Press, 1977.

NEWSON, J. Dialogue and development. In A. Lock (Ed.), *Action, gesture and symbol: The emergence of language.* London and New York: Academic Press, 1978.

PHILLIPS, J. Syntax and vocabulary of mothers' speech to young children: Age and sex comparisons. *Child Development, 1973, 44,* 182–185.

PIAGET, J. *The origins of intelligence in children.* (Margaret Cook, translator). New York: International Universities Press, 1952.

PIAGET, J. *The construction of reality in the child.* New York: Basic Books, 1954.

PIAGET, J. *Play, dreams and imitation in childhood.* New York: W.W. Norton, 1962.

PREMACK, D. A functional analysis of language. *Journal of Experimental Analysis of Behavior, 1970, 14,* 107–125.

REES, N. Bases of decision in language training. *Journal of Speech and Hearing Disorders, 1972, 32,* 283–304.

REES, N. Pragmatics of language: Applications to normal and disordered language development. In R.L. Schiefelbusch (Ed.), *Bases of language intervention.* Baltimore: University Park Press, 1978.

RICE, M. *Cognition to language: Categories, word meanings, and training.* Baltimore: University Park Press, 1980.

RICHARDS, M.M. First steps in becoming social. In M.P.M. Richards (Ed.), *The integration of a child into a social world.* London: Cambridge University Press, 1974.

RICHARDS, M.M. Come and go reconsidered: Children's use of deictic verbs in contrived situations. *Journal of Verbal Learning and Verbal Behavior,* 1976, *15,* 655–665.

RUMBAUGH, D.M. (Ed.) *Language learning by a chimpanzee: The LANA project.* New York: Academic Press, 1977.

RYAN, J. Early language development: Towards a communicational analysis. In M.P.M. Richards (Ed.), *The integration of a child into a social world.* London and New York: Cambridge University Press, 1974.

SCHIEFELBUSCH, R.L. (Ed.) *Language intervention strategies.* Baltimore: University Park Press, 1978.

SCHIEFELBUSCH, R.L., & Bricker, D.D. (Eds.) *Early language: Acquisition and intervention.* Baltimore: University Park Press, 1981.

SCHIEFELBUSCH, R.L., & Hollis, J.H. *Language intervention from ape to child.* Baltimore: University Park Press, 1979.

SCHLESINGER, I.M. The role of cognitive development and linguistic input in language acquisition. *Journal of Child Language,* 1977, *4,* 153–169.

SEARLE, J. Indirect speech acts. In P. Cole & J. Morgan (Eds.), *Speech acts.* New York: Academic Press, 1975.

SINCLAIR-DeZWART, H. Language acquisition and cognitive development. In T.E. Moore (Ed.), *Cognitive development and the acquisition of language.* New York: Academic Press, 1973.

SKINNER, B.F. *Verbal behavior.* New York: Appleton-Century-Crofts, 1957.

SLOBIN, D.I. Universals in grammatical development in children. In G.B. Flores d'Arcais and W.J.M. Levelt (Eds.), *Advances in psycholinguistics.* New York: American Elsevier, 1970.

SNOW, C. Mothers' speech to children learning language. *Child Development,* 1972, *43,* 549–565.

SNYDER, L. Cognitive and communicative abilities and disabilities in the sensorimotor period. *Merrill-Palmer Quarterly,* 1978, *24,* 161–180.

STAATS, A.W. (With contribution by Staats, C.K.) *Complex human behavior.* New York: Holt, Rinehart & Winston, 1963.

WELLS, G. Learning to code experience through language. *Journal of Child Language,* 1974, *1,* 243–269.

WITTGENSTEIN, L. *Philosophical investigations.* New York: Macmillan, 1953.

CHAPTER TWO

REVIEW OF NORMAL LANGUAGE ACQUISITION

Linda McCormick

Why is study of normal language acquisition important?

This chapter provides a brief overview of how normal children learn to understand and use language. There is every reason to think that children with deficient language: (a) need language learning experiences at least as rich as those provided normal language users, (b) will attend to, understand, and talk about many of the same objects, events, and relations as typical learners, and (c) want and need to experience the same control over their environment as their more competent peers at the same stage of development. Three questions to address to developmental findings are: What linguistic and social elements of the environment contribute to early language learning? What non-linguistic phenomena do very young children attend to, understand, and talk about? How do children learn to use language to affect their environment?

To impose some order on the data, we have chosen to highlight those areas where there are significant regularities and points of agreement. An unfortunate consequence of this type of selective review is that many controversial (and often interesting) issues are slighted. For those interested in pursuing these controversies, several references for normative reviews are listed at the end of the chapter.

This chapter is divided into three major sections: The first considers language development of children from birth to age 2, the second looks at attainments from ages 2 to 4, and the third provides a synthesis of the environmental variables which significantly contribute to how and what children learn in these important years.

Biological factors receive relatively little attention in this chapter, but it is not because we consider these factors irrelevant to language-learning ability. The problem is a lack of definitive data demonstrating the relation between specific activities in the brain and concurrent language behavior. Teachers and specialists interested in reading about relations between language development and central nervous system maturation are referred to Lenneberg (1967, 1975), Lecours (1975), and Fodor (1981).

The three elements—content, form, and use—introduced in Chapter 1 organize the discussion in this chapter. Although related and interdependent, the somewhat different knowledge and skill requirements of each element facilitate partitioning. The following general themes recur frequently throughout the literature on normal development. Because each has important implications for practitioners concerned with language intervention, they introduce and summarize the chapter.

There are four important themes in literature on normal development.

1. *There is enormous variability in "normal" language learning styles and patterns.* The considerable heterogeneity within the population of "normal" language learners precludes development of a single set of standards against which to judge the development of language deficient children. However, this heterogeneity should not be dismissed as simply a troublesome feature of early language; it has important implications for assessment and remediation. In fact, study of the ways in which normal learners differ from each other can be more useful than documenting the ways in which they are similar.

2. *Children are active participators in the language learning process; they are actors long before they are reactors.* At birth, the orienting reflex is already functional in both visual and acoustic modalities, and very soon thereafter the infant begins actively to analyze, structure, and store information in a highly differentiated manner. The persistence, attentiveness, and desire to manipulate objects that we see in infants are evidence of what Hunt (1965) has called the motivational characteristic of infancy. The caregiver's role is essentially one of following the baby's lead and orchestrating the dynamics of the exchange process.

3. *The caregiver role is critically important in early language learning.* That adults are generally responsive to infants is commonly observed, but until recently the significance of this responsiveness was not fully realized. Caregiving rituals such as feeding, joint action routines like playing peekaboo, and the natural propensity of caregivers to treat babies as if they were intentional communicators (long before they actually are) play a significant role in early development. Without a listener there can be no communication; unless there are "significant others" willing to interact socially and linguistically with an infant, language learning will be profoundly hindered. Caregivers are the mediators, facilitators, and determiners of all infant learning activities.

4. *The interactionist perspective provides the best framework for understanding normal language learning.* The basic premise of the interactionist perspective is twofold: (a) infants are born with some general tendencies to perceive, organize, and interact with their world in certain ways, and (b) the amount and variety of experiences that infants are provided will significantly affect the realization of their predispositions. There is little doubt but that

they come prepared to learn to talk; however, the environment must teach them about talking. An analogy is the child who comes to school with books, paper, and pencils, as well as the ability and motivation to learn. There is little question that preparedness is necessary. It is not, however, sufficient for learning to occur. Appropriate learning experiences must be provided.

The interactionist position is supported by the observations that: (a) all children, unless limited by sensory, neuromuscular, or cognitive impairments, become competent communicators when provided with a reasonable amount and variety of linguistic and social experiences, and (b) all normal learners acquire the particular language system of their linguistic environment. The first observation, that all nonhandicapped children acquire language, is evidence of some innate predisposition; the second, that they acquire the language of their culture, confirms environmental impact on these mechanisms.

The interactionist perspective as introduced in the previous chapter reflects a rapprochement between cognitive, pragmatic, and behavioral theories as encouraged by Staats (1974), Moerk (1977), and Bricker, Macke, Levin, and Campbell (1981). The Piagetian viewpoint is heavily emphasized in this chapter because Piaget's writings are the most comprehensive and detailed account of early cognitive development available. However, many of the concepts can be encompassed by learning theory and translated into behavioral terms. For example, compare Piaget's description of the development of concepts—a progressive structuring so that later structures subsume earlier structures on a new level of functioning (Furth, 1970)—with a behavioral description of response class formation—a progressive series of differentiations producing a terminal response quite different from any of the responses previously exhibited (Staats, 1966). Note that both deal with learning, one from an internal viewpoint, the other from an external viewpoint. But in both cases, the product is the same—a concept. From a practical standpoint, Piaget's conceptualization can aid teachers and communication specialists in *describing* cognitive development; functional analyses lead to empirical research and formulation of intervention strategies.

See Tables 2–1, 2–3, and 2–6 for material adjunctive to the following discussion. Tables 2-1, 2-3, and 2-6 provide adjunctive material for the following discussion. These tables are a useful reference for developing individualized checklists as described in Chapters 4 and 5. Table 2-1 pinpoints the development of content (sensorimotor/cognitive) skills. Table 2-3 pinpoints achievements in the development of form and form/content (auditory-vocal) skills. Table 2-6 charts the emergence of use (social-interactive) skills.

DEVELOPMENT FROM BIRTH TO AGE TWO

At 0;1 (10) he alternately looks at his nurse and at me and, in examining me, his eyes oscillate between my hair and my face.... At 0;1 (25) he looks in turn at his nurse, his mother, and myself with a change of attitude when confronted by each new face and an abrupt and spontaneous moving of his glance from one face to the other. (Piaget, 1952, p. 69)

As Piaget observed, and as anyone who has had any experience with infants can testify, they are anything but passive, helpless, and undemanding. Seemingly "tuned" to understanding, sharing, and communicating, infants invariably elicit these same types of behaviors from their caregivers. Given this responsiveness, it is not surprising that infants show more interest in people than in inanimate objects (Stern, 1974).

> Infants are "tuned" to understand, share, and communicate, and they elicit the same from their caregivers.

The newborn's potential for organization and development within his environment is shown, among other things, by his ability to quiet himself to pay attention to his caregivers and by his obvious preference for faces and human voices (Brazelton, 1979). When he hears a human voice, he searches for the face, and when he finds it, his face brightens and his eyes become wide, soft and eager. He may even crane his neck and lift his chin gently toward the source of the voice, and his body tension visibly increases. It is a rare adult who can resist picking him up and cuddling him. The baby then responds, in turn, and molds his body to the caregiver's, clinging gently with his legs and possibly even grabbing hold of the adult's clothing. The interaction continues as the adult, naturally reinforced by these responses, cuddles some more, often engaging in face-to-face contact and perhaps rocking and singing. Thus, caregiver-child communications begin and so they will continue, with both partners participating, until such time as the child learns conventional language symbols to replace cooing, crying, quieting, looking, and cuddling.

PRECURSORS TO LANGUAGE CONTENT

This section specifies the cognitive achievements of children before they begin to produce syntactic constructions. Recent studies of early cognitive and semantic development and early diary studies (Piaget, 1952, 1954, 1970, 1980) have provided some answers to several provocative questions about the construction of meaning.

1. How do infants learn about the functional properties and states of animate and inanimate objects?

2. How do infants learn the ways objects can properly relate to one another?

3. What criteria do infants use when they select some objects, events, and relations to learn before others?

4. How does an infant categorize and store experiential knowledge so that he can retrieve it and talk about it?

5. How and when do infants come to realize that something can "stand for" something else—that signals and symbols represent ideas?

40

These important questions have been particularly difficult to answer because the primary data are not directly observable. Answers must be inferred from secondary data sources, e.g., the child's actions with animate and inanimate objects, and the way he uses and misuses words when he begins talking. You can get some idea of how difficult this task is if you imagine yourself trying to discover how a library is organized and what it contains without ever entering the building. You could query everyone leaving and note the books they are carrying so your description would be *relatively* accurate, if you asked the right questions. But there will also be many inconsistencies, gaps, and presumably, inaccuracies in such a description. This is precisely the situation confronting researchers attempting to describe language acquisition.

How do children learn to organize their sensory impressions in a meaningful way?

To introduce our discussion of the enormous organizational task facing the infant, we begin with this rather esoteric statement: *Children learn about objects and events through a process of progressive, qualitative organization and reorganization of their own actions and perceptions.* Organization is the key word in this statement; it is also the key process in cognition. Consider the following scenario to appreciate what "organization" means in this context.

Imagine that you have just moved to a new house or apartment. The movers have unpacked the boxes marked "kitchen" and you must now make some kind of order out of the chaos. You are faced with the task of sorting and storing a variety of items so that they will be easily retrievable when you want to prepare a meal. You may try a number of ways to do this, possibly with some help from another person. Eventually you will come up with categories of items that should be stored in close proximity to each other for maximum efficiency during meal preparation, baking and clean-up times.

The task you are faced with in organizing your kitchen is similar to the one facing the young child who is organizing sensory information and constructing meanings. He must come up with a classification and storage system so that he can understand what others are talking about when they address him and so that he will be able to retrieve meanings when he wants to talk about something. Prior to grouping his countless experiences with the world so that they will be retrievable, the child must first determine their relevant characteristics. Just as you will group all glasses and baking pans together in your kitchen because they have common perceptual and functional properties, the infant will group according to perceptual and functional similarities (when he can figure out what these are). If you leave items scattered wherever the movers happened to place them, you would find preparing a meal difficult, if not impossible. By the same token, if the child does not come up with a system for classifying the sensory information he receives, language will be impossible.

We might add that the infant's task is made exceedingly more complicated by the fact that the categorizations are not totally left to his discretion. Decisions regarding how the world is to be divided up for the purposes of language have already been made by the particular language community in which he finds himself. The child must discover the principles that govern the form in which each meaning is expressed in his language culture. In other words, different cultures generate different "meaning potentials" and categorizations because the purpose of language can be strikingly different across cultures. Consider how much more difficult your kitchen organizing task would be if some categorizations were dictated by our culture rather than left totally to your discretion.

According to Piaget, organization is one of the tendencies which exert the greatest influence on learning. Organization is the tendency to systematize and combine processes into cohesive, orderly, and ultimately, smoother functioning patterns. Consider looking and grasping, two of the infant's earliest means of operating on the environment. Initially, each functions independently; the infant can grasp an object, or he can look at it, but he cannot manage both at the same time. In time, after considerable practice grasping and looking, he will be able to combine the two. He will learn to look at what he grasps, and grasp what he is looking at.

Infants become aware of regularities related to objects and events (e.g., that they exist even when not directly perceivable) through repeated action upon and with the stimuli in their environment (Piaget, 1952, 1954, 1970). They learn, for example, that "things" can cease to exist and then recur, that people (including themselves) can relate to objects in certain prescribed ways such as owning them, locating, and relocating them, and that objects also relate to themselves and each other in a relatively consistent manner.

Infants learn about objects and events by repeatedly experiencing them.

The infant decides which among the myriad objects and events in his environment he will turn his attention to and learn about. Probably, as the "moderate novelty principle" predicts, this selection depends on how discrepant from the familiar the objects and events are. Those that are moderately novel are most likely to attract the infant's attention and therefore have the greatest probability of being learned.

In addition to organization, there must be adaptation. Adaptation has two parts, *assimilation* and *accommodation*. *Assimilation* is the process through which new information and new experiences are incorporated into the organism's existing cognitive repertoire. The other side of the coin, *accommodation,* is the process through which the organism's existing cognitive repertoire changes in accordance with the new and different information. The end result of these two processes, which never occur in isolation, is a more complex and sophisticated repertoire. Consider this scenario as an example of the adaptation process. A 4-month-old encounters a new object, a small teddy bear. He applies his limited "knowing strategies"—grasping, mouthing, hitting, and shaking—to the strange new "thing." Two properties of the teddy bear, presumably novel to the infant, are softness (for cuddling) and furriness (for stroking). If he attends to these properties and begins to cuddle and/or rub the teddy bear, he has learned something from this experience with a new object; he has assimilated and accommodated. Adaptation has occurred. For Piaget, all learning from birth to death reflects the dynamic fluctuations of assimilation

Part of the child's adaptation to a new object is to assimilate it; the other part is to accommodate to the object's unique features.

and accommodation. When either one dominates, there is disequilibrium which incites the organism to go beyond its present state in search of new knowledge.

Learning, bringing assimilation and accommodation into balance, requires (a) attending to apparently discrepant elements in the environment, (b) interpreting and appreciating them as discrepant, (c) responding to the discrepancy by trying to explain or resolve it, and (d) coming up with a reconceptualization of the situation that resolves the apparent conflict. A nonsense analogy will help you see how this works.

As an adult, you have a firm and broad concept of grass. Among its myriad properties you have perceptual attributes such as its usual color, green. Imagine that you go outside one morning and find, to your amazement, that all the grass in your neighborhood is purple. After you recover from this startling discovery, you assure yourself that the purple stuff growing from the ground is indeed grass, and, perhaps, checking a nearby neighborhood, you assimilate the information that grass can be purple as well as green. As your concept for grass changes to conform to this new information (accommodates), learning occurs.

Learning occurs when there is disequilibrium.

Your cognitive system moves from a state of equilibrium (relative to the concept of grass) to one of disequilibrium, or cognitive conflict, and then adjusts back to a state of harmony. According to Piaget, the state of disequilibrium or cognitive conflict impels humans to make cognitive progress—to learn. New, more intellectually advanced states are achieved by conceptualizing discrepant perceptual information. Piaget argues that all significant cognitive advances are made through this kind of adaptation or self-regulation process. Throughout life there is a give-and-take between perceiving and adapting (conceptualizing and reconceptualizing), the important processes through which meanings (concepts) are formed.

Cognitive development undoubtedly influences language development. Precise relationships, however, are not clear.

Something to keep in mind when reading about prelinguistic concepts is that there are not, as yet, enough solid data to argue *unequivocally* for a *causal* relationship between specific cognitive structures and language attainments. That cognition in some way and to some extent *influences* language development must be considered a rational, rather than an empirical, consensus at the present time. This is the reason we use the more cautious term *precursor* in place of *prerequisite.* Although many investigators suggest using Piaget's theory of cognitive development as a guide for the precursors of language development (e.g., Bates, 1976; Bloom, 1973; Bloom and Lahey, 1978; Ingram, 1976; Sinclair-deZwart, 1969, 1971; Robinson and Robinson, 1978), there is little empirical verification of direct relationships between specific cognitive attainments (e.g., object permanence) and subsequent language variables, such as vocabulary growth or semantic categories. Two-way relationships between thought and language and language and thought are assumed, and certainly are logical; but they have not yet been empirically demonstrated. Whether the attainment of any one or of any known combination of cognitive structures assures language acquisition is, at best, a questionable assumption. Teachers and clinicians cannot assume that language is being facilitated when only perceptual and cognitive processes are targeted. These processes are only one piece of an enormously complex puzzle. At this point, we are not sure of the size of this piece or, for that matter, even its exact shape.

TABLE 2-1   Emergence of language content from birth to age 4

Age Range	Sensorimotor/Cognitive Skills
0–1 month	Visually follows some objects (if supine) Orients to light and some sounds Practices innate reflexes (sucking, prehension)
1–4 months	Follows slowly moving object through 180° arc Continues to look at point where slowly moving object disappeared Coordinates action schemes (e.g., vision + hearing, sucking + grasping, vision + grasping) Holds and briefly inspects two objects and alternately mouths them
4–8 months	Continues manual search for an object *if* grasping is interrupted by removal of the object Looks at the point where a moving object should reappear Searches for partially hidden object Behaves as if an object no longer exists when it drops out of sight Bangs objects together Shakes "shakeable" objects (e.g., rattle, bell) Performs some *differentiated* actions with objects—crumbling (paper), sliding (toys on surface), tearing, stretching, rubbing, mouthing Finds object hidden under one of 3 screens (*if* hiding is visible)
8–12 months	Finds object hidden under a number of superimposed screens Demonstrates new actions on objects (related to object properties) Drops and throws objects/toys intentionally Uses objects in socially relevant manner (e.g., puts necklace on, hugs doll, dresses doll) Searches for and finds object under a single screen after invisible displacement (object not directly visible during the hiding) Combines functional relationships (e.g., cup on saucer) to some extent Places one cube in cup and removes it (on command)
12–16 months	Searches for object after invisible displacement under one of two screens (later, with three screens) Varies actions on objects to "experiment with different effects" (e.g., explores gravity) Links more objects in functional relationships Shows/offers objects to others to look at Can place 6–9 cubes in a cup and then remove them (after demonstration) Pulls out and replaces one peg in peg board Puts pellets in and then removes them from a bottle Places round shape in three shape formboard Builds tower of 2–3 blocks

TABLE 2-1 (continued)

Age Range	Sensorimotor/Cognitive Skills
16–24 months	Finds object hidden by a series of successive invisible displacements (knows it must be there someplace) Demonstrates understanding of the functions and social meanings of a large number of objects Performs several action patterns in sequence with familiar objects (e.g., places cup in saucer, stirs imaginary drink, drinks from cup) Puts 6 pegs in peg board Places 2 round and 2 square blocks in form board Places triangle, square and circle correctly on form board Builds tower of 4–6 blocks Indicates knowledge of the whereabouts of familiar persons and recognizes current absence Matches on the basis of color Demonstrates understanding of reflexive object relations (relations of object to itself or to an equivalent object of the same class)—that an object can exist, cease to exist or disappear and then reappear or recur Demonstrates understanding of the following agent-object relations (meaning usually encoded with single word): a. agent bringing about an action b. object affected by agent's action c. action Demonstrates understanding of simple locative relations (the location of two objects in relation to one another) Demonstrates understanding of state relations: a. possession—that objects belong to, or are associated with, particular persons b. attribution—that certain attributes (shape, size, color, etc.) distinguish among like objects from an object class
2–3 years	Enjoys simple pictures and stories Performs more realistic and expanded action series (4-5 appropriately chained actions) Indicates object missing from a small array of familiar objects Recognizes (points to) and names colors Solves match-to-sample problems (with shapes, objects, pictures, colors) Groups objects by single dimensions (color, shape, size) Uses newly acquired behaviors in varied settings Engages in prolonged domestic make-believe play Builds tower or bridge with 7–9 blocks Applies previous experience to solving new problems Demonstrates the ability to remember absent objects and events
3–4 years	Places as many as 10 shapes in place Makes tower or bridge with 9 or more blocks Remembers daily routine sequences Knows shapes, sizes, positions and colors Knows number symbols 1–10 Knows time (day-night) and seasons

The cognitive universals alleged to have a precursive relationship to the emergence of language in the second year are object permanence, schemes for relating to objects, means-end behavior, causality, and imitation. The infant begins constructing some concepts (Piaget calls these early schemes *preconcepts*) at birth. These concepts become more sophisticated, refined, and better organized during the 18 to 24 months which follow. Finally, in the last half of the second year, the infant begins to use words and some word combinations consistently and meaningfully. Symbolic skills, as first shown in symbolic play, do not begin to emerge until near the end of the sensorimotor period (about 18 to 24 months of age), so they will be discussed in the next section. Table 2-2 presents an overview of the development of object permanence and schemes for relating to objects. Achievement of these two concepts appears related to language learning, particularly the construction of meanings.

Object permanence is defined as the understanding that objects continue to exist even when not immediately perceptible. For example, you know that your car will be where you left it. Although you cannot see or touch it right now, you know that it will still be there, unless it has been towed away or stolen. Construction of this concept means that the child is learning to separate himself from his environment and to analyze it into separate objects which still exist when they are out of sight.

Definition of *schemes for relating to objects* is a little more involved. In the Piagetian literature, the term *scheme* is used in reference to specific actions or action sequences consistently and habitually carried out with, or applied to, particular classes of objects and situations. The scheme itself is the mental (internal) organization of the overt actions or action sequences arising from the child's individual experience. The cognitive capacity makes organized, object-specific behavior patterns possible. For example, the very young infant who sucks everything that finds its way into his mouth would be said to have a sucking scheme. He has the ability and inclination to apply a specific action, sucking, in response to particular objects ("suckables"). Similarly, we talk about listening, grasping, looking, hitting, kicking, etc. schemes. An important property of schemes is that they can be combined, recombined, and coordinated in various ways to form larger action patterns. At first all objects elicit the same schemes (e.g., sucking, grasping) which happen to be in the infant's reflexive repertoire. Gradually, schemes become differentiated and under the control of object properties (e.g., the child throws a ball, drinks from a cup, shakes a rattle).

As noted above, *means-end behavior* and *causality* also appear to influence language acquisition. Because they are considered precursors of language use, they are presented in a separate table in that section. The development of *imitation* is presented as a precursor to language form. Age ranges for the various attainments are designated in all of the tables, but they should not be considered inviolate; some infants move through the substages more rapidly than others. What is considered to be inviolate

Certain cognitive attainments are posited as necessary to the emergence of language.

1. Object permanence

2. Schemes for relating to objects

3. Means-end behavior

4. Causality

is the sequence. A substage is never skipped. Following is a description of behaviors demonstrating object permanence and schemes for relating to objects—two of the four constructs presumed to be precursive to the developing language content. Table 2-2 includes more recent findings of other investigators that support Piaget's clinical observations of the development of perceptual and cognitive structures in the first 18 to 24 months.

By the latter half of their second year, children are attending to and learning about the properties of objects (see Table 2-2). They are demonstrating relatively efficient and usually accurate categorization of new concept exemplars as reflected in production of an increasing number of concept labels (e.g., "pencil," "cow," "apple").

One way to get some clue about how children are progressing in their organization of internal representations of the world (their semantic "groupings") is to analyze their errors in word usage. The kinds of mistakes young children make tell us how they are categorizing nonlinguistic objects, events, and relations, and what hypotheses they have formed about concept-word associations. This information is useful when planning intervention targets.

The word usage error which has generated the most research attention is *overextension*. A child overextends (overgeneralizes) a word when he uses it to refer to objects and events or in contexts where an adult would not use it. Use of the word "doggie," for example, to refer to a four-legged animal other than a dog represents a guess by the child that the four-legged animal is a member of the category which his culture refers to as dogs. He has taken what preliminary information he has gleaned about what the word means and guessed (tested the hypothesis) that it can be used to refer to this new creature. Such overgeneralization errors give us information about how children relate form and content and the extent to which their semantic organization matches that of an adult.

The opposite of overextension is *underextension*—the use of a word for only a subset of the objects, events, or relations for which an adult would use the word, e.g., "cookie" used only for round cookies or "juice" only for orange juice. A third type of mistake is overlap, where the child's usage of a word demonstrates both overextension and underextension: "cookie" for round cookies and round crackers, but not for cookies of other shapes. When a child makes an overlap error, we can assume that he has not yet established a stable, adult-like semantic concept.

The hypothesis-testing process manifest in overextensions, underextensions, and overlaps appears to be an effective learning strategy for the child. When adults make appropriate responses to children's guesses, they contribute to vocabulary growth. It is not difficult to see the importance of both linguistic and nonlinguistic experiences to language learning and the difficulties children encounter grappling with organization of reality and form-content (word-meaning) linkages.

Environmental input interacts with cognitive developments and activities to produce higher-order concepts. What seems clear is that children are from the very beginning active explorers and fairly competent or-

> The word errors children make tell us something about how they are organizing what they learn.

TABLE 2-2 Representative behaviors in the development of object permanence and the schemes for relating to objects (Suggested precursors to language content)

	Object Permanence	Schemes for Relating to Objects	Related Findings
Birth–1 month Stage 1: Modification of Reflexes	Continuously practices innate reflexes such as sucking, vocalization, and some eye, hand, arm and leg movements until they become refined Orients in response to voice on both sides and light stimuli Demonstrates some visual pursuit when lying on back	No discernable separation in development from object permanence at this stage	Rudimentary ability for depth discrimination evident in differential responses to spheres and circles (Kessen, Haith, & Salapatek, 1970) Attraction to light, sharp edges, and contours (Salapatek & Kessen, 1966)
1–4 months Stage 2: Primary Circular Reactions	Gradually coordinates schemes—vision and hearing, sucking and grasping, and vision and grasping become related Able to visually follow a slowly moving object through a 180 degree arc in a smooth tracking response Very little, if any, visual or manual search for a vanished object—"out of sight is out of mind" Lingers with only a brief glance at the point where a slowly moving object disappears	Shows *incidental* object use in the process of practicing different behaviors such as grasping and looking Mouths some objects Holds and briefly inspects various objects Tactually explores objects to some extent	Shifts from attending to contours and movement to preference for complex and moderately novel objects (Kagan, 1971) Able to focus both eyes on near objects with well-developed depth and size perception (Bower, 1965, 1974)

TABLE 2-2 (continued)

	Object Permanence	Schemes for Relating to Objects	Related Findings
4–8 months Stage 3: Secondary Circular Reactions	Visually anticipates the future positions of objects—looks at the point where a moving object should appear Continues manual search for an object *if* grasping movements are interrupted while in process Recognizes and obtains an object which is *partially* hidden Behaves as if an object no longer exists when it is *completely* covered or drops out of sight	Shows *systematic* object use in practicing different behaviors Bangs objects together Shakes a rattle, bell, and other objects Visually inspects an object *while* tactually exploring it Displays other differentiated actions with objects including: crumpling (of paper) sliding (of toys on surface) tearing stretching rubbing mouthing	Understands object identity but *not* object constancy (Bower, 1965) Searches *only* around the point where an object disappears (Miller, Cohen & Hill, 1970) Exhibits facial and vocal surprise when a hidden toy is uncovered (Bower, 1974)
8–12 months Stage 4: Coordination of Secondary Reactions	Looks for an object after it has vanished behind a screen and reliably retrieves it Reacts with only mild surprise/puzzlement when object retrieved differs from the one hidden Continues searching for an object at point A (where it is usually found) even after watching it being hidden at new location B Toward the end of this stage, infant's search becomes more persistent and he will find the object hidden alternately under any one of three screens	Demonstrates new actions on objects resulting from (related to) object properties Intentionally drops and throws objects Uses objects in a socially relevant manner: Puts a necklace around his neck Pretends to drink from a cup Hugs doll or stuffed animal Tries to dress a doll Sniffs flowers Builds structure with blocks Pretends to drive a toy car Combines functional relationships such as placing cup in saucer to some extent	Attends to objects that offer manipulative possibilities and more than one perceptual dimension; prefers objects that make noise, have texture as well as pattern and color, and come apart (Kagan, 1971) Searches successfully for hidden objects but still depends more upon searching skills than memory of the hidden objects (Gratch, 1972)

TABLE 2-2   (continued)

	Object Permanence	Schemes for Relating to Objects	Related Findings
12–16 months Stage 5: Tertiary Circular Reactions	When the hiding is visible, infant will search in the place where it was last seen (even with three screens) Not successful at retrieving objects if hiding is not visible because he cannot yet "think" where an object *might* be	Varies actions on objects to "experiment" with different effects (such as dropping objects to study their trajectory) Links more objects in functional relationships: Puts cup on saucer and pretends to drink from cup Slides brush or comb over his hair Pushes truck/car back and forth Places as many as nine cubes in cup Builds a two block tower Stacks cups	Searches for a hidden object in the place where it was last *seen*, rather than the place where it was last found (Gratch & Landers, 1971) Changes actions on objects to produce variations (Lowe, 1975)
16–24 months Stage 6: Invention of New Means through Mental Combinations	Systematically searches for an object that has undergone as many as three invisible displacements—searches each hiding place (sometimes in reverse order)	Demonstrates understanding of the functions and social meanings of a large number of objects: Holds telephone to ear and vocalizes Tries to put shoes and socks on Lines truck and trailer up as if truck is pulling trailer (Lowe, 1975) Names familiar objects	Attention attracted by things that move and can be acted upon (Nelson, 1973) Actions with objects reflect the unique functional properties of the objects (Lowe, 1975)

ganizers of their environment. They seem intent upon, or perhaps even somehow preprogrammed for, discovering regularities in their perceptions of the world and in relations between their actions and the objects upon which they act. They apply what they discover about regularities and relations to productive adaptations of their behavior for different purposes at different stages.

That children's behavior in some way draws upon and is influenced by past experiences is unmistakably clear. Precisely how experiences are internally represented and organized is difficult to establish but we can be confident that they are somehow organized in meaningful and accessible ways. Otherwise the child could not, as all children eventually do, communicate his experiences through the formal system of language. Returning to the kitchen analogy, it can be said that the child begins "organizing his kitchen" almost at birth, and by the time he is approaching age 2, he has sufficient organization to express a range and variety of meanings.

Precisely what the child will attend to and learn about at any point in time depends upon at least four variables.

As teachers and clinicians, our concern is with influencing achievement of the cognitive precursors of language. The cognitive development research suggests some direction for our efforts. What is meaningful for infants and very young children—what they will attend to and ultimately learn about—depends upon at least the four following child and environmental variables (Wells, 1974):

1. *The child's deprivation state relative to certain needs.* The child's reasons for engaging in a particular environmental interaction will affect whether he pays attention to that interaction. According to Hunt (1965) and Bruner (1969), earliest interactions are stimulated by and have a physiological base in avoidance of thirst, hunger, and discomfort and by an innate drive for action and learning. The need for social interaction also motivates early interactions with the environment (Schaffer, 1971, 1977; Uzgiris, 1981). In either case, whether the reasons are biological or social, which elements of the environment are meaningful to the child will depend on his deprivation status relative to these variables. If he is hungry, food will attract and hold his attention; if he is bored, a musical mobile may be meaningful. Eventually, language is the instrumental means by which these purposes are realized, but the child must first attend to, construct, and organize the meanings language will communicate. When he moves into his second year, the meaningfulness of different aspects of the environment will undoubtedly be determined by more complex and sophisticated purposes than by the relatively primitive "drives" noted above. But initially physiological states, boredom, curiosity, and the need for social interaction will determine attention, actions and, consequently, learning.

2. *How caregivers structure and selectively direct the child's attention.* Gaining attention, with both verbal and nonverbal devices, is an important element of early caregiver-child interactions (Ratner & Bruner, 1978). Kagan (1971) delineates three variables

related to environmental structure that influence children's selection of what they will attend to and subsequently process: (a) the range of objects and events that are available, (b) the number of routines and rituals, such as feeding, which permit the child to experience different events repeatedly occurring in relation to one another, and (c) the amount of encouragement the child receives to act upon and with those aspects of the environment which interest him. Because these variables are all under caregiver, teacher, or clinician control, they have enormous significance for intervention planning and implementation.

3. *The information processing strategies that are available to the child.* Information about processing strategies is the area about which we know the least and over which we have the least direct control. The processing strategies children bring to the task of constructing meaning are difficult, if not impossible, for clinicians and teachers to directly observe or manipulate. Somehow the normal child filters incoming information, reduces it to manageable proportions, stores what he finds useful in a retrievable form, and links it with established knowledge categories. The task of teachers and clinicians is to help handicapped children accomplish these processing strategies (see Chapter Five).

4. *What the child already knows.* What objects, events, and relations are salient and meaningful to a child at any given time depends upon how he has organized his established meaning categories. What he notices and tries to understand depends, to some extent, on what he already knows. With practice, clinicians and teachers can make some felicitous deductions about the child's extant organizations. Keep in mind that early concepts go through frequent modifications during the course of sensorimotor development. An experience may be uninterpretable and therefore essentially meaningless to an infant at, say, 3 months, but salient and "useable" at 9 months because of new concepts constructed from many actions upon and perceptions of the objects and events in his environment between 3 and 9 months. The newly constructed concepts may provide relevant criteria for assignment of meaning to the new experience.

This section has considered the precursors to language content—how very young children, prior to any considerable mastery of syntax, acquire and organize their experiences so that they can talk about them. Because the present state of our judgments depends more on inferences and intuition than on empirical data about the relationships between perceptual and cognitive development and language acquisition, we have cautioned against assuming that cognition determines language. However, cognitive achievement is certainly necessary for language acquisition. Language specialists and teachers cannot afford to gloss over these important normative findings.

PRECURSORS TO LANGUAGE FORM

A child's ultimate mastery of functional language depends in part upon his ability to discriminate and learn conventional linguistic devices, including sounds, words, manual signs (or other meaning representations), and syntatic rules. While they serve the very young infant quite well, crying and cooing soon become inadequate to express more sophisticated needs and desires. If speech is to be his language mode, he must learn to produce acoustic signals; if, for some reason, oral language is not feasible, he must learn to form manual or other visual signs. In either case he must also learn the morphological markers (prefixes and suffixes) of his language culture and, eventually, its syntax to convey a rapidly accumulating store of meanings and intentions.

Phonological Development   As emphasized in Chapter One, the precise physiological and neuromuscular coordination required by speech is exceedingly complex. In addition to precise control of the lips, tongue, teeth, and hard and soft palates, oral language requires coordinations of respiration, phonation, and resonance. The normal infant begins learning these coordinations from the moment of his first cry. During the early months of life, through exercise and refinement of his eating-related reflexes (rooting, sucking, swallowing, etc.) and crying and vocalization, he gradually gains control over breathing and the oro-facial structures required for speech sound production.

> Development of the child's sound system begins at birth. In the first phase of phonological development the child produces some segments of speech-like sounds and discriminates certain features of adult speech.

Vocalizations (crying and noncrying sounds) which are initially reflexive soon become intentional until, by about the fifth or sixth month, the infant is producing long streams of playful squeals, screams, coos, and babbles. During this babbling period there is a noticeable increase in the number and kinds of sounds made by the hearing child (in contrast to the deaf or hearing-impaired infant). Babbling sounds begin to resemble the consonants and vowels of adult speech in the child's language culture. In time, consonant-vowel sequences are identifiable as the infant begins to imitate specific sounds of the adults in his environment (Ingram, 1976; Ferguson, 1976). An overview of the development of imitation, based primarily on Piaget's work, is presented in Table 2-4.

Table 2-4 shows that imitation is not a simple construct. The infant does not acquire this skill without considerable practice over a period of approximately 18 months. It is important for teachers and language specialists to keep this developmental progression in mind when imitation training is being considered. Guidelines for imitation training are provided in Chapter Six.

In the seventies there was particularly rapid growth in our understanding of the perceptual abilities of infants. The fact that all sensory organs are functional at birth is in itself an impressive finding. In a summary of the first decade of research in infant speech perception, Morse (1979) concludes that for almost all of the discriminations tested, the infants' perceptions are surprisingly similar to those of adults. However, while they

TABLE 2-3 Emergence of language form and form/content linkages from birth to age four

Age Range	Auditory-Vocal Skills
0–1 month	Reacts (startles, stops movement, shifts eyes) to sharp/loud auditory stimuli Vocalizes occasionally (other than crying)
1–3 months	Reacts (stops whimpering, startles, turns head) to voice, rattle of spoon, and bell sounds Vocalizes (babbles, coos) in play and when spoken to Demonstrates mutual imitation (responds to model of own sounds) Produces single vowel sounds (*ah, eh, uh*)
4–6 months	Localizes source of voice sounds and noisemakers Attends and responds to voice affect (anger, playfulness) Babbles repetitive syllable series (e.g., *da-da-da*)
7–9 months	Responds to simple requests (e.g., "wave bye-bye") Selectively attends to familiar words (e.g., "no-no," "daddy," own name) Imitates speech sounds (*if* already in his vocal repertoire) Imitates nonspeech sounds (cough, tongue click, lip smacking) Says "da-da" and/or "ma-ma" Vocalizes in recognition of familiar persons
10–12 months	Responds to inhibitory words (e.g., "no-no") Responds to simple action requests Responds immediately to own name Gives objects on request (e.g., cup, spoon, ball, car) Says three or more words (other than da-da and ma-ma) Vocalizes familiar sounds on hearing novel ones (begins to approximate novel sounds)
13–15 months	Points to familiar persons, animals, toys on request Imitates novel sound sequences Locates familiar objects on request (if kept in a predictable location) Says 5 to 10 words (usually nouns referring to animals, food, and toys) Uses two-words (noun phrases or verb phrases) to express semantic relations previously encoded by single words (see Table 2-5) a. existence b. negation c. recurrence d. attribution e. possession f. location g. agent-action h. action-object i. agent-object Begins to name absent objects and events
16–18 months	Responds to requests for play actions ("push the truck," "kiss the baby") Points to three named body parts (on self or doll) Follows one-step directions

TABLE 2-3 (continued)

Age Range	Auditory-Vocal Skills
19–22 months	Points to pictures of familiar objects (2–5) on request Responds to simple two-step directions with an object Responds to the following two-term relations: possessor-possessed, entity-locative, agent-action, and action-object Produces successive single-word utterances coding different aspects of same event (e.g., "car . . . see," "juice . . . mommy") Uses some two-word combinations to code relational meanings (e.g., "more cookie") Produces approximately 50 single words Says "What's that" to elicit object names At least 25% of speech is intelligible
2–2½ years	Produces simple noun phrases (modifier + noun) Produces simple verb phrase with main action verb unmarked (no inflections) Answers yes/no questions that deal with familiar events At least 60% of speech is intelligible
2½–3 years	Produces expanded noun phrases (demonstrative + modifier [or articles] + noun) Produces verbs marked with the present progressive grammatical inflection (-ing) Uses -s to mark plurality Uses the preposition "in" Indicates negation by inserting "no" or "not" after the simple noun phrase ("mommy no") or before noun phrase or verb phrase ("not baby," "no kiss") Answers "what doing?", "what is this?", and "where?" questions dealing with familiar objects and events Uses more and different words to encode the same semantic relations (see above) At least 75% of speech is intelligible
3–3½ years	Produces further expanded noun phrases (demonstrative + article + adjective + noun) Uses "to be" as copula but *not* as auxiliary Uses the preposition "on" Uses possessive -s consistently Uses *wh*- word to introduce questions Uses "can't" and "don't" to mark negatives Answers "whose?", "who?", "why?", and "how many?" questions Imitates sentences up to 6 words in length At least 85% of speech is intelligible
3½–4 years	Expands noun phrase to include prepositional phrase Interchanges auxiliary and subject noun phrases in producing yes/no questions ("I am big" = "Am I big") Uses "cannot" and "do not" (as well as "can't" and "don't") Answers "how?" questions Begins to use past tense At least 95% of speech is intelligible

TABLE 2-4 Development of sensorimotor imitation

Stage 1 (Birth to 1 month):	**Vocal contagion.** Infant is incapable of "true" imitation, but acts that appear to be imitative do occur. One crying newborn is likely to stimulate the other infants to cry. Piaget describes this phenomenon as the triggering of existing response patterns through external stimulation.
Stage 2 (1–4 months):	**Mutual imitation.** The infant will often repeat a habitual response (gestural or vocal) if someone has immediately mimicked the production. Reproductions are limited and are only gross approximations of the model.
Stage 3 (4–8 months):	**Systematic imitation.** Since the child is now able to coordinate vision and prehension, he can imitate many more acts. He can now imitate movements such as opening and closing the fist but cannot imitate acts, such as opening and closing the eyes, that he cannot see himself performing. The child apparently needs a visual impression that matches that which he has seen the model create in order to duplicate the model. Also, the child will imitate only those sounds and movements that are already in his repertoire. Thus, imitation at this stage is less a learning strategy than a strategy to prolong or continue those events the child finds meaningful.
Stage 4 (8–12 months):	**Imitation of new behaviors.** The ability to imitate movements that he cannot see himself, and produce and imitate some acts that are not already known emerge simultaneously. Imitation undergoes a transition from being a means for continuing interesting events, to being a means for learning new ones. However, only actions and vocalizations *similar* to those in the child's repertoire are imitated.
Stage 5 (12–18 months):	**Expanded imitation of new behaviors.** Reproductions of new models are immediate, deliberate, and usually quite accurate. Imitation is used in a trial-and-error fashion to discover the properties of objects. Novel vocalizations will be imitated repeatedly as if to perfect the reproduction.
Stage 6 (18–24 months):	**Deferred (or representative) imitation.** Imitation no longer requires that the model be immediately present. The child is now capable of mental representation and long term memory for what was modeled. He is also capable of imitating complex new acts and objects as well as persons.

have been shown to be sensitive to speech sounds in a particular way which is appropriate for linguistic processing (e.g., Juszczyk, Rosner, Cutting, Foard & Smith, 1977), it remains unclear to what extent these abilities reflect innate predisposition or the effect of the linguistic environment.

There is considerable controversy as to precisely *how* phonological development and perception proceed from the babbling stage, but *what* occurs is clear. First, around the third or fourth month, cooing and babbling monologues become more frequent, and the sounds used, more varied (Ferguson, 1976). By 7 or 8 months the infant is regularly responding with his own babbling when an adult imitates him. A few weeks later he is babbling when someone speaks to him, and by about 10 months specific vowel sounds are being produced. Clear consonant-vowel syllables with occasional vowel or consonant-vowel-consonant syllables (*mammam, papapa, dadada, nonono, anna*) are evident by around the first month of the second year. Ferguson suggests three general characteristics of phonological development during this period:

1. *The child is very active and creative.* He creates sound sequences from the sounds surrounding him (e.g., animal cries, sounds of cars).

2. *Early vocables (repetitive sound syllables) appear to link babbling and speech.* Early vocables such as "mama," "tata," "dada," are used meaningfully, though not always conventionally, and continue into the stage of adult-modeled words as a link to speech. The child begins to get the idea that certain sound sequences are consistently associated with particular objects and specific routines—that different sound sequences (e.g., *bye-bye*) are appropriate at different times.

3. *The child's perceptual and production systems appear to be relatively independent in the early stages.* This observation is based on the fact that childrens' first meaningful vocables usually consist of repeated vowels, syllabic consonants, and other sounds that do not exist as words in adult speech. In building up sound sequences for production, the child initially seems to proceed independently, without reference to the adult words he hears. Soon, however, he seems to realize the enormity of the task of constructing his own productions and begins selecting some words used by the adults in his environment to imitate.

Ingram (1976) divides the sensorimotor period into two stages based on phonological development. In the first stage, from birth until about 10 to 12 months, the infant (a) learns important perceptual discrimination skills, (b) "plays" with the sounds (babbling) which will later constitute some of his first words such as "mama" and "baba," and (c) increases his ability to imitate. During the second stage, which lasts from about a year until 18 months, first words are acquired. Phonology is still primitive and, because the child does not yet have the representational

During the second phase the child attempts to produce target utterances in the adult language.

ability to associate sound sequences consistently with specific meanings, "words" are often over- or underextended.

Form-content linkage   By about 15 months of age, the child is using ten different "words." By 18 to 20 months, most children have acquired an additional 40 words. The vast majority of the first set of 10 words, for most children, are names for specific objects or persons (e.g., "mommy") and classes ("doggie" referring to any dog). Action words such as "up" and "bye-bye," modifiers such as "pretty," and grammatical function words such as "what" are represented, but much less frequently. In the second set of 40 words, two-thirds are nominals; but action words, modifiers, and function words are more frequent (Nelson, 1973).

> Names for specific objects or persons and classes predominate in the child's earliest vocabulary.

It is interesting to note that in Nelson's (1973) listings of the nominals used by her 18 subjects, there was no noun that was used by all the children. The fact that very few words were shared by even half the children is among the most impressive pieces of evidence for the influence of environmental differences. Children learn names for different objects and events because they encounter different objects and events. However, *labels for objects which move or can be acted upon are most frequent.* Such common nouns as stove, lamp, tub, etc., labeling objects which are simply "there"—not acted upon by the young child in any significant way—are absent from early vocabulary lists. Instead, we find many words for food and drink, animal names, clothing, and toys—objects children directly experience and objects that move.

Nelson also found that the children in her sample could be differentiated according to the *types* of words in their vocabularies. One group used a proportionately greater number of nouns, or object references while others used more social or expressive words such as "thank you," "hi," and "bye-bye." Interestingly, first-born children were more likely to be "referential" while later-born children were more likely to be "expressive."

Another way of differentiating words is according to the type of information conveyed. As discussed in Chapter One, a word can convey two distinct types of information, depending on its function or its semantic role (Bloom, 1973). Every word may be categorized as "substantive" or "relational." Substantive words refer to particular objects such as "baby" (used by a child to refer to a specific doll) or "Daddy," or classes of objects ("juice," "dog"). These words are usually nouns in the adult grammar, and their function is to name or make reference. Relational words (sometimes called function words) play a different but equally important role. They include such parts of speech as verbs, prepositions, and adjectives and refer to object state, attributes, actions, and interactions. Relational words such as "this," "there," "gone," "no more," "again," are numerous in children's early expressive vocabularies. Because they refer to many different objectives and events and function to control the environment, relational words are used more frequently than substantive words. However, early vocabularies do not contain as many different relational words as substantive words.

> Words can convey two types of information—substantive or relational information.

Although a single word may code a relational meaning, it is often difficult for the listener to interpret the message correctly without an additional element. Consider the word "more," for example. If the child with a half-eaten meal simply says "more" and does not point to or otherwise indicate his drinking cup or the cookie jar, the intent of the utterance might not be accurately decoded. However, if he combines the word with a gesture (holding up his cup), or a second word ("juice"), it becomes clear that he desires more juice. When a child uses a single word to communicate what an adult would say with a sentence (e.g., "I'd like more juice") the one-word utterance may be termed *holophrastic.* Note, however, that use of this term assumes there is such a thing as a "one-word sentence," which many researchers dispute (e.g., Crystal, Fletcher, and Garman, 1976).

At the point when the child begins to demonstrate some knowledge of syntax—that there are rules governing word order, for example—it becomes increasingly more difficult to discuss content and form separately. Meaning and structure become closely intermingled.

Early multiword utterances   Whether syntax officially begins when the infant uses single sentence-like words (holophrases) to express relationships or when he first strings two words together under one intonation contour, is an area of considerable controversy. Greenfield and Smith (1976) argue the former position, that some syntactic knowledge can be inferred even before the child produces multiword combinations. They contend that the infant who says "Daddy" while pointing to his father's shoes should be credited with understanding the relational meaning *possession.* According to this holophrastic view, the child's single-word utterance, along with the nonlinguistic context, constitutes a multi-element syntactic construction. The child is producing a single word which is really a little sentence. Bloom (1973) takes an opposing position, contending that children should not be credited with syntactic knowledge until the latter part of their second year. She argues that until multiword utterances provide evidence of knowledge of sentence structure (word order) as well as relational meanings, they cannot be properly classified as syntactic.

There are two indicators of early syntactic knowledge.

At the two-word stage, two types of evidence indicate early syntactic knowledge (de Villiers and de Villiers, 1978). If a child uses consistent word order to encode meanings and if his two-word constructions have a single prosodic contour (no pauses), it is generally agreed he should be credited with at least some grasp of the notion of syntax. However, early multiword utterances are probably governed more by semantic than by syntactic knowledge. They are often referred to as *telegraphic speech,* described in Chapter One, because the same types of words (articles, prepositions, and conjunctions) typically omitted from telegrams are noticeably absent in these constructions.

There are two stages in the progression from single-word to multiword utterances.

Children seem to begin the gradual progression from single-word utterances to "real sentences" in the last half of their second year. The first step in this transition, the *successive single-word utterances* stage, begins between 18 and 21 months (Bloom, 1973). The child uses two words together (separate one-word utterances) to comment on two aspects of an ongoing event. The child begins to perceive relations among persons and objects, but he does not yet sufficiently understand language to express these relationships properly.

The second step in the transition to syntactic constructions is encoding of *two-word semantic relations.* Semantic relations are combinations of two or more words which convey more and different meaning than any one of the involved elements (words) could convey in isolation. Semantic relations incorporate two types of meaning: the meaning of the individual words *plus* the meaning implicit in the way the words are combined. This stage is particularly significant for two reasons. The child's encoding of semantic relations is evidence of expanded awareness and understanding of different types of nonlinguistic relationships. Now he is beginning to convey this understanding of relationships linguistically. However, because the range and variety of ideas and relational concepts the child has acquired by this age exceed his expressive abilities, the same word combinations will frequently be used to express different intentions. For this reason, we have to know where he is, what he is doing, and what others in the setting are doing and saying to understand the intent of many of his utterances.

> Encoding of semantic relations is evidence that the child understands the meanings of the separate words *and* the relationship between the two words.

Semantic relations can be explained better by considering some examples from Bloom's (1970, 1973) research. A famous example is the utterance "mommy sock." When the child says "mommy sock" as his mother is putting on his sock, the utterance conveys understanding of the relationship between an agent (mommy) and an object (sock). When expressed while holding up his mother's stocking, the same utterance is evidence that the child understands the relationship between a possessor (mommy) and a possession (sock). Note that each of these different relational meanings is expressed with the same two-word utterance.

In both instances the child is demonstrating two types of knowledge: knowledge of the meanings of the separate words (the child must know who Mommy is and what a sock is) and knowledge of the relationship between the two. He is telling us much about his understanding of relationships and something about his emerging knowledge of how people talk about these relationships. He knows that mommys can affect (act upon) socks in ways that socks cannot affect mommys (agent-object relationship) and that mommys can own socks, but that socks cannot own mommys (possession). Equally significant is the suggestion of some knowledge of word order. The child knows that the word order to express these relations is agent-object and possessor-possession, not vice versa.

Considering the many things that children could talk about, it is amazing that the types of content represented in children's earliest word combinations are as easily defined as they are. Equally remarkable is the evidence of universality; there are striking parallels among children from such widely different language communities as Germany, Russia, Finland, and Samoa (Brown, 1973). The fact that all over the world children attend

> There are striking similarities in what children of different cultures talk about with their earliest word combinations.

TABLE 2-5 Stage 1—Semantic relations: Prevalent meanings expressed in early two-word combinations

Semantic Relation	Form	Possible Context	Example
Existence	relational word + object name (introducer + entity)	child calls attention to an object or picture of an object by pointing	"this car"
Negation (three meanings) non-existence, rejection, denial	relational word + object name (negation + entity)	if indicating *nonexistence*, child may be searching for lost cookie; if *rejection*, child may be refusing an offer of a cookie; if *denial*, child may be responding to the question "Is this your cookie?"	"no cookie"
Recurrence	relational word + object name (more + entity)	child indicates awareness of the reappearance of an object *or* the desire for an additional amount (a new instance) of something	"more juice"
Attribution	adjective + noun (attribute + entity)	child calls attention to some characteristic of an object	"big ball"

TABLE 2-5 (continued)

Semantic Relation	Form	Possible Context	Example
Possession	noun + noun or pronoun + noun	child indicates (pointing to or holding up) someone's property	"mommy sock"
Locative (two types) action entity	verb + noun/pronoun, noun/pronoun + verb (action + locative) or noun + noun (entity + locative)	child indicates a movement occurring in a specific place or child indicates an object as existing in a particular place	"sit beach" or "sweater chair"
Agent — action	noun/pronoun + verb	child indicates the initiator of an action and the movement	"mommy go"
Action — object	verb + noun/pronoun	child indicates a movement or process with someone or something receiving it	"hit ball"
Agent — object	noun/pronoun + noun/pronoun	child indicates someone or something in direct interaction with another person or thing	"daddy ball"

to and talk about basically the same things—objects, events, people, and the relations among them—with their first words and word combinations is persuasive evidence of universal human perceptual-cognitive predispositions.

Three prominent psycholinguists, Brown (1973), Bloom (1970), and Schlesinger (1971), have studied data describing children's utterances at Stage I (MLU something less than 2.0). Each of these researchers independently compiled a list of the most prevalent semantic relations at this stage. It is significant that they agreed upon so many of the categories. Table 2-5 presents the most prevalent Stage I meanings.

This list provides criteria against which to judge the language development of a child in the two-word speech stage (Stage I). Keep in mind, however, that it cannot be determined whether the child is expressing a semantic relation, or which one he is expressing, without knowledge of the context of the utterance. The form alone does not provide sufficient information to determine intended meaning and assign the utterance to a particular category. Unless the nonlinguistic context is taken into account, it is impossible to determine whether an utterance like "more milk" means that the child has drunk all the milk and wants more, or whether mother has given the child a glass of milk and poured one for herself, prompting the comment that additional milk has appeared.

The next development in the form domain, which is discussed later in this chapter, begins around age 2. The central feature of this more advanced stage is production of longer utterances. Two-term semantic relations—agent-action, action-object, or agent-object—are combined and expanded to yield three-, and eventually, four-term semantic relations. Where, prior to age 2, the child might say "Mommy book" or "Mommy read" or "read book" to comment on his mother's activity, he will now use a three-term relation, "Mommy read book," in the same context. During this stage, the child also begins to use word endings, such as those signifying the tense of verbs or plurality of nouns, and function words such as articles and prepositions.

PRECURSORS TO LANGUAGE USE

The relationship between rules of grammar and communication strategies (or rules of usage) can be compared to the relationship between the rules for a game and strategies for playing that game. The rules of backgammon are relatively simple and easy to learn. However, whether or not a person wins the game depends on how well he learns and exploits certain playing strategies. These strategies are more difficult to explain than the rules because they depend on such variables as the stage of the game, the other player's positions, etc. As in learning the backgammon strategies, learning to be a competent communicator requires many years and much "playing" experience.

A number of theorists have attempted to account for how infants begin to learn rules of usage, or communication strategies (e.g., Bruner, 1975; Bates, 1976; Dore, 1974; Halliday, 1975; Ryan, 1974). Before con-

TABLE 2-6 Emergence of language use from birth to age 4

Age Range	Characteristics
0–1 month	Regards persons momentarily Quiets/responds to voice Eyes follow moving person
1–4 months	Smiles/coos in response to voice and adult smiling Becomes "excited" when caregiver approaches Quiets upon seeing or hearing caregiver Shows anticipatory response upon seeing bottle Shows anticipation when about to be picked up Shows awareness of strange situation or strange persons Cries in reaction to physiological distress (hunger, fatigue, discomfort) Repeats actions that accidentally produce interesting results
4–8 months	Continues to attend to and repeat actions that produce interesting results Discriminates strangers and withdraws Requests continuation of a play activity by touching adult's hand, smiling or performing some motor element of the activity Vocalizes states such as pleasure, satisfaction, anger Follows adult gaze (if adult breaks contact to look elsewhere) Takes turns in familiar action games with caregiver Removes cloth placed over head to reinstate visual contact Responds to being called by name Extends arms to be picked up
8–12 months	Demonstrates goal-directed behavior by releasing or pushing aside one object to grasp another and moving to retrieve a desired object Pulls a support to obtain desired toy Vocalizes deliberately to initiate interpersonal interactions Shouts to attract attention, listens, then shouts again Shakes head for "no" Gives affection to caregiver and familiar adults Waves "bye-bye" Repeats a behavior which others laugh at Anticipates the occurrence of events from signs (e.g., cries when caregiver puts her coat on) Expresses anger and distress when a toy is taken away Looks at caregiver's face when receiving an object (as if to acknowledge receipt)
12–18 months	Uses an attached string or stick to obtain desired toy Indicates wants by gesturing and vocalizing Hands mechanical toy to adult to "request" reactivation Shows/offers objects to "request" social interactions Tries to turn doorknob and looks at adult to "request" outside play Uses gestures such as pointing to direct adult attention Hands book to adult to "request" a story Pulls adult to certain locations to "request" attention to an object or event Gestures and vocalizes loudly to "request" desired objects and events

TABLE 2-6 (continued)

Age Range	Characteristics
18–24 months	Gestures and vocalizes loudly to "request" proximity of familar adult Uses words to request desired objects and events Says "what's that?" to elicit adult attention Names objects spontaneously in the presence of others Vocalizes immediately following the utterances of another (but vocalizations are not necessarily contingent or related to the prior utterances)

2–3 years	Vocalizes about objects and events that are not immediately present
	Vocalizes about the actions of others
	Initiates spontaneously vocal interactions
	Adds information to the prior utterances of communication partner
	Answers simple questions appropriately
	Asks increasing numbers of questions (particularly about location and identity)
	Uses increased number of utterances that serve the interpersonal functions
	    a. calling attention to self or objects and events in the environment
	    b. regulating the behavior of others
	    c. obtaining desired objects or services
	    d. participating in social interaction rituals (e.g., "Hi", "Bye")
	    e. commenting about objects and ongoing events
	    f. engaging in vocal play

3–4 years	Refers more frequently to the activities of others Refers more frequently to objects and events removed in time Changes tone of voice and sentence structure to adapt to listener's level of understanding Uses some alternative forms that take context differences into account (e.g., speaker/hearer pronoun distinctions, definite/indefinite articles, and ellipsis based on shared information) Elaborates and expands the prior utterances of another

sidering how the infant masters these strategies however, we need to discuss the strategies themselves. What do competent communicators know that allows them to play the communication game appropriately and effectively?

There are certain strategies a child must learn before he can play the communication game well.

Adult speakers of a language have implicit knowledge of many devices other than words and sentences for getting across what they mean, and they are sensitive to the use of these devices by others. Hymes (1971, p. 12) describes this as "tacit knowledge of who can say what, in what way, where and when, by what means and to whom." It goes beyond the understanding and production of meaningful linguistic forms and structures (grammatical knowledge) to their appropriate and effective use.

In addition to knowing when meaning is shared, the child must learn to set up a mutual field of attention and establish reciprocity.

Shared meaning assumptions are one of the most important requirements for successful communication. At the very least, a speaker assumes that his listener (a) has auditory perception, (b) shares the same language code, (c) can identify the source of the message, (d) is able to interpret the message with regard to its frame of reference, (e) is able to interpret the intentions of the message, and (f) can act or react to the message in the way the speaker expects (Shields, 1978). The competent communicator also has strategies for setting up a mutual field of attention (e.g., "You won't believe who I saw last night!") and the ability to establish and maintain reciprocity through such devices as taking turns and acknowledgement ("Is that so?"). Every communication context dictates the strategies to apply in that particular situation. Generally, the more accurate a speaker's "reading" of his listener and the context, and the more sophisticated he is in using standard discourse strategies for realizing his intentions, the more successful the communication.

The fact that normal learners acquire use strategies in addition to, and almost simultaneously with, a range and variety of other cognitive and linguistic skills is one of the most impressive feats of language acquisition. Paralleling development in the content and form domains, the learning of communication strategies begins almost at birth. Infants signal hunger, discomfort, excitement, pleasure, and boredom with reflexive sounds (e.g., crying) and movements. Not only do they signal the desire to eat, sleep, play, or be left alone, but they also let their caregivers know if the signals have been responded to as intended. The striking fact is that primitive signals usually *are* answered as the baby intends. Caregivers inevitably attend to and treat their infants' communications as significant, and all indications are that they respond in a manner the baby finds satisfying (Newson, 1978). From the beginning, caregivers assume that the infant is attempting meaningful dialogue and act accordingly. The caregivers impute meaningful intentions towards other objects and towards themselves long before the infant is intentionally communicating. You have undoubtedly heard caregivers remark "He's hungry" or "She wants to play" in response to crying or cooing. The baby is credited with having thoughts, feelings, and intentions even though these human qualities and sensitivities are only in an embryonic stage. As a consequence, by the age of 2 the child has begun to form some ideas about controlling his world and some assumptions about the internal representations of other persons.

> Caregivers credit the infant with having thoughts, feelings, and intentions and respond accordingly.

Caregivers seem to coordinate their behavior in a nonpredictable, but by no means random, way with infant activities and spontaneous reactions. Ritualistic interaction games played by caregivers and children (e.g., peekaboo) appear to be key teaching techniques. Shared meanings gradually develop between caregiver and infant because caregivers assume that any event that has significance and meaning to them naturally has the same significance and meaning to their baby. When a baby smiles, the assumption is that he is pleased; when he yawns, he is prepared for sleep. When caregivers talk to a baby, their movements are regular and subdued. They are highly attentive, and they speak quietly and gently with a rhythmic, almost musical patterning. As much time is spent waiting and watching the baby as is spent in actually speaking.

Caregiver-infant interactions play a critical role in facilitating this learning. They provide the context for learning how to express needs and desires long before the infant is capable of producing speech. In the context of routine "action dialogues" with his caregiver, the infant discovers the predictable structure of communication exchanges and comes to realize that others are responsive to his signals. Over time he becomes more adept at exploiting these exchanges and this rather amazing "power game." He begins to use vocal and nonverbal signals to intentionally direct the attention and actions of others. This is early evidence of the *directive function* of language. He also learns to exchange information; he points out and, later, names objects, actions, and states, demonstrating use of the *referential function* of language. Both of these functions are typically demonstrated about his first birthday.

By the time the infant produces his first words he is already familiar with the expressive, directive, and referential functions of communication.

When the infant begins to use his first words, around the end of his first year, there is no need to acquire any profound new principles about using language; he simply substitutes conventional symbols for gestures and vocalizations. He is already familiar with at least three of the functions of communication—*expressive, directive* and *referential* (Moerk, 1977). Since birth he has been demonstrating the *expressive function*. He has been using both gross and fine motor behaviors and vocalizations to express his intentions and desires. All that is required at this point is to substitute or add a word or words in place of the less conventional devices. The *directive function* is evident from the time he first recognizes the temporal if-then sequence of his signals and caregiver responses, and begins to use his crying, facial expressions, gestures, and vocalizations to direct intentionally the behavior of others. Early evidence of the *referential function* can be seen toward the end of the first year when pointing replaces reaching and grasping as the first step toward ostensive definition.

Bates describes three stages of communicative development and relates them to cognitive development.

Bates (1976) describes and labels the three functions—expressive, directive, and referential—somewhat differently from Moerk and places them in a developmental sequence. Using speech act terminology derived from the work of Austin (1962) and Searle (1969) as a heuristic framework, she delineates three phases of communicative development during infancy and relates these developments to the child's cognitive development. The first phase, called the *perlocutionary stage,* corresponds to Piaget's sensorimotor stages one through four. (Perlocutions are defined as signals which, though unintentional from the infant's standpoint, produce a systematic effect.) The next phase of communicative development is the *illocutionary* stage which corresponds to sensorimotor stage five. In this phase, the child intentionally uses conventional, socially recognized nonverbal signals to convey requests and to direct adult attention to objects and events. The third phase, the *locutionary* stage, corresponds to sensorimotor stage six. The child uses conventional utterances (words and sentences) in a meaningful way to perform the same functions for which he previously used illocutions—to direct adult attention to objects and events.

Bates emphasizes the importance of two "performatives": commanding and declaring (similar to Moerk's directive and referential functions). She describes commanding (the imperative) as the use of an adult to obtain a desired object; declaring (the declarative) is the use of an object as the means to obtain adult attention. The preverbal precursors of these functions are termed the "protoimperative" and the "protodeclarative" respectively. Presumably, the child progresses through the same restructuring, elaboration, and coordination processes in acquiring these intentional communicative functions as in the acquisition of nonlinguistic constructs such as object permanence and the object concept.

Bates links attainment of the illocutionary and locutionary stages to the sensorimotor learning Piaget calls "means-end behavior" and "causality." She argues, however, that progress in communicative development is more closely tied to construction of means-end and causality concepts (the appreciation of cause and effect relationships) than to constructing object permanence or the object concept. Table 2-7 depicts the development of means-end behavior and causality with some examples of parallel communication strategies (from Bates and others). Because they are so closely related, means-end differentiation and causality are displayed as a single developmental series.

Based on an extensive diary-type study of his son, Nigel, Halliday (1975) factors speech acts into even narrower categories than Bates or Moerk. He labels communicative functions as (a) the *instrumental* function ("I want" use of language), (b) the *regulatory* function (to direct adult attention and actions, and (c) the *interactional* function (to establish and maintain social contact). Described as emerging in the fourth stage of the sensorimotor period (at about 9 or 10 months), these three functions closely resemble Bates' "protoimperative" function and Moerk's directive function. Somewhat later, the *heuristic, imaginative,* and *informative* functions (similar to Bates' protodeclarative and Moerk's referential functions) appear. The last, the informative function, which appears around 18 months, is associated with the transition to "true" language.

> According to Halliday, the child has learned seven communicative functions by 18 months of age.

The terminology used to label the various communications functions is relatively unimportant. What is significant is that communicative intentions are basic and universal and that there is an orderly and predictable progression from (a) primitive communications, without intention or conventional form, to (b) intentional use of language, still without conventional form, to (c) intentional communication with conventional forms and arbitrary symbols. By the time a child begins producing words and sentences, he already knows many strategies for playing the communication game. At that point he is ready to go on and learn when and how different forms are appropriate and most effective: which forms are polite and which are insulting, how to talk to younger and older children, and how to communicate with familiar and unfamiliar persons. In other words, by the end of his second year, the young child is ready to learn the important subtleties of communicative exchanges. Mastery of these constructs is presented in a subsequent section when later attainments in language use are discussed.

The implications of these data for early identification and intervention with language deficient children are discussed in other chapters. Most important to remember is the context of this learning. Communication is a

TABLE 2-7 Parallels between means-end and causality development and emergence of communicative functions

Sensorimotor Stages	Means-End Behavior-Causality Development	Interaction-Communication Strategies
Stage 1 (Birth to 1 month)	Repeats/practices reflexes	*Perlocutionary acts* Quiets and responds to human voice
Stage 2 (1–4 months) Primary Circular Reactions	Gradually coordinates schemes (e.g., hand-watching, thumb/hand sucking) Grasps toy *if* both hand and toy are in view Immediately repeats behaviors that have *accidentally* produced interesting results (e.g., attempting to keep a mobile in motion)	*Perlocutionary* (unintentional) Smiles and coos in response to adult smiling and/or vocalization Shows anticipation when about to be picked up Emits distinguishable cries for anger, hunger, pain, etc.
Stage 3 (4–8 months) Secondary Circular Reactions	Continually repeats actions which have accidentally produced interesting results but no effort to explore the cause of the effect Uses such behaviors as consistent vocalization, kicking, waving, etc as if attempting to "cause" continuation of an interesting sight Attempts to "cause" resumption of a play activity by touching the adult's hand or the toy, or performing some motor element of the activity	*Perlocutionary acts* Shows enjoyment when played with Vocalizes states such as pleasure, satisfaction, anger Follows adult gaze (if adult breaks eye contact to look elsewhere) "Recognizes" caregiver Performs joint action "rituals" with caregiver (turn-taking routines)
Stage 4 (8–12 months) Coordination of Secondary Circular Reactions	Intentional, goal-directed behavior apparent in: releasing or pushing aside one object to grasp another pulling a support to obtain a desired toy moving to retrieve a toy needed in play Appreciation of causality outside himself demonstrated by: pushing adult's hand to continue an interesting sensory effect anticipating the occurrence of events from signs (e.g., crying when mother gets her coat out)	*Perlocutionary acts*[1] Extends arms to be picked up Withdraws from approach of a stranger Reacts negatively when a toy is taken away Waves "bye-bye" Shows affection to parents and other adults Looks at caregiver's face when receiving an object *as if* to acknowledge receipt Plays peekaboo, hiding his face for another to watch

TABLE 2-7 (continued)

Sensorimotor Stages	Means-End Behavior-Causality Development	Interaction-Communication Strategies
Stage 5 (12–18 months) Tertiary Circular Reactions	Experiments with means and ends as if to see what will happen and learn about the inherent properties of objects Demonstrates considerable interest in novelty for its own sake Uses an attached string or a stick to obtain a desired toy without demonstration (and even if toy is not in direct view) Hands a mechanical toy to an adult to be reactivated (a "request" for the adult to "cause" it to run again) Shows object to others to instigate social interaction	*Illocutionary acts* Tries to turn doorknob as a request to "go outside" Uses gestures such as pointing to direct adult attention Hands book to adult to request reading of a story Pulls adult to view certain situations or a new location Shows/displays/points out objects to others to elicit attention and social interaction
Stage 6 (18–24 months) Invention of New Means through Mental Combinations	Ability to evoke internal representations of absent objects and events evident in mental problem solving (mental foresight of effects): solves problems when unseen obstacle blocks a gate Immediately looks for causes of his actions Attempts to activate toy himself When faced with putting a long necklace in a tall container, takes unsteadiness of container into account and adopts a successful approach Sets aside solid ring immediately rather than trying to force it into a peg	*Locutionary acts* Asks for desired objects (with conventional symbols) Uses words to make wants/desires known Names objects in the presence of others Says "what's that?" for adult attention

[1]Some Stage 4 behaviors appear to be illocutionary (intentional communicative) acts.

dyadic phenomenon; communication strategies are acquired, practiced, and ultimately applied in the context of ongoing encounters with significant others. From a very early age, the infant has a contribution to make, stemming from his own interests and directed by his own purposes.

ATTAINMENTS BY AGE 2

Following is a summary of the attainments of a child by age 2 in the areas of content, form, and use.

Summary of language attainments at age 2.

Content   By age 2 the child is capable of representational thought in preparation for the period Piaget calls "preoperational thought." He knows that object existence is absolute—that objects continue to exist even when not immediately visible—and that different objects have different perceptual and functional properties. Some one-word functional relations (words such as "more," "no," "allgone" that depend on the context for interpretation) are still being used, but the range of two-term semantic-syntactic relations is becoming prevalent (see Table 2-5). Comprehension continues to depend heavily on contextual cues, and some overextension and underextension may still be evident.

Form   The 2-year-old's vocabulary includes two to three hundred words, and is increasing rapidly. Two-word utterances are used to express the meanings that were, for the most part, encoded by single words until around 16 to 18 months. The fact that words are linked in particular ways and the order in which they are sequenced may be evidence of at least some syntactic knowledge, but, as yet, there is little evidence of grammatical markers (e.g., tense markers, plural markers).

Use   Attainment of Piaget's Stages 5 and 6—the ability to use gestures and symbols for achieving desired ends (the tool-use capability)—parallels the emerging use of conventional language forms for intentional control of the social environment. The 2-year-old is using language for reference (to comment about objects and ongoing events), for vocal play, to regulate the behavior of others (e.g., "more milk"), obtain objects, call attention to himself or objects, and for social interaction purposes (e.g., "Hi," "Bye-bye") (Bloom and Lahey, 1978). He is ready to learn more sophisticated conversation strategies.

It is important to keep in mind that there are a wide range and variety of factors contributing to the child's ability to understand and use language during this period (Bridges, Sinha, & Walkerdine, 1981). The child is aided by the way in which adults orient towards and respond to his needs, as well as by the physical context. Caregivers' responses are adjusted to the gap in communication skills between themselves and the child and oriented to the child's present and anticipated needs. Patterns of family life involve the child from the start as a conversational partner. These contextually-bound patterns and routines deserve major credit for the child's ability, at age 2, to "break the linguistic code" and attribute meaning to a significant proportion of the words, phrases and sentences addressed to him.

AGES 2–4—ELABORATION AND EXPANSION

Imagine a toddler trying to report to his mother about the events which just transpired between two of his playmates. Both are wailing, and pieces of a toy truck are scattered on the floor. Mother asks what happened, and the child blurts out "broke," "Janie," "truck," "Mark." He repeats the four words several times but the mother is still not sure what happened. She notes that Mark and Janie apparently had a dispute involving the truck, which probably belongs to one of them, but the relationships of actors, actions and object are not clear to the mother from her son's report.

After a little more experience with language, the youngster will learn that in English the initiator of an action is before the action, the thing affected is after the action, and the possessor precedes the possession. As emphasized earlier, word order is extremely important. It allows a speaker to go beyond the words alone to convey the relationships holding between the events—to say, for example, "Mark broke Janie's truck" which conveys the intended complaint. When words are sequenced in the proper order, it is more than a sum of the parts, it is a new entity—a sentence. Grammar provides a structure which allows the speaker to communicate relational meanings and the listener to understand the meanings the speaker wishes to convey.

CONTENT-FORM LINKAGES—THE DEVELOPMENT OF GRAMMAR

During the early preschool years, children advance from a rudimentary and idiosyncratic semantic organization to a system that begins to resemble that of the adults in their language culture. Around age 2 they begin to use proper word order consistently to talk about what is happening around them in a relatively sophisticated manner. Major accomplishments during this period include the expression of (a) three and, soon, four term relations (e.g., agent-action-object), (b) morphological inflections (e.g., plural morpheme), and (c) interrogative and negative sentences. Most children master the basic structures of language and are able to express themselves quite well by age 3. Objects and events that are not immediately present in the nonlinguistic context are talked about more often as the months pass. By age 4, they have attained a productive vocabulary of about 1,500 words (Smith, 1926).

Basic differences among children at this stage continue to be rate-related rather than sequence-related. The order in which they learn to produce increasingly longer and more complex utterances is generally consistent. Keep in mind, however, that, although there are many ways that children learning language are similar, there are also important differences in the paths they take to arrive at the same goals. Recognizing this considerable variation among different children who can be called "normal language learners" is particularly important for potential interventionists. It is very useful to view language difficulties as another form of varia-

Major accomplishments include expanded length, morphological inflections, and negative sentences.

tion rather than as a deviance. A major factor contributing to variations in language development is the increasing complexity of the process and products.

You remember that the ability to symbolize, to represent meaning with linguistic forms, is a significant development during the latter months of the child's second year. This accomplishment signifies movement from sensorimotor intelligence, which operates on immediately present stimuli, to mental representation or imagery (thought). Mental representation has definite advantages over sensorimotor intelligence because thinking is faster and more flexible than action. For example, you can think about tying your shoes much faster than you can do it. Thinking is freed of the constraints of time and specific situations. You can think about tying your shoes even when they are home in your closet.

The emergence of symbolic play in sensorimotor Stage 6 has particularly important implications for the development of mental representation. In symbolic play the child represents absent objects and events with substitutes and/or overt copies. To illustrate this, Piaget describes his 18-month-old daughter "pretending" to wash her hands by rubbing them together and saying "soap." At 20 months, she pretended to eat bits of paper and other inedibles, saying "very nice." The symbolic quality of this behavior is obvious. The child is learning that objects and events can symbolize, or function in place of, other objects and events.

During symbolic play, the child confers the meaning of a particular object, event, or relationship to a different object, event or relationship. When a child uses one element in place of another he is demonstrating "distancing", the understanding that meaning can be differentiated from the specific object, event or relationship. When a child uses a block for a car he is demonstrating that he knows what a block is and what a car is, and that the one can substitute for the other. This knowledge transfers to the understanding that a word can be used for a concept.

Early symbolic abilities are evident around 17 to 19 months when the child pretends to go to sleep, drinks from an imaginary cup, or pushes a block around while making a motor sound. That pretending is involved is unmistakable from the child's playful manner. At about the same time marked vocabulary growth takes place.

At around 20 to 22 months, symbolic play is extended to include more sophisticated relations. At this age children are spending considerable time playing with toys such as dolls, toy cars, and trucks which require some imagery. The child remembers, and imitates, caregiver actions with a doll; he manipulates toy cars and trucks as he remembers the actual vehicles being moved. By age 2 the child is re-enacting a greater variety of daily routines in play and assuming different agentive functions (e.g., daddy, mommy, baby).

The 3-year-old demonstrates an ability to create even more involved scenarios (mixing, baking, and serving cake) that may be less frequently experienced or observed. This ability to pretend sets the stage for, and appears to parallel, expanded sentence constructions, grammatical inflec-

One skill that may underlie both play and language is the ability to establish a relationship between a sign and its referent.

tions, interrogative structures and negation functions. These four areas are highlighted because they permit a fairly accurate picture of progress during this period.

Sentence Expansion   By age 3, children understand and express the functional relationship among subjects, predicates, and objects. They are able to expand a simple subject into a noun phrase, a verb into a verb phrase with auxiliaries, and an object into a noun phrase and a verb phrase (Menyuk, 1969). These expanded constructions provide the listener with more accurate and precise information. This means that even though the child at age 3 is expressing many of the same intentions he expressed at 2, they are now less dependent on listener interpretation. At about 18 months he said, "want more," and his listener had to consider the context (pointing to the cookie jar) to interpret the request. At 30 or 36 months he says, "I want more cookies." Two important processes for combining simple sentences (conjunction and embedding) also are learned so that by age 3 the child is able to express more than one idea in a sentence.

The 3-year-old is producing considerably longer and more complex sentences.

Grammatical Morphemes   Grammatical inflections have an extended period of development. Some are acquired as early as 2½ and others are not mastered until 6 or 7 years of age. Although the rate of development varies, the order is fairly constant and agreed upon among many researchers. The order of acquisition is probably controlled by both semantic and syntactic complexity. The order of acquisition of the first 13 morphemes, as ranked by Brown (1973), is:

1. *-ing* marking the present progressive tense (children first use this without auxiliary verb).
   Example: "I runn*ing*."
2. "in" and "on" used in locative state utterances
   Example: "Cookie *in* there."
3. *-s* marking the regular noun plural (and some irregular forms)
   Example: "That doll*s*"
4. some past tense irregular verbs such as "went" and "came"
   Example: "She *went*."
5. *-'s* marking the noun possessive
   Example: "Daddy*'s* shoe."
6. "am," "is," "are," "was," and "were," the uncontracted copula[2] forms of *to be* (contracted forms are acquired much later)
   Example: "Here *is* my book."
7. "a" and "the" to distinguish between definite and indefinite referents.
   Example: "That *a* doggie."

---

[2]The copula is a "to be" verb used to connect subject and object. Uncontractible forms are those that do not use contractions.

8. *-ed* marking the regular past tense
   Example: "She cook*ed*."
9. *s* endings on third person regular verbs
   Example: "He move*s*."
10. third person irregular verb forms
    Example: "is," "has," "does"
11. uncontractible auxiliary verbs
    Example: "He *is* going to school."
12. contractible copula forms
    Example: "It's my book."
13. contractible auxiliary verbs
    Example: "He's reading a book."

This listing is valuable as a reference to measure mastery of these important grammatical markers. Instruction should focus first on those inflections that are used in some, but not all, contexts.

Questions   The development and refinement of questioning skills is a particularly interesting sequence. Children do not learn to ask some types of questions until they have learned to answer questions of the same kind (Soderbergh, 1974). For example, they typically do not ask "why" questions until they are able to answer "why" questions appropriately (Hood, 1977). Ervin-Tripp (1970) found that the sequence in which five children responded to different questions after the age of 21 months was "where," "what," "whose," and "who" (in that order). "Why," "how," and "when" were responded to somewhat later.

Children first learn to answer and ask "where," "what," "whose," and "who" questions.

McNeill (1970) has identified three stages in the development of questions:

Stage 1:   Most questions are more like statements with a rising intonation (e.g., "Me eat cookie?") but child may use a few *wh*-words.

Stage 2:   *Wh*-forms ("why," "where," "what") are used to introduce statements (e.g., "why you smiling?").

Stage 3:   Auxiliary verbs are now used, but in *wh*-questions subject and verb are not transposed (e.g., "What baby will eat?"). Another variation at this stage is use of the carrier phrase "do you want" to introduce many questions (Dale, 1976). At the same time, however, the child is producing correctly inverted yes/no-type questions (e.g., "Can I ride in it?").

By about age 4 the child's questions resemble adult forms with most of the necessary auxiliary verbs and pronouns in place (Brown, 1968).

Negation   At about age 2, negatives are formed by tagging "no" or "not" onto simple phrases. Sentences like "not more juice" (said while holding up an empty cup) and "no can do it" (said while trying to force a puzzle piece on the board) are prevalent. The function usually intended by these early negative forms is nonexistence. Rejection is the next category of negation expressed, and denial is the last (Bloom, 1970). All negative functions may initially be expressed by tagging on "no" or "not" in one way or another. However, it is quite clear that the child has different intentions even though he uses the same negative form. Rejection, for example, might be expressed "not meat." Denial (negating the truth of a statement made by someone else or an event) may also be expressed by using "not" (e.g., when offered a blanket with the statement "Here's your teddy," the child says, "not teddy").

Expression of negation begins with the meaning of nonexistence and progresses to rejection and denial.

Children are able to understand all of the basic functions of negation almost from the start (despite limited production capabilities) and progress relatively soon to more conventional and differential expressions of negation. By the age of 3 or 3½, the contracted forms "can't" and "don't" are used, although in a restricted fashion to code negative imperatives (e.g., "don't break that"), negative interrogatives (e.g., "why me can't eat?"), in addition to their use to negate affirmative statements (e.g., "me can't do it"). The conspicuous absence of "can not" and "do not" during this same period is evidence that "can't" and "don't" have been learned, and function as single unanalyzed wholes. Initially, they cannot be considered as evidence of advanced negative constructions (where the negative element is attached to the auxiliary verb).

By 3½ or 4, children have an extensive repertoire of negation possibilities. Negative utterances now contain "can not" and "do not" as well as "can't" and "don't." Other negative forms, such as "won't" and "isn't," are beginning to be used. It will be many years, however, before they master the use of negation with indefinites such as "some," "none," and "any."

EXPANSION OF USE STRATEGIES

Language development permits the child to understand different social and linguistic contexts. At the same time, experiences with communication strategies in different social contexts contribute to his production of language; there is a reciprocal influence.

At about 2 years it becomes apparent that the child is not so tied to the present. Gradually, temporal references are expanded in both directions until, by school age, he is able to talk about the distant past and the distant future. In addition to learning to talk about events other than those that are occurring at that moment, the child learns to use language devices such as word order, stress and intonation to accomplish specific functions. Messages are modified to fit different social contexts (called alternation), and there is evidence of expanded knowledge of the rules and conventions of dialogue. The child learns to use his listener's knowledge in selecting and modifying the meanings to communicate.

The child begins using alternative forms to achieve the same purpose.

Because the many contexts and environments in which language is used continue to expand and change throughout the human life span, learning the rules for changing message forms according to the different ways in which they need to be used is extremely important. As the child learns more about the language code and develops conceptually and socially, he begins to realize that different forms of messages have different effects on different listeners. For example, to ask for a cookie, he could say, "Give me a cookie," "I'm hungry," "Do you have any cookies?" or simply "I'd like a cookie." The effectiveness of the form to obtain the desired treat depends upon the listener and the context. "I'm hungry" may work with grandmother when she is baking cookies, but may not be effective with a parent if it is right before mealtime. "Give me a cookie" might work with another child, but not with a parent who insists on a more proper form. In the second and third years children begin to learn how to select different forms to encode their intentions, depending on the requirements of the situation. They learn the rules for deciding when and how to say what to whom, and where different forms are appropriate and effective.

Early development of communication strategies for meeting different needs in different situations with different people is also reflected in the young child's ability to infer what his listeners already know, or do not know, and to take this listener knowledge into account in forming messages. There is evidence that children from 2 to 5 ask significantly more questions when interacting with an adult than when interacting with children their age (Smith, 1926), simplify their speech when talking to younger children (Shatz and Gelman, 1973) and whine only with their parents (Berko-Gleason, 1973). Additional documentation of alternation is found in research indicating that there are differences both in the initiation of topics and in message complexity in situations that differ according to activities, people present, and the extent to which the child feels in control (Shatz, 1974; Corsaro, 1981).

> Children ask significantly more questions of adults than of peers, simplify their speech for younger children, and whine *only* with adults.

Another type of alternation is *shifting reference.* From about the age of 3 on through the school years, children gradually begin using "shifters." These are words such as kinship terms, personal and demonstrative pronouns (e.g., "I"/"You," "this"/"that," "here"/"there") definite and indefinite articles ("the"/"a") and deictic verbs ("come"/"go," "bring"/"take"). These are difficult words because they do not have a stable reference: their use depends on the orientation of the speaker, and orientation varies among speakers and within and across situations.

> Around age 3 the child begins to use "shifters."

The correct use of shifters tells us that the child is taking his listener's knowledge and perspective into account, but precisely how he learns to do this is unclear. Prior to this time, research (Bloom, Lightbown, and Hood, 1975; Brown, 1973; Haviland and Clark, 1974) has simply documented that shifters begin to be used in the preschool years. Total mastery takes much longer. In fact, until around age 10, the child does not appear to fully understand that others do not have complete access to his thoughts and experiences, and that meaningful conversation requires him to share his thoughts explicitly.

Conventions of dialogue have to do with the mechanics of discourse —the structural organization or rules for conversation. Children must learn how to enter or initiate conversation, how to leave or terminate conversation, how to take turns, shift topics, handle digressions, ask questions, and temporally space their speech with pauses. All of these devices are essential to appropriate and effective discourse. Some are demonstrated as early as age 3 (Garvey, 1975; Keenan, 1974). By this age children have already learned to use repetition and contingent queries (e.g., "What?" "Where did he go?"), establish that someone is listening before continuing a linguistic interaction, and sequence their contributions (taking turns) to discourse. These skills are learned in early nonlinguistic interaction games/routines with caregivers, as described earlier in this chapter.

Children have learned many of the conventions of dialogue by age 3.

ENVIRONMENTAL VARIABLES WHICH CONTRIBUTE TO LANGUAGE LEARNING

The discussion of language acquisition to this point has centered primarily on *what* is learned. However, if you review the preceding sections you will find repeated references to environmental variables affecting acquisition. Because the following factors have the potential to affect design and development of intervention procedures, they are presented separately. The focus in this section is on *how* children learn.

An impressive amount of evidence accumulated since the late 1960s and the early 1970s has led to reasonably clear and detailed descriptions of the language addressed to infants and young children by adults in their environment and the context in which it is provided. We are not suggesting that the conditions responsible for normal language learning will always function in the same way for children who, for one reason or another, are not developing language in a normal manner. However, these data provide essential theoretical and conceptual background for professionals.

COMPREHENSION-PRODUCTION RELATIONSHIP

Researchers, parents, and clinicians have generally assumed that children understand much more than they produce. This premise recently has been qualified. It is necessary to have heard a word before it can be used, but the child need not necessarily understand the word before producing it; understanding may come through use. For example, some recent data document the use of object labels and color terms prior to discrimination and recognition of the represented concepts (Bartlett, 1977; Nelson and Bonvillian, 1978).

Understanding does not always precede production.

The traditional view that understanding consistently precedes production in both semantic and syntactic areas is further challenged by evidence that children produce some grammatical structures reflecting rules which they do not understand (Chapman, 1981). They may produce sentences with subject and verb agreement before they understand what such agreement designates (Keeney and Wolfe, 1972). They seem to use situational cues and their knowledge of probable meanings to give the appearance of understanding these syntactic devices when, in fact, they do not.

Also, there is recent research demonstrating that children may produce sentences with correct word order before they apply word order strategies to processing the sentences of others (Chapman and Miller, 1975; de Villiers and de Villiers, 1973).

These data highlight the need to be cautious in estimating a child's semantic and syntactic knowledge from responses to comprehension tasks. The interaction between comprehension and production is more dynamic and complicated than previously thought. It may be that some children will show the expected accurate comprehension before correct production, although for others the reverse will be true. There even may be variability in production and comprehension performance within the same child, as well as among children. Still another possibility is that age and experience with language influence the kinds of information a child uses and the extent to which he uses different kinds of information.

IMITATION

Imitation appears to be important to language acquisition but how important is not clear.

Without question, children imitate. The issue is whether imitation is important to the language learning process. If it is, how important? One reason investigators have not always agreed on this question is that their operational definitions of imitation often differ (Moerk, 1977). Because children in some cases may fail to produce exact repetitions of modeled utterances does not necessarily mean they are nonimitators or that they have not learned from the process, as some have contended. Less than exact imitations still may result in the acquisition of new grammatical rules and increased vocabulary. At the very least, they acknowledge that the child is attending to the speaker (Keenan, 1974; Shipley, Smith, and Gleitman, 1969; Bloom, Hood, and Lightbown, 1974; Uzgiris, 1981).

Investigators have found that children differ in the extent to which they imitate; for those children who do imitate, imitation appears to be selective (Bloom, Hood & Lightbown, 1974; Ramer, 1976; Moerk, 1977). Imitating children reproduce linguistic segments they are in the process of learning, but they do not imitate words and syntactic structures that are entirely familiar or new. At least for these children, imitation seems to function as a facilitator for processing difficult material.

Data indicating that mothers frequently imitate their children during certain developmental stages provide another perspective on the role of imitation in language learning (Slobin, 1968; Cross, 1975). When the mother imitates and expands the child's utterance, the child often imitates the mother's expanded imitation. This circular feedback exchange obviously performs an instructional function because the mother's expanded model, which the child has imitated, is several complexity units advanced from the child's original utterance (Folger and Chapman, 1978).

SOCIAL PLAY ACTIVITIES

Child-caregiver play activities (imitative routines, ritualized games, and pretend actions) provide an ideal context or scaffold for teaching and practicing communicative devices. Taking turns, role differentiation, and the important notion that vocalizations and words are actions that can "do things" appear to have their ontogenetic origins in these interactions. One reason for their effectiveness as contexts for language learning may be the playful and familiar atmosphere surrounding social games; this permits the child to innovate and rehearse different forms and structures he might not attempt in more formal scenarios. Another reason may be the special stimulus and reinforcement value of caregivers (both fathers and mothers), which undoubtedly enhances their effectiveness in eliciting and maintaining attention and participation routines.

Child-caregiver play provides a context for language learning and language use.

The reasons are less important than the reality that social play activities facilitate the attainment of communicative competence. This learning begins at a very young age. Infants as young as 3 to 4 months are already engaging in simultaneous and alternating patterns of joint action and shared vocalizations in social play activities (Bruner, 1975; Sterne, Jaffe, Beebe, and Bennett, 1975; Ratner and Bruner, 1978).

At least three characteristics of social play activities seem to assist this learning. The first is the familiar and highly restricted nature of the semantic situation in which the play occurs. Early games, such as peekaboo, hide-and-seek, and build-and-tear-down, involve a limited number of exchange elements. In peekaboo, for example, one partner hides and then peeks, and then the other hides and peeks, etc. A second supporting feature of early games is their predictable and clear-cut structure. Each action sequence has a clearly marked beginning, middle, and end, and the order of events rarely varies (e.g., the partners take turns hiding and peeking in peekaboo) and vocalization is interspersed at predictable and regular points in the exchanges to mark different actions. Thirdly, these games have a clearly demarcated and reversible role structure. In peekaboo, for example, sometimes the baby hides, and sometimes the parent hides. In build-and-tear-down, parent may stack and baby knock down, or vice versa. The important aspect is that both partners participate: a double cause-effect relationship exists with the infant participating as an active and, after some practice, equal partner.

Three characteristics of interactive play appear to facilitate learning of communication skills.

CAREGIVER-CHILD DISCOURSE

What forms and structure a child understands and what he talks about when he begins producing first words depends, to a very large extent, on his linguistic environment. Whether the intention of caregivers is specifically to instruct or simply to be understood, the effect is the same: linguistic input aids and guides language learning. The linguistic environment of the infant and young child has been described as uniquely suited for language instruction (Newport, 1976; Phillips, 1973; Snow, 1972; Chapman, 1981).

Caregivers continuously adjust the phonological, semantic, syntactic, and pragmatic characteristics of their linguistic input to the child's developmental level. Phonological alterations include exaggerated pitch (a

Caregivers speak differently to children from the way they address other adults.

considerably higher fundamental frequency and greater frequency range), intensity variations (marked intensity shifts including whispering), duration differences (longer duration of content words, particularly in commands), more stress (two primary stresses in sentences where one would suffice), and rate differences (slower speech both within and between utterances). The majority of utterances addressed to language-learning children are shorter, simpler, and better-formed syntactically than those addressed to older children and other adults. They are usually adjusted to a level approximately two to three words beyond what the child is producing.

The semantic adjustments caregivers make when talking to young language learners are especially interesting. The child-directed vocabulary is less diverse (a fewer number of different words), more concrete (fewer abstract terms), and higher frequency (the same words are used more often). Shifts in form classes are evident as the child's development advances. Caregivers use more modifiers, and the frequency and diversity of *wh*-questions increases. The semantic roles and relations used typically include those the child is in the process of acquiring. Pragmatic characteristics associated with caregiver-child interactions that are likely to enhance the child's learning include: (a) the immediate presence of the object or event being talked about; (b) the apparent salience of the object or event to the child; (c) the incorporation of comments on what the child is attending to within a conversational routine, and (d) lexical expansion of the child's utterances to confirm that he has been understood and to model small additions to his utterances.

The following summarizes the more common strategies used by caregivers to teach language:

The child's major source of knowledge about his language is the conversations directed at him by caregivers.

1. *Talking about shared perceptions at the time the objects or events are the focus of the child's attention.* Caregivers talk in the "here and now," as they should, because the infant has little, if any, capability to remember even the most recent past or to anticipate the future. They play a naming game, supplying the label of an object, event or picture that has attracted the child's attention, or they ask "What is this?"

2. *Providing models for the child to imitate and expanding the child's imitations and spontaneous utterances.* Not only do caregivers model words and sentences for their children to reproduce, but also they specifically direct the child to imitate ("Say _____"). When repeating and expanding the child's utterances, caregivers take care not to change the intended meaning. Mothers who frequently expand and extend their children's utterances are likely to have linguistically accelerated children (Cross, 1977).

3. *Asking questions.* With infants as young as 3 months old, caregivers have already begun to ask questions, for which they supply their own immediate answers (Snow, 1975, 1976; Stern, 1974). Detailed and precise knowledge of the child's vocabulary is evident in the questions caregivers select to ask. Sure that the child

knows and is capable of answering, they reformulate and "break down" the structure of the question if he does not respond to the original form. Caregivers are likely to address questions about internal states ("Do you have a tummy ache?") to 2-year-olds. They address questions seeking new information about the external world to older children (Sachs and Devin, 1976). Requests for action, including inquiries of the child's willingness to carry out the action, almost double between the ages of 23 and 30 months (Rondal, 1978).

4. *Using incomplete sentences.* Caregivers will begin a sentence and then pause for their children to supply the final element (Moerk, 1977). If the required word or phrase is not immediately forthcoming, the adult will model it. What seems uppermost in the mind of the caregiver is maintaining the interaction at a level which will allow the child to participate and keep the conversation going.

5. *Being repetitive.* Much of the speech addressed to young children is repetitive. Caregivers are especially likely to use repetitions when children seem unable to understand a word or statement or to comply with a request (Messer, 1980). About the role of input frequency in overall language development, recent though still tentative data indicate that the more input the child receives, the faster his acquisition rate. Furthermore, children are prone to attempt those constructions first that their caregivers use most frequently (Forner, 1977; Moerk, 1980). There appears to be a positive relationship between input frequencies and acquisition rate and sequence.

6. *Positioning forms and structure the child should attend to first in sentences.* Children appear to have a bias toward processing constructions that are in the initial position. Caregivers somehow realize this and appropriately highlight important words and/or phrases accordingly (Newport, Gleitman, and Gleitman, 1977; Furrow, Nelson, and Benedict, 1979).

7. *Using a less complex communicative style.* Caregivers simplify their linguistic input semantically, syntactically, and stylistically (Furrow et al., 1979). Semantic simplification refers to the use of "here and now" language as noted above: talking about those aspects of the world which the child can readily understand. Syntactic simplification takes the forms of brevity, concreteness, and a reduced number of contractions and pronouns. Stylistic simplification is more difficult to define, but generally involves increased sensitivity to the child's attention span, interests and cognitive level.

Data indicating that caregivers systematically, though unintentionally, modify their linguistic input to children and the growing appreciation and understanding of the influence that this modified speech (sometimes called "motherese") has on language development have profound implications for language training. Though much remains to be established about precisely what caregivers do that makes a difference at different points, there are sufficient data already available to help professionals arrange an optimal language learning environment for the language-delayed child. This objective is developed further in later chapters.

SUMMARY

1. Children learn about objects and events through a process of progressive, qualitative organization and reorganization of their actions and perceptions.

2. Cognition requires assimilation (adapting external stimuli to internal mental structures) and accommodation (adapting these mental structures to the structure of the external stimuli).

3. Two-way relationships, between thought and language and language and thought, can be logically assumed, but empirical verification of the precise nature of these relationships is not yet available.

4. The sensorimotor attainments alleged to be *precursive* to the emergence of language are object permanence, schemes for relating to objects, means-end behavior, causality, and imitation.

5. Children make such errors as overextension, underextension, and overlap because their early concepts are not yet stable.

6. There are at least four variables which will influence what a child attends to and learns at any point: (a) state of deprivation, (b) caregiver structure and direction, (c) available information processing strategies, and (d) level of cognitive development.

7. Phonological development in the sensorimotor period can be divided into two distinct stages: a first stage when the child produces speech-like sounds and discriminates certain aspects of adult speech, and a second stage when first words are acquired.

8. Most of children's first words are labels for objects which move or can be acted upon; action words, modifiers, and function words are represented, but much less frequently.

9. Credit a child with some syntactic knowledge when he uses consistent word order and when his two-word constructions have a single prosodic contour.

10. There is striking evidence of universality in what children attend to and talk about with their first words and word combinations.

11. Paralleling development in the content and form domains, the child begins at birth to form some ideas about using language to control his world and the internal representations of other people.

12. Communication strategies are acquired, practiced, and ultimately applied in social and caregiving contexts; the infant's contributions to this process stem from his unique interests and purposes.

13. Major accomplishments (in the content-form domain) after age 2 include: (a) understanding and use of three- and four-term relations, (b) morphological inflections, and (c) interrogative and negative sentences.

14. Major accomplishments (in the use domain) after age 2 include (a) the ability to talk about events other than those that are "here and now," (b) use of alternative forms to achieve the same purpose, (c) the ability to take listener knowledge into account, and (d) the use of "shifters."

15. Use caution in estimating semantic and syntactic knowledge from either comprehension or production tasks because the interaction of these two processes is not altogether clear.

16. Children differ in the extent to which they imitate but, at least for some children, imitation appears to function as a facilitator for processing difficult material.

17. There are at least three characteristics of social play activities that appear to assist learning: (a) the familiar, highly restricted nature of the play situation, (b) the predictable and clear-cut structure, and (c) the clearly demarcated and reversible role structure.

18. The linguistic environment (caregiver speech) of the infant and young child seems ideally suited for language instruction.

19. There are at least seven common teaching strategies caregivers apply to enhance language learning.

REFERENCES

AUSTIN, J.L. *How to do things with words.* Cambridge, Mass.: Harvard University Press, 1962.

BARTLETT, E.J. *Semantic organization and reference: Acquisition of two aspects of the meaning of color terms.* Paper presented at biennial meeting, Society for Research in Child Development, New Orleans, March, 1977.

BATES, E. *Language and context: The acquisition of pragmatics.* New York: Academic Press, 1976.

BERKO-GLEASON, J. Code switching in children's language. In T.E. Moore (Ed.), *Cognitive development and the acquisition of language.* New York: Academic Press, 1973.

BLOOM, L. *Language development: Form and function of emerging grammars.* Cambridge, Mass.: The MIT Press, 1970.

BLOOM, L. *One word at a time: The use of single-word utterances before syntax.* The Hague: Mouton, 1973.

BLOOM, L., HOOD, L., & LIGHTBOWN, P. Imitation in language development: If, when, and why. *Cognitive Psychology,* 1974, *6,* 380–420.

BLOOM, L., & LAHEY, M. *Language development and language disorders.* New York: John Wiley and Sons, 1978.

BLOOM, L., LIGHTBOWN, P., & HOOD, L. Structure and variation in child language. *Monographs of the Society for Research in Child Development,* 1975, *40,* 2.

BOWER, T.G.R. Stimulus variables determining space perception in infants. *Science,* 1965, *3,* 323–324.

BOWER, T.G.R. *Development in infancy.* San Francisco: W.H. Freeman & Co., 1974.

BOWER, T.G.R. Infant perception of the third dimension and object concept development. In L. Cohen (Ed.), *Infant perception: From sensation to cognition.* New York: Academic Press, 1975.

BRAZELTON, T.B. Evidence of communication during neonatal behavioral assessment. In M. Bullowa (Ed.), *Before speech: The beginning of interpersonal communication.* New York: Cambridge University Press, 1979.

BRECKER, W.A., MACKE, P.R., LEVIN, J.A., & CAMPBELL, P.H. The modifiability of intelligent behavior. *Journal of Special Education,* 1981, *15,* 145–163.

BRIDGES, A., SINHA, C., & WALKERDINE, V. The development of comprehension. In G. Wells (Ed.), *Learning through interaction.* New York: Cambridge University Press, 1981.

BROWN, R. The development of Wh questions in child speech. *Journal of Verbal Learning and Verbal Behavior,* 1968, *7,* 279–290.

BROWN, R. *A first language, the early stages.* Cambridge, Mass.: Harvard University Press, 1973.

BRUNER, J. Eye, hand and mind. In D. Elkind & J.S. Flavell (Eds.), *Studies in cognitive development: Essays in honor of Jean Piaget.* Toronto: Oxford University Press, 1969.

BRUNER, J. The ontogenesis of speech acts. *Journal of Child Language,* 1975, *2,* 1–19.

CHAPMAN, R.S. Mother-child interaction in the second year of life: Its role in language development. In R.L. Schiefelbusch & D.D. Bricker (Eds.), *Early language: Acquisition and intervention.* Baltimore: University Park Press, 1981.

CHAPMAN, R. S., & MILLER, J.F. Word order in early two and three word utterances: Does production precede comprehension? *Journal of Speech and Hearing Research,* 1975, *18,* 355–371.

CROSS, T. Some relationships between mothers and linguistic level of accelerated children. *Stanford University Department of Linguistics, Papers and Reports in Child Language Development,* 1975, *10,* 117–135.

CROSS, T. Mother's speech adjustments: The contributions of selected child listener variables. In C. Snow & C. Ferguson (Eds.), *Talking to children: Language input and acquisition.* Cambridge: Cambridge University Press, 1977.

CRYSTAL, D., FLETCHER, P., & GARMAN, M. *The grammatical analysis of language disability: A procedure for assessment and remediation.* London: Edward Arnold, 1976.

de VILLIERS, J.G., & de VILLIERS, P.A. A cross-sectional study of the acquisition of grammatical morphemes. *Journal of Psycholinguistic Research,* 1973, *2,* 267–278.

de VILLIERS, J.G., & de VILLIERS, P.A. *Language acquisition.* Cambridge, Mass.: Harvard University Press, 1978.

DORE, J. A pragmatic description of early language development. *Journal of Psycholinguistic Research,* 1974, *4,* 343–350.

ERVIN-TRIPP, S. Discourse agreement: How children answer questions. In J.R. Hayes (Ed.), *Cognition and the development of language.* New York: John Wiley & Sons, 1970.

FERGUSON, C. *Learning to pronounce: The earliest stages of phonological development in the child.* Paper presented to the Conference on Early Behavioral Assessment of the Communicative and Cognitive Abilities of the Developmentally Disabled, Orcas Island, Washington, May 1976.

FODOR, J.A. The mind-body problem. *Scientific American,* 1981, *244,* 114–123.

FOLGER, J.P., & CHAPMAN, R.S. A pragmatic analysis of spontaneous imitations. *Journal of Child Language,* 1978, *5,* 25–38.

FORNER, M. *The mother as LAD: Interaction between order and frequency of parental input and child production.* Paper presented at the sixth annual University of Minnesota Linguistics Symposium, 1977.

FURROW, D., NELSON, K., & BENEDICT, H. Mother's speech to children and syntactic development: Some simple relationships. *Journal of Child Language,* 1979, *2,* 423–442.

FURTH, H.G. *Piaget for Teachers.* Englewood Cliffs, N.J.: Prentice-Hall, Inc., 1970.

GARVEY, C. Requests and responses in children's speech. *Journal of Child Language,* 1975, *2,* 41–63.

GRATCH, G. & LANDERS, W. Stage IV of Piaget's theory of infants' object concepts: A longitudinal study. *Child Development,* 1971, *42,* 359–372.

GRATCH, G. A study of the relative dominance of vision and touch in six-month-old infants. *Child Development,* 1972, *43,* 615–623.

GREENFIELD, P.M., & SMITH, J.H. *Communication and the beginnings of language: The development of semantic structures in one-word speech and beyond.* New York: Academic Press, 1976.

HALLIDAY, M.A.K. Learning how to mean. In E. Lenneberg & E. Lenneberg (Eds.), *Foundations of language development* (Vol. 1). New York: Academic Press, 1975.

HAVILAND, S.E., & CLARK, H.H. What's new? Acquiring new information as a process of comprehension. *Journal of Verbal Learning and Verbal Behavior,* 1974, *13,* 512–521.

HOOD, L. *A longitudinal study of the development of the expression of causal relations in complex sentences.* Unpublished doctoral dissertation, Columbia University, 1977.

HUNT, J. McV. Intrinsic motivation and its role in psychological development. In D. Levine (Ed.), *Nebraska symposium on motivation.* Lincoln: University of Nebraska Press, 1965.

HYMES, D. Competence and performance in linguistic theory. In R. Huxley & E. Ingram (Eds.), *Language acquisition: Models and methods.* New York: Academic Press, 1971.

INGRAM, D. *Phonological disability in children.* London: Edward Arnold, 1976.

JUSCZYK, P.W., ROSNER, B.S., CUTTING, J.E., FOARD, C.F., & SMITH, L.B. Categorical perception of nonspeech sounds by two-month-old infants. *Perception and Psychophysics,* 1977, *21,* 50–54.

KAGAN, J. *Change and continuity in infancy.* New York: John Wiley & Sons, 1971.

KEENAN, E. Conversational competence in children. *Journal of Child Language,* 1974, *1,* 163–183.

KEENEY, T., & WOLFE, J. The acquisition of agreement in English. *Journal of Verbal Learning and Verbal Behavior,* 1972, *11,* 698–705.

KESSEN, W., HAITH, M.M., & SALAPATEK, P. Infancy. In P.H. Mussen (Ed.), *Carmichael's manual of child psychology* (3rd Ed.). New York: Wiley, 1970.

LECOURS, A.R. Methods for the description of aphasic transformations of language. In E. Lenneberg & E. Lenneberg (Eds.), *Foundations of language development:* Vol. II. New York: Academic Press, 1975.

LENNEBERG, E. *Biological foundations of language.* New York: John Wiley & Sons, 1967.

LENNEBERG, E. The concept of language differentiation. In N. O'Conner (Ed.), *Language, cognitive deficits and retardation.* London: Butterworth, 1975.

LOWE, M. Trends in the development of representational play in infants from one to three years: An observational study. *Journal of Child Psychology,* 1975, *16,* 33–48.

McNEILL, D. *The acquisition of language: The study of developmental psycholinguistics.* New York and London: Harper & Row Publishers, 1970.

MENYUK, P. *Sentences children use.* Cambridge, Mass.: The MIT Press, 1969.

MESSER, D.J. The episodic structure of maternal speech to young children. *Journal of Child Language,* 1980, *7,* 29–40.

MILLER, D.J., COHEN, L.B., & HILL, K.T. A methodological investigation of Piaget's theory of object concept development in the sensory-motor period. *Journal of Experimental Child Psychology,* 1970, *9,* 59–85.

MOERK, E.L. *Pragmatic and semantic aspects of early language development.* Baltimore: University Park Press, 1977.

MOERK, E.L. Relationships between parental input frequencies and children's language acquisition: A reanalysis of Brown's data. *Journal of Child Language,* 1980, *7,* 105–118.

MORSE, P.A. The infancy of infant speech perception: The first decade of research. *Brain, Behavior and Evaluation,* 1979, *16,* 351–373.

NELSON, K. Structure and strategy in learning to talk. *Monographs of the Society for Research in Child Development,* 1973, *38* (149).

NELSON, K., & BONVILLIAN, J.D. Early language development: Conceptual growth and related processes between two and 4½ years of age. In K. Nelson (Ed.), *Children's language* (Vol. 1). New York: Gardner Press, 1978.

NEWPORT, E.L. Motherese: The speech of mothers to young children. In N.J. Castellan, D.B. Pisoni, & G.R. Potts (Eds.), *Cognitive theory* (Vol. 2). Hillsdale, New Jersey: Lawrence Erlbaum Associates, 1976.

NEWPORT, E.L., GLEITMAN, H., & GLEITMAN, L.R. Mother, I'd rather do it myself: Some effects and non-effects of maternal speech style. In C.E. Snow & C.A. Ferguson (Eds.), *Talking to children: Language input and acquisition.* London: Cambridge University Press, 1977.

NEWSON, J. Dialogue and development. In A. Lock (Ed.), *Action, gesture and symbol: The emergence of language.* New York: Academic Press, 1978.

PHILLIPS, J. Syntax and vocabulary of mothers' speech to young children: Age and sex comparisons. *Child Development,* 1973, *44,* 182–185.

PIAGET, J. *The origins of intelligence in children.* (Margaret Cock, translator). New York: International Universities Press, 1952.

PIAGET, J. *The construction of reality in the child.* New York: Basic Books, 1954.

PIAGET, J. *Genetic epistemology.* New York: Columbia University Press, 1970.

PIAGET, J. The psychogenesis of knowledge and its epistemological significance. In M. Piattelli-Palmarini (Ed.), *Language and learning: The debate between Jean Piaget and Noam Chomsky.* Cambridge, Mass.: Harvard University Press, 1980.

RAMER, A. Syntactic styles in emerging language. *Journal of Child Language,* 1976, *3,* 49–62.

RATNER, N., & BRUNER, J. Games, social exchange and the acquisition of language. *Journal of Child Language,* 1978, *5* (3), 391-402.

ROBINSON, C., & ROBINSON, J.H. Sensorimotor function and cognitive development. In M. Snell (Ed.), *Systematic instruction of the moderately and severely handicapped.* Columbus, Ohio: Charles E. Merrill, 1978.

RONDAL, J. Maternal speech to normal and Down's syndrome children matched for mean utterance length. In C.E. Myers (Ed.), *Quality of life in severely and profoundly mentally retarded people: Research foundations for improvement.* Washington, D.C.: American Association on Mental Deficiency, 1978.

RYAN, J. Early language development: Towards a communicational analysis. In M.P.M. Richards (Ed.), *The integration of a child into a social world.* London and New York: Cambridge University Press, 1974.

SACHS, J., & DEVIN, J. Young children's use of age-appropriate speech styles. *Journal of Child Language,* 1976, *3,* 81–98.

SALAPATEK, P., & KESSEN, W. Visual scanning of triangles by the human newborn. *Journal of Experimental Child Psychology,* 1966, *3,* 155–167.

SCHAFFER, H.R. *The growth of sociability.* Harmondsworth: Penguin Books, 1971.

SCHAFFER, H.R., *Studies in mother-infant behavior.* New York: Academic Press, 1977.

SCHLESINGER, I. Production of utterances and language acquisition. In D. Slobin (Ed.), *The ontogenesis of grammar.* New York: Academic Press, 1971.

SEARLE, J. Speech acts: *An essay in the philosophy of language.* London: Cambridge University Press, 1969.

SHATZ, M. *The comprehension of indirect directives: Can two year olds shut the door?* Paper presented at the summer meeting, Linguistic Society of America, Amherst, Mass, 1974.

SHATZ, M., & GELMAN, R. The development of communication skills: Modifications in the speech of young children as a function of listener. *Monographs of the Society for Research in Child Development,* 1973, *38* (152).

SHIELDS, M.M. The child psychologist: Construing the social world. In A. Lock (Ed.), *Action, gesture and symbol: The emergence of language.* New York: Academic, 1978.

SHIPLEY, E., SMITH, C., & GLEITMAN, L. A study in the acquisition of language: Free responses to commands. *Language,* 1969, *45,* 322–342.

SINCLAIR-deZWART, H. Developmental psycholinguistics. In D. Elkind & J.H. Flavell (Eds.), *Studies in cognitive development.* New York: Oxford University Press, 1969.

SINCLAIR-deZWART, H. Sensorimotor action patterns as a condition for the acquisition of syntax. In R. Huxley & E. Ingram (Eds.), *Language acquisition: Models and methods.* New York: Academic Press, 1971.

SLOBIN, D.I. Imitation and grammatical development in children. In N. Endler, L. Boulter, & H. Osser (Eds.), *Contemporary issues in developmental psychology.* New York: Holt, Rinehart & Winston, 1968.

SMITH, M.E. An investigation of the development of the sentence and the extent of vocabulary in young children. *University of Iowa Studies in Child Welfare,* 1926, *3,* 5.

STAATS, A.W. *Complex human behavior.* New York: Holt, Rinehart and Winston, 1966.

STAATS, A.W. Behaviorism and cognitive theory in the study of language. In R.L. Schiefelbusch and L.L. Lloyd (Eds.), *Language perspectives—acquisition, retardation, and intervention.* Baltimore: University Park Press, 1974.

UZGIRIS, I.C. Experience in the social context. In R.L. Schiefelbusch and D.D. Bricker (Eds.), *Early language: Acquisition and intervention.* Baltimore: University Park Press, 1981.

CHAPTER THREE

PERSPECTIVES ON CATEGORIZATION AND INTERVENTION

Linda McCormick

Most professionals disapprove of present classification procedures. There is general agreement with Hobbs (1975) that special education services should be made available to students on the basis of *educational* deficits and needed remedial services. Nevertheless, the practice of assigning labels based on etiological categories continues. Public Law 94-142 requires disability classification prior to assignment to a special services arrangement and most funding in the field is closely tied to the etiological categories (Hobbs, 1978).

The basic presumptions of the present classification system are (a) that differential diagnosis is possible, (b) that disabilities and aptitudes within a category are consistent, and (c) that lumping similar aptitudes together will result in more efficacious programming. We will not pursue a discussion of the errors in these assumptions. It is enough to say that labels (e.g., phsically impaired, learning disabled, mentally retarded, etc.), while they may aid placement decisions in the present system, do *not* predict the nature or severity of children's language difficulties. Category labels convey little, if any, instructionally relevant information because children sharing the same classification often exhibit markedly different language and communication abilities.

We essentially agree with the philosophical and practical arguments of opponents of labelling, arguments based on the fact that this practice invites overgeneralizations concerning individual children. However, we cannot avoid discussion of subgroups within the larger population of atypical learners because much of the research concerned with language and communication disorders has focused on groups of children assigned to one or another of the disability classifications. Rather than identifying and describing their subject population with more relevant variables such as developmental age, sensory acuity, past linguistic experiences, and mean length of utterance (MLU) researchers have generally concentrated on trying to define linguistic parameters (e.g., echolalia, deviant articulation) associated with the various etiological categories. While these studies have

Assignment to etiological classifications tends to obscure the fact that children within a category have very different language characteristics.

generally failed to show significant correlations between specific language characteristics and disability designations, they *have* generated a considerable amount of interesting, if not always useful, data.

The first part of this chapter will present a brief overview of these categorical research findings. Then we will propose an alternative, program-relevant classification system. This system was introduced in Chapter One as an interactionist perspective. It is based on the content-form-use organization suggested by Bloom and Lahey (1978). The primary advantage of this system is its ability to pinpoint language deficits so that remedial procedures can be specified. The last section of this chapter is a preface to some of the more practical concerns dealt with in the remainder of the book. It identifies the context within which assessment, program planning, and service delivery constructs are presented.

LANGUAGE AND COMMUNICATION PROBLEMS ASSOCIATED WITH MOTOR DISORDERS

Children with motor disorders form one of the largest and most educationally heterogeneous disability subgroups. The National Advisory Committee on the Handicapped estimated in 1976 that approximately 9% of the total number of handicapped children being served at that time had a crippling or other health-impaired condition. Instructional goals for these youngsters range from accelerated programming (e.g., for the gifted child with muscular dystrophy) to basic skill development (e.g., for the multiply handicapped child with severe developmental delays resulting from central nervous system damage). Intensive physical, occupational, and speech and language therapy are usually essential to the educational management of this latter group. However, most of the less severely involved children with motor disorders participate in regular classrooms.

CEREBRAL PALSY

Among the numerous conditions included under the rubric of motor impairment, cerebral palsy accounts for the largest number of children in special education programs. The term, which refers to a general category of motor handicaps, is applied to a broad range of syndromes with quite different etiologies and manifestations. Definitions abound, but generally include three elements: (a) motor deficits as the most prominent symptom, (b) some form of brain pathology as the etiology, and (c) insult to the brain occurring prior to age 6.

Cerebral palsy is the result of damage to the brain prior to age 6.

Speech, language, and communication disorders occur with high frequency among children with cerebral palsy. The inability to coordinate resonation, articulation, and respiration mechanisms causes dysarthria, which is the primary speech deficit. "Dysarthria" is a technical term referring to a disturbance in voluntary control over the speech musculature. These children cannot speak with normal muscular speed, strength, precision, or timing. In some children, dysarthria may be relatively mild; but the speech of others, because of severe muscular weakness and

Children with cerebral palsy generally demonstrate dysarthria and, sometimes, mental retardation.

incoordination, is all but unintelligible. Children with severe dysarthria are prime candidates for alternative communications systems (as described in Chapter Ten).

In addition to the motoric difficulties demonstrated by children with cerebral palsy, there are often associated disabilities such as mental retardation. Severe and profound retardation is most commonly found in rigid, ataxic, and spastic quadriplegic groups. Many also demonstrate some form of seizure disorder, visual difficulties, hearing loss, secondary spinal curvature deformities, and perceptual processing difficulties in addition to their speech, language, and communication problems (Verhaaren & Connor, 1981). The multiplicity of secondary functional deficits hampers development of normal language-learning strategies.

The speech, language, and communication problems of children with cerebral palsy will vary, depending upon the degree of involvement, but some specific characteristics usually associated with the different types can be enumerated. The spastic child may develop a slow, labored speech; the athetoid, jerky speech; and the ataxic, a tremorous, quavering voice.

> Augmentative communication systems are described in Chapter Ten.

Children with spastic or athetotic forms of cerebral palsy perform poorly on visual perception and visual-motor tasks (Cruickshank, Bice, & Wallen, 1957). These processing problems, along with a lack of motivation (because attempts at vocalization may not be rewarded) combine to increase the child's difficulties and frustrations. Too often people simply nod when they do not understand, try to talk for the child, or ignore unintelligible utterances. These responses impede rather than facilitate language and communication.

SPINA BIFIDA

Children with spina bifida usually have normal intelligence. However, damage to the developing nervous system may result in multiple physical handicaps, including varying degrees of paralysis, bowel and bladder incontinence, and hydrocephalus (accumulation of fluid around the brain).

> Hydrocephalic and spina bifida children often exhibit "cocktail party" language.

Some display a language pattern called the "chatter-box" or "cocktail party" syndrome (Swisher & Pinsker, 1971; Lawrence, 1971). They will converse readily with anyone who will listen, but their language reflects disorganized thought processes and conceptual weaknesses. Many vocalizations are illogical and lacking in content. They do well repeating stories from memory, but cannot explain the meaning of what they have recited; they usually perform well on picture-vocabulary items, but poorly on verbal tasks requiring reasoning and comprehension. Younger children may demonstrate impaired auditory association and reception abilities (Spain, 1972).

MUSCULOSKELETAL DISABILITIES AND OTHER HEALTH IMPAIRMENTS

Orthopedic disabilities—disabilities related to maintaining a straight and normal skeletal and muscular state—include amputation (the absence at birth, or later removal, of a limb or limbs), arthrogryposis (persistent flexure or joint contractures present at birth), Legg-Perthes disease (a degenerative disease of the head of the femur), muscular dystrophy (progressive and continuous weakening of voluntary muscles), and osteogenesis imperfecta (a condition manifested in abnormally brittle bones). Health impairments which restrict the physical well-being and physiological functioning of children include asthma, cardiac disorders and hemophilia. These conditions do not affect learning *unless* mobility is severely restricted prior to ages 2 to 3.

In summary, there is little evidence that motor disorders alone (unless there are accompanying perceptual and/or sensory impairments) account for specific language problems. But there is no question that the restricted mobility they imply affects the rate of language learning. As infants, these children do not have the same access to physical and social stimuli as their more active healthy peers. If we continue to restrict their learning opportunities by placing them in classrooms with less competent peers, this disadvantage will be compounded (Duncan, Sbardellati, Maheady, & Sainoto, 1981). Ultimately, the impact of the disability on language learning depends on mobility and socialization restrictions, and on the amount and quality of early intervention services provided.

Restriction of physical activity can affect rate of language learning.

LANGUAGE AND COMMUNICATION PROBLEMS ASSOCIATED WITH SENSORY DEFICITS

HEARING IMPAIRMENT

A child who has difficulty hearing speech naturally will have difficulty acquiring oral language. Rather than being a learning device, language becomes a barrier, preventing full realization of academic, intellectual, and social potentials. About 5% of school-aged children have some hearing loss (Davis & Silverman, 1970). This percentage increases steadily to over 17% for persons aged 65 and over. The total number of persons with a significant bilateral (both ears) hearing loss is about seven million.

The severity of a child's language difficulties depends on the age of onset of the hearing loss and the degree of loss. Of the two major sources of hearing impairment, genetic conditions account for 40 to 60% of all causes of deafness. Of the 57 identified forms of genetic deafness, 10 also involve visual problems (Larson & Miller, 1978). Disease and trauma are the second major contributors to deafness. Among the most prevalent diseases are bacterial and viral infections, such as maternal rubella, meningitis, and serious otitis media. Trauma, usually resulting from blows to the head, birth complications, and exposure to sounds of great intensity and duration also account for some damage to the auditory system.

The age at which a hearing loss occurs is critical.

Each of the major types of hearing loss, conductive, sensorineural, and mixed, has a different prognosis and a somewhat different effect on language and communication.

Conductive hearing losses Conductive hearing losses are due to abnormalities or problems associated with the outer or middle ear. The problem is usually a malformation or blockage that prevents clear transmission of sound waves to the inner ear. Examples are impounded wax, infections in the middle ear, excess fluid in the eustachian tube, or interruptions in the middle ear bones. The primary effect of a conductive problem is loss of hearing sensitivity due to the fact that the level of sound reaching the inner ear is reduced. Conductive impairments are usually amenable to medical intervention (removal of the blockage) or amplification (a hearing aid).

Sensorineural hearing loss   Sensorineural hearing loss is the result of damage or disease in some portion of the inner ear, auditory nerve, and/or the neural pathways. The signal may not reach the brain at all or may arrive in a highly distorted form. Usually sound impulses remain unclear and distorted even when amplification is provided. Medical and surgical procedures are of limited usefulness with this type of hearing loss.

A mixed hearing loss is a combination of sensorineural and conductive losses. The two exist simultaneously. There may be some benefits from amplification if the conductive loss is the greater; but even then, the prognosis for sound discrimination is generally poor.

In addition to understanding the *type* of hearing loss a child has, a clinician must determine the *degree* of loss and the potential effects of the loss on the child's ability to hear everyday speech. Sharpness and range of hearing are measured by a device called an audiometer. Threshold measurements, the faintest level of sound that the child can reliably detect, are recorded on an audiogram.

Sound intensity is measured in decibels (dB). (The softest sound a normal hearing child can perceive is defined as 0 dB; a rock concert would measure about 100 dB). Larger dB numbers represent increasingly louder sounds. Children with mild hearing losses (15–40 dB) may have a mild auditory learning dysfunction with resulting inattention, mild language delay, and mild speech problems. The child hears the louder, voiced speech sounds, but may miss some of the less intense speech sounds, like voiceless stops and fricatives. She may have to work harder in school to hear relevant instructions and thus may be subject to fatigue and erratic academic performance. The term "deaf" is usually reserved for those children with over a 70 dB loss through the speech range. If the loss is present before 1 year of age, these children will not develop speech and language spontaneously (Northern & Lemme, 1982).

Differences among children due to such factors as intelligence, emotional stability, and socialization, plus variations attributable to age of onset and degree and type of impairment, preclude description of the language learning characteristics of an "average" hearing-impaired child. Knowing that a child is hearing-impaired does not tell a teacher or clinician the quality or quantity of language to expect or the child's programming needs.

The greatest controversy in the area of educational programming for the hearing-impaired concerns the extent to which deaf children should be taught to produce and understand speech. Some insist that a "purely

The severity of a hearing loss is described in terms of decibels; the larger the number, the more severe the loss.

oral" method is best for helping deaf children develop speech and language skills and discourage the use of signs and gestures. Other educators feel that manual systems should be used along with speech to facilitate more "natural" communication. Despite a considerable volume of research addressing the issue, little progress has been made towards its resolution, especially regarding children with severe impairments. Most advocate a multisensory approach called *total communication.* These programs use a variety of methods to teach students to express themselves by speaking and signing (supplemented with fingerspelling as needed), and to understand others through speechreading, auditory training, signs, and fingerspelling.

Very little specific information about the rates or stages of language acquisition for hearing-impaired children is available. When language is significantly delayed, it is undoubtedly an effect of deficiencies in both linguistic and cognitive experiences. When all other factors are equal, the hearing impairment is diagnosed early, and the quality and quantity of home communication experiences approach normal standards, language performance (oral and/or manual) and achievement in other areas may parallel *or even exceed* that of hearing youngsters (Moores, 1974, 1977; Wilbur, 1976). Exactly how hearing-impaired children integrate whatever they do hear with their visual and tactile input is not clearly understood, but we can assume that tactile modalities play an important role.

Hearing-impaired children require precise and systematic instruction in all language domains.

The vast majority of hearing-impaired students, over 70%, are being educated in regular classrooms (Nober, 1982). However, the combination of visual and hearing impairments, with or without other physical problems, calls for a highly individualized approach to programming and transdisciplinary decision making. The intellectual level of these children may range from gifted to profoundly retarded, and the vast majority experience severe communication difficulties.

VISUAL IMPAIRMENT

The language development of visually impaired children has not been investigated as extensively as that of hearing-impaired children. Most blind children eventually develop skills comparable to those of their sighted peers (Warren, 1977), but some rather significant differences in learning rate are evident prior to age 5.

Delays in attaining the object concept and object permanence (stemming from the blind child's immobility and inability to engage in sustained search behavior) undoubtedly play some role in the reported early language delay. Fraiberg (1968) noted that some blind children do not construct these sensorimotor concepts until 4 or 5 years of age, in contrast to 18 to 24 months for the sighted child. Early vocalizations and imitation, on the other hand, emerge at the expected ages. In fact, some blind babies begin imitating sounds earlier than their sighted peers (Fraiberg, 1977).

The inability to see limits a child's sensory experiences and, consequently, impacts learning.

Spontaneous word production generally is delayed at least four months. This delay is probably attributable to delayed cognitive development stemming from a deprived experiential base. Restricted mobility affects experiences with objects and, therefore, opportunities to learn word-concept linkages. Likewise, delay in producing word combinations can be explained by lack of exposure to attributes, actions, and qualities. Impaired vision interferes with the child's perception of object and event relations.

The ability of visually impaired children to understand and express language content often lags behind their development of form and use skills. Because wants and needs derive from internal rather than external states, their expression is not as hampered by restricted ability to explore the environment.

LANGUAGE AND COMMUNICATION PROBLEMS ASSOCIATED WITH CENTRAL NERVOUS SYSTEM DYSFUNCTION

Myers and Hammill (1976) posit a possible range of impairment, from mild to severe, of central nervous system dysfunction assumed to be associated with language and communication problems. *Learning disability* is a complex impairment of functions that seems to indicate a mild central nervous system disorder. *Aphasia* is assumed to be a more severe central or congenital disorder that produces severe problems in developmental language functions. Observable differences among children with these possible causal conditions, however, are not easily specified.

LEARNING DISABILITIES

Of all the problems demonstrated by children with learning disabilities, language and communication difficulties are among the most serious and the most pervasive. The relationship between language disorders and learning disabilities is apparent in the widely accepted definition from section 5(b)(4) of P.L. 94–142 of learning disabilities as "a disorder in one or more of the basic psychological processes involved in understanding or in using language, spoken or written, which may manifest itself in an imperfect ability to listen, think, speak, read, spell. . ." Conservative prevalence estimates based on this definition range from 1% to 8% of all school children (Hare & Hare, 1979). It is reasonable to assume that the majority have language deficits of one type or another (Marge, 1972; Lerner, 1981).

The range and variety of complex, language-related difficulties demonstrated by children identified as "learning disabled" have attracted considerable attention. Areas of deficit may include visual and auditory perceptual difficulties, motor incoordination, problems integrating information from two or more sensory sources, and storage and retrieval problems (Wiig & Semel, 1980). However, the single most significant deterrent to educational progress seems to be their inability to use oral and written language effectively. Studies have consistently found learning disabled children to be deficient on measures of linguistic structure: syntax, semantics, morphology, and phonology (e.g., Vogel, 1977; Wiig & Semel, 1980).

In a review of an important series of recent studies considering the possibility that learning disabled children have deficits in pragmatics, the understanding of the rules governing language use in social context, Bryan, Donahue, and Pearl (1981) concluded:

1. *Learning disabled children have more difficulties than nondisabled children in ambiguous or socially complex situations.* They appear to lack such pragmatic skills as asking questions, responding to inadequate messages, disagreeing and supporting an argument, sustaining a conversation, holding the conversational floor, and monitoring a conversation.

2. *Learning disabled children appear to elicit different responses from their peers, compared to nondisabled children.* Peers, in addition to evidencing some discomfort in the interaction, tend to ask them simpler questions and provide fewer elaborative responses.

3. *Learning disabled children appear to be less able to adapt their speech to the needs of their listeners and less cooperative conversation partners.* Girls performed more poorly than boys in responding to subtle facial feedback from listeners and they were also less proficient in judging the adequacy of the speaker's message.

There is evidence that learning disabled children have deficits in pragmatic competence.

Learning disabled children usually demonstrate average or above average IQ scores, but their learning difficulties (including language) are so pervasive that most will require many hours of special instruction to keep up with their peers. The young learning disabled child usually stands out from her preschool peers because of an inability to name colors and/ or to arrange two or three objects in a size progression. She is likely to be slow in following verbal directions (if she responds at all), unable to count in sequence, name the days of the week, or identify items belonging to the same semantic class. Misarticulations, nonfluency, and baby talk may persist well beyond the period normal for young children. In addition to this multiplicity of problems, the learning disabled preschooler may demonstrate sound, sequencing, and word discrimination deficits. Her speech may be rapid and jerky, and it may be difficult to determine the intention of her utterances because of inappropriate prosody. Generally, the impression one gets when interacting with a learning disabled child is of a youngster who is confused, inattentive, slow to respond, and (at the same time) impulsive. As demands for language and other reading-related skills increase, her problems (and her frustrations) multiply.

Preschool teachers are often the first to recognize that the child's speech, language and communication skills fall outside the normal range.

Wiig and Semel (1980) provide excellent recommendations for assessment and day-to-day programming for the elementary school-aged learning disabled child with a language disorder. Though not nearly as helpful to preschool personnel, this volume is highly recommended as a resource for teachers and speech/language clinicians.

APHASIA

The term aphasic was first applied to adults who had lost language skills because of some traumatic event, such as an accident or a stroke. Noting similar behaviors in children, physicians began to use the term *childhood aphasia* to describe severe receptive and expressive language problems resulting from dysfunction in the central nervous system. Acquired aphasia, loss of established language skills, is usually differentiated from congenital or developmental aphasia, cases where normal language skills have not developed. Notions concerning the etiology of congenital aphasia are, for the most part, speculative; but it is usually attributed to pathology in the central nervous system (specifically the left hemisphere of the brain). In acquired aphasia, if injury occurs early enough in the normally dominant left hemisphere, the right hemisphere will take over the language functions. After a transient period of aphasia, the child will usually repeat the stages of language development that she has already passed through and reacquire adequate language skills.

Aphasia is often difficult to differentiate from other severe language disorders.

Precisely how childhood aphasia differs from other severe language disorders is not altogether clear. Eisenson (1972) describes childhood aphasia as including such behaviors as perseveration, inconsistent responses, hyperactivity, emotional lability, auditory inefficiency, and perceptual and intellectual inefficiencies. However, all these behaviors are also evident in children labelled mentally retarded, deaf, or autistic. Also, it is rare to find a child labelled as aphasic who does not demonstrate some hearing impairment and/or motor impairment (Eisenson & Ingram, 1972), so perhaps these children could be more accurately designated as multiply handicapped when classification is necessary.

LANGUAGE AND COMMUNICATION PROBLEMS ASSOCIATED WITH SEVERE EMOTIONAL-SOCIAL DYSFUNCTION

Controversy about precise definition and diagnosis within the exceptional subcategory labelled *severely emotionally disturbed* (SED) has raged for several decades. Rutter (1968) provides the clearest available differentiation of subclassifications. He recommends reserving the term *psychosis* for disturbances which begin in adolescence and resemble adult schizophrenia and using the term *childhood schizophrenia* for disturbances evident between the ages of 3 and 5. *Autism* is evident at birth or, at least, by age 2 or 3. Kauffman (1977) suggests that 0.1% of all children (1 in 1,000) are severely disturbed.

Although personal characteristics of diagnosis, age, and social skills vary, the majority of children labeled "severely emotionally disturbed" have one characteristic in common—a profound disruption in the development of verbal and nonverbal interaction skills. Because there has been considerably more research in the area of autism, we shall concentrate on describing the language characteristics of autistic children. Children identified as displaying childhood schizophrenia share some, but not all, of these characteristics.

The language characteristics of children with mild behavior disorders are not addressed. The reason is a total absence of research data in this area. Behaviorally disordered children are generally poor achievers who appear to share many of the learning problems associated with the categories "learning disabled" and "educable mentally retarded," most notably problems in attention and problem solving (Kauffman, 1977). If, as is now generally accepted, the process of language development rests on social-affective development as well as linguistic and cognitive variables, then some language deficits would be expected in this population. However, researchers in this area have been so concerned with defining and classifying the behavior problems of this population (i.e., aggression, hyperactivity, withdrawal) that the question of language and communication skills has not surfaced.

AUTISM

Autism is the term used to describe a syndrome of developmental disabilities involving multiple perceptual and cognitive impairments and extreme social and behavioral maladjustment. Disturbances in the development of speech and language skills and poor communication skills are commonly singled out as diagnostic (and prognostic) indicators (Rutter, 1978; Wing, 1969; Lovaas, Koegel, Simmons, & Long, 1973). Autism is also characterized by disturbances of relating, mobility, and developmental rate (Ornitz & Ritvo, 1976). These children show little, if any, inclination to interact socially with peers, family, or caregivers. Many engage in such stereotyped, repetitive, self-stimulatory behaviors as body-rocking, twirling, and spinning objects. The best evidence to date suggests that autism is associated with severe brain disorders (Rutter & Schopler, 1978).

Two groups of autistic, or autistic-like, children can be differentiated (Bartak & Rutter, 1976). One group, the majority, is comprised of mentally retarded children; the other includes children with borderline or normal IQ scores. The two groups share many autistic characteristics, but, as would be expected, the prognosis is much better for the latter group. The effects of intellectual retardation on learning and performance are clearly more influential than are the effects of the autistic behaviors (Bartak & Rutter, 1976; Hermelin & O'Connor, 1970).

Most autistic children have subnormal intelligence.

Whether the language processes of autistic children are deviant (qualitatively different) or delayed (quantitatively different) remains a point of some disagreement. (A parallel to this argument can be found in the literature dealing with the language disorders of the retarded.) The possibility that both positions are correct should not be discounted, though most investigators maintain that the evidence points to aberrant language processes and products in autistic children (e.g., Cunningham, 1968; Rutter, 1966; Rutter & Schopler, 1978; Ward & Hoddinott, 1968; Weiland & Legg, 1964).

Echolalia (the meaningless repetition of previously heard words, phrases, and/or sentences) is one of the most perplexing and frequently cited characteristics of the language of autistic children. Some distinguish between immediate and delayed echolalia, with immediate echolalia referring to the literal repetition of the utterances of others immediately after their occurrence, and with delayed echolalia referring to a literal repetition sometime later (Ricks & Wing, 1976).

Apart from attempts to compare the speech and language disorders of autistic children with the language of other atypical groups and *explain* the inevitable speech and language differences of autistic children, there are numerous detailed, but less formal, reports describing their language and communication difficulties. Not only echolalia, but also pronoun reversals, mutism, inappropriate and noncommunicative utterances, comprehension problems, invented words (called neologisms), and articulation difficulties are common. A lack of questions and informative statements, frequent use of imperatives, deviations in pitch, rhythm, and inflections, muddled sequencing of sounds and words, confusions of related words, and problems with function words are also noted (Savage, 1968; Hingtgen & Bryson, 1972; Wing, 1972). Interaction deficits (lack of facial gestures; preferences for inanimate contacts) have the potential to negatively influence nonverbal communications (Lovaas, Koegel, Simmons, & Long, 1973; Hicks, 1972).

The communicative behavior of autistic children seems largely nonsymbolic; if they do develop speech, it is rarely used for communicative purposes.

Although by no means conclusive, research to date seems to suggest that a number of the cognitive skills necessary for language are impaired in autism. For those autistic children who are testable on standard IQ measures, a particular and idiosyncratic performance pattern—verbal subtests invariably below performance subtests—has been noted. They perform well on block design, object assembly, digit span, similarities, and picture completion tasks and poorly on comprehension, vocabulary, picture arrangement, and digit or symbol coding tasks (Simmons & Tymchuk, 1973). The former abilities, where functioning is least retarded, are those believed to reflect right-hemisphere-mediated skills. Autistic children seem to perform best on items that suggest their own solution and thus do not require analytic skills or sequential processing.

The extent to which autistic children exhibit deficiencies of communicative behavior rather than more specific language deficits is addressed by Schuler (1980). She notes that much of the speech and many vocalizations of autistic children are self-stimulatory rather than communicative. Those utterances that do have communicative intent consist largely of concrete requests. Even when appropriate, the speech of autistic children is often mechanistic and flat. Poor conversation skills may be an effect of their inability to take listener perspectives into account. All of these deficits are undoubtedly related to, if not a consequence of, the autistic child's characteristic avoidance of social interactions. The context of social interactions, where normal learners acquire communication skills, is not a learning sphere for these children.

The important issue to remember about autistic children is that they represent a highly variable exceptional subgroup and are diagnosed according to diverse criteria. Most are functioning significantly below their age peers in social and cognitive development, as well as in language.

LANGUAGE AND COMMUNICATION PROBLEMS ASSOCIATED WITH COGNITIVE DISORDERS

Unless accompanied by markedly disturbed social interactions or specific evidence of sensory or motor impairment, the primary label applied to children with limited cognitive abilities is *mental retardation*. Problems of definition and classification, plus diagnosis and assessment limitations, make it difficult to estimate the prevalence of speech and language disorders among the retarded population, but extremely high figures would be expected. One reason it is difficult to estimate prevalence is that language performance is one of the behaviors tapped by IQ tests to arrive at a diagnosis of mental retardation in the first place. Secondly, language learning is undoubtedly linked to, if not dependent upon, cognitive attainments. Generally the more severe the retardation, the greater the language and communication problems.

> The more severe the retardation, the greater the language and communication problems.

Paralleling the same controversy in other areas of exceptionality are differing viewpoints on whether the language deficiencies of retarded children should be classified as deviant or delayed. Although a few researchers (notably Cromer, 1974) have contended that retarded children learn language differently from children with normal cognitive development, most argue that retarded children acquire language skills in much the same fashion as their more competent peers, but at a slower rate and perhaps at a lower ceiling (Evans & Hampson, 1968; Lackner, 1968; Ryan, 1975).

The main factor hampering comparisons of the language skills of retarded and nonretarded populations and accurate estimation of the prevalence of the language and communication problems among the retarded population has been reliance on IQ as the single criterion for definition and classification of mentally retarded persons. Studies comparing the language performance of retarded and normal learners have generally matched their subjects on the basis of mental age. This procedure places the validity of their findings into question because mental age is computed from performance on an IQ test and IQ tests are acknowledged to be heavily loaded with language factors. (In fact, the Stanford-Binet is sometimes used in preschool programs that emphasize language development because it is considered a particularly good measure of language skills.) After samples of retarded children are matched with normal learners on the basis of mental age scores (derived from what are essentially language tests), the two groups are then compared on the same variable—language.

> Reliance on IQ as the single criterion for classification of the mentally retarded has hampered efforts to estimate the prevalence of language and communication problems.

The fallacy of this procedure is obvious. It is something like matching two groups of children on the basis of their scores on a motor development test and then turning around and looking to see how much they resemble one another in motor development. Certainly more similarities than differences would be predicted. This is the reason for caution when interpreting the results of research studies comparing the language abilities of retarded and nonretarded populations (if mental age scores are used as a basis for matching).

MLU is a better measure of a child's language development than mental age.

One way to avoid the problems inherent in comparing children matched by the controversial mental age criterion is to match children on the basis of MLU (as discussed in Chapter One). Since most early language attainments, at least until about age 4, result in increased *length*, MLU is an appropriate alternative to mental age. A higher MLU reflects increased sophistication. When two children have the same MLU, the quality of their utterances (e.g., semantic functions, grammatical inflections) should be very similar.

Most data (e.g., Ryan, 1975; Duchan & Erickson, 1976) indicate that the primary differences between the language processes of retarded and nonretarded children are rate-related. However, whether the language development of retarded children is simply delayed or qualitatively different from that of nonretarded children will undoubtedly continue to be an issue.

The precise relationship of cognitive deficits with communicative competence is not clear because there has been little research on the development of pragmatic skills by retarded children. One exception is a report by Longhurst (1972) that retarded adolescents' referential communication is often incomplete or idiosyncratic and that they do not change their message even when it is clear that the listener has misunderstood the intent.

AN INSTRUCTIONALLY RELEVANT CLASSIFICATION SCHEME

As suggested in the introduction, disability definitions and classifications may serve a placement function but they are virtually useless for instructional purposes. In the area of language and communication, as well as in other educational domains, there is a need for careful differentiation and profiling of strengths and deficits. Ideally, such a classification scheme would have educationally relevant categories (without the potential for stigma) and there would be little or no overlap across and variability within categories. Mutually exclusive categories would facilitate generalizations about how to approach assessment and programming for children in the various subgroups.

The content-form-use organization proposed by Bloom and Lahey (1978) at least approximates this ideal. Certainly, content, form, and use are not discrete domains any more than motor impairments or cognitive deficits are discrete diagnostic categories, but this scheme does permit focus on the independent and dependent variables relevant to language assessment and intervention. Placement in one or another of the subgroups described below has implications for formulating appropriate assessment questions and determining objectives for language intervention.

At this point you may want to refer to Chapter One and review the full explanations for the terms *content, form,* and *use.* Understanding these terms is critical for application of the proposed classification scheme.

1. **Content** refers to the semantic or meaning dimension of language. What children talk *about*—the objects, events, and relations in their environment—comprises the content of language.
2. **Form** refers to the phonological, morphological, and syntactic dimensions of language. What children talk *with*—sounds, words, phrases, and sentences—comprise the form of language. An important property of form is its linkage to content. If sound, words, phrases, and/or sentences do not convey meaning (content) they cannot be considered language.
3. **Use** refers to the "why," "when," and "where" aspects—the functional dimensions of language. Pragmatic skills, or how children use language for various purposes, are essential for communicative competence.

Bloom and Lahey differentiate five subgroups within the very large population of language-disordered children:

> There are at least five subgroups within the population of language disordered children.

1. Children who exhibit problems in formulating and conceptualizing ideas about objects, events, and relations (a **content problems** subgroup)
2. Children who demonstrate problems in learning the code and linking the code to what they know about the world (a **form** or, more precisely, a **form/content problems** subgroup)
3. Children who have difficulties speaking or understanding in certain contexts or adjusting their language for certain purposes (a **use problems** subgroup)
4. Children who have a problem with associations between content, form, and use (an **association problems** subgroup)
5. Children who demonstrate language and communication abilities similar in all aspects to those of a younger child with normal development (a **delayed language development** subgroup)

Each subgroup is described in more detail below with generalizations about the language behaviors that suggest assignment to the category. Additional suggestions to aid category assignment will be presented in Chapter Four.

CONTENT PROBLEMS

Children whose level of cognitive functioning is significantly less advanced than their form and use skills may be said to have content difficulties. Relatively few children, except for blind children and children with spina bifida, will qualify for this subgroup. The disparity between their form and use skills and their content skills may be explained by reference to a smaller range and variety of experiences which, in turn, is attributable to restricted mobility. Researchers have found significant cognitive delays in young visually impaired children (Warren, 1981). They may develop little understanding of spatial relationships, faulty impressions of distance, and problems with form, size, and position relationships as well as lags in the acquisition of various conservation abilities. They are unable to learn through imitation of what they see, and so must rely on direct experiences, which, unfortunately, may be limited.

The spina bifida, hydrocephalic youngster with "cocktail party speech" provides another example of content difficulties. Children with hydrocephalus associated with myelomeningocele (the most severe type of spina bifida) generally exhibit some mental retardation which may be masked by excessive verbalization and what appear to be advanced social skills. Most utterances will be well-formed and seemingly appropriate to the context, but the content is superficial and irrelevant.

As noted above, relatively few children demonstrate content problems. Conceptual development does not usually lag far behind form and use abilities because cognitive development plays a significant role in learning forms, rules of grammar, and pragmatic skills. When they do occur, content problems are an effect of not learning the perceptual and functional characteristics of objects, actions, and/or events and their relations. These youngsters need intervention directed towards construction and organization of the meanings which necessarily underlie language.

Warren (1981) suggests several strategies for enhancing the cognitive abilities of visually impaired children:

1. Train the child with partial vision to use it effectively
2. Focus on training verbalization, identification, manipulation and recognition of changing spatial relationships
3. Provide training in classification tasks including verbal and tactile discovery of class problems, and form, orientation, texture, and size classification problems
4. Provide conservation and formal operations training tasks

FORM DISORDERS

Children with form disorders score much higher on nonverbal intelligence measures than on language tests. Further, there is evidence of relatively advanced communication skills, though they may rely on gestures and such primitive devices as tantrums and whining to control the environment. Their problems are related to learning the surface aspects of language, phonology, morphology, and syntax, to represent their ideas and intentions.

Children described as aphasic may fall into this subgroup. Neurological defects and brain damage (associated with disease or injury) can impair auditory perception, the ability to recognize written or verbal symbols, and the muscle coordination necessary for speech. The problems these children experience are somewhat analogous to the problems we experience when trying to communicate in a foreign language. We know what we want to say and where and when to say it. The problem is *how* to say it. Aphasic children are unable to express what they know. In some cases they may not know, or be able to recall, the right word or words; in other cases, the difficulty may be a linkage problem—they have not made the necessary connections between forms and concepts.

Speech disorders, either organic or functional, would also be classified as form difficulties. Organic problems (articulation, voice, and fluency disorders) are caused by physical or neurological abnormality; functional problems are attributed to improper learning, short auditory memory span, and discrimination problems.

The four types of articulation errors are substitutions (using one phoneme for another), distortions (mispronouncing the sound), omissions (leaving out a sound), and additions (putting in an extra sound) (Van Riper, 1978). Voice disorders include pitch, intensity and voice quality problems. Fluency problems include stuttering and cluttering. The age of onset of stuttering is typically between 2 and 7 years, and it affects about 1% of the total population (Milisen, 1971). Cluttering is often confused with stuttering. Van Riper (1978) has compared the clutterer's speech to what happens when a beginning typist's speed exceeds control and the keys pile up on top of each other. It is fast speech garbled with extra sounds or mispronounced sounds and sometimes mixed-up sentence structure.

Most children with hearing impairments will also be classified as having form problems. Their speech difficulties, articulation, voice quality, and fluency problems, result from not hearing well enough to learn conventional symbols and patterns. As discussed earlier in the chapter, the age of onset and severity of hearing loss will determine the effect on speech and language development. A child with mild to moderate loss will probably develop language skills slowly, but will usually learn to speak effectively with therapy and adequate amplification. A child born deaf may never acquire functional oral language skills.

Many learning disabled children also demonstrate form disorders or, more accurately, form-content linkage problems (others are more appropriately classified as use disorders). Affirmative answers to the following questions suggested, in part, by Vitter (1982), assist determination of whether a child has exhibited a form disorder:

Phonology
1. Has the child learned the rules governing sounds? (Or does she make different articulation errors each time she speaks?)
2. Does the child discriminate among words that differ only in respect to initial or final consonants? (Or does she confuse such words as "cat" or "rat?")
3. Are the child's spoken utterances intelligible?

Morphology and Syntax
1. Has the child learned the rules governing word order and other aspects of grammar, such as subject-verb agreement?

2. Does the child appear to understand the grammatical form used in instructional directions?
3. Has the child mastered the grammatical morphemes for her MLU stage?

   Stage II (MLU = 2.0–2.49)   *ing*, plural, *in*
   Stage III (MLU = 2.50–2.99)   *on*, possessive
   Stage IV (MLU 3.0–3.74)   no new acquisitions
   Stage V (MLU = 3.75–4.50)   regular and irregular past tense, regular third person singular, articles *a, the,* and the contractible copula *be*
   Stage V + (MLU = 4.51 +)   contractible and uncontractible auxiliary *be,* uncontractible copula *be,* and the irregular third person

USE PROBLEMS

Some children have constructed meanings and they demonstrate knowledge of the code and rules for expressing meanings, but their communicative competence is not commensurate with their content and form knowledge. (Recall from Chapters One and Two that a speaker's ability to express intentions to alter the listener's attitudes, beliefs, and/or behaviors is termed *communicative competence.*) Returning to the analogy suggested in the last chapter of learning and playing backgammon, we can say that the child who has not developed successful playing strategies has language use problems.

These children may talk about things that are out of context, and string together ideas tangentially without regard for the listener's perspective. Many utterances seem to have a bizarre quality. Rees (1978) describes a child who, when asked, "What's this?" and shown a cup, responds *"That* is a red cup." Compared to the normal response to such a question, "A cup," this response, which had been laboriously trained, sounds stilted and inappropriate. A child who routinely greets visitors with, "How are you, I am fine today, isn't it a lovely day" without pauses or intonation contours has use problems. You cannot quarrel with the form or the content of the utterance (if it is, in fact, a nice day) but it is immediately recognizable as inappropriate. Both of these examples reflect a training problem. They are the result of misdirected training efforts on the part of teachers and/or clinicians.

Other use problems are not so easily explained. However, it is logical to assume that the inappropriate utterances of many severely emotionally disturbed children may be related to deviations in primary socialization processes. These children often appear to have difficulty receiving and/or interpreting conversational cues; they fail to adjust their language to the cues provided by others. Their communication is often predominantly in a motoric-gestural mode, if they attempt communication at all. There appears to be no motivation for reciprocal eye contact and other nonlinguistic interactions. Problems dealing with deixis—particularly the distinction between when to use *I* and when to use *you*—are common. Whether these atypical behaviors so often observed in autistic children are due to an unwillingness to learn communication skills, or to an inability, is not clear. This is one of the many questions to be answered on an individual basis as part of the assessment-intervention process.

As discussed earlier in this chapter, use problems among learning disabled children are common. In situations that require them to initiate a verbal interaction or situations where the context does not precisely specify what an appropriate communication strategy might be, they seem to evade conversational responsibilities. One consequence of this type of evasion is avoidance by their peers and by adults which, in turn, leads to fewer opportunities to learn appropriate conversational strategies. The use problems demonstrated by learning disabled children have been attributed to lack of verbal fluency, overuse of a limited concrete vocabulary, use of only a concrete vocabulary, use of pronouns without antecedents, and failure to understand the need to clarify information (Wiig & Semel, 1980). Whether these problems derive from attention, perception, or memory deficits cannot be determined, but all three have the potential to affect acquisition of language use knowledge and skills.

CONTENT-FORM-USE ASSOCIATION PROBLEMS

Some children demonstrate adequate development in each of the language domains, but associations between and among the three appear to be either weak or disrupted. The child may have a concept to communicate about, and there may be evidence (from observations and documentation of past productions) that she knows the form with which to express the concept. However, instead of associating the concept with the correct form, she produces an inappropriate utterance that does not function as desired. An inability to represent meaning with relevant, meaningful and/or functional linguistic forms, in spite of evidence that the form ability has been acquired, indicates association difficulties. It shows weak or distorted associations, or transfer difficulties, among the three domains.

Children with association or transfer difficulties produce age-appropriate forms and structures, but these structures are not used in the appropriate context to convey the intended meanings. Unlike children with content difficulties, they have attained sufficient cognitive-semantic concepts; they simply do not code them appropriately. Unlike children with use difficulties, children with association problems use language for interpersonal interactions. But there is a contradiction between the content of the message and its use. An example is the seriously disturbed child who recites nursery rhymes or television commercials in a conversation.

PARALLEL CONTENT-FORM-USE DELAY

Where a child's language and communication skills resemble those of younger children with normal development, her difficulty reflects either onset of language later than normal or development proceeding at a slower rate. An example would be a 3-year-old Down Syndrome child whose language closely resembles that of a normal 2-year-old. There are many mildly and moderately retarded children who do not demonstrate content, form, and use skills at the ages when they ordinarily appear. They may have deficits in any or all of the processes necessary to learn language—attention, hearing, auditory perception, memory, and an output capability. The effect is a generally depressed performance level.

PERSPECTIVES ON INTERVENTION

The remainder of this book focuses upon language assessment and intervention. Since the material to this point has dealt primarily with research reports and theory, this section is a bridge from theoretical to practical issues. A reasonable way to begin construction of this bridge is to present some recently altered perspectives on intervention. In addition to describing the context of subsequent chapters, these assumptions reflect the progress that has been made in special education and language intervention over the past decade.

THE RIGHT TO EDUCATIONAL INTERVENTION

Passage of Public Law 94-142 (The Education for all Handicapped Children Act) in 1975 was evidence of recognition by the federal government that millions of handicapped children were being denied their full rights as citizens. Many of these youngsters were excluded from any public education service, and others were receiving only partial services. Because it accelerated concern for and focus on the unique characteristics and needs of the handicapped, this legislation is one of the most significant and influential laws ever passed in this or any other country.

With the enactment of P.L. 94-142, educators became one of the first professions in the history of our nation to be given legislative direction on the conduct of their professional practices. Among other directives designed to safeguard the rights of handicapped children, the law mandates development of an individual education program (IEP) for each handicapped child and specifies the components this instructional plan should include. It also identifies the sequence of events that should lead to IEP formulations. States are to provide appropriate instruction, related services, teacher training, and improved diagnostic procedures to remedy the inequality of past practices. These benefits are to be made available to preschool children with special needs (unless inconsistent with state law or practice), as well as to elementary and secondary students. Students with the most severe handicaps within each disability area are designated as service priorities.

The IEP process is described in Chapter Five.

Public Law 94-142 is a commitment to assure handicapped children the rights that nonhandicapped children have taken for granted. The implicit intent of the legislation is to enable handicapped children to grow up and live in "normal" environments, with "normal" activities and "normal" friends. They are to be regarded as individuals, treated fairly and humanely in school, and to be provided with the special services and special attention that their special needs require. The IEP is a contract between the school district and handicapped child's parents to assure that this occurs.

CONCERN FOR FUNCTIONAL AND AGE-APPROPRIATE SKILLS

Since the mid-1970s Lou Brown and his colleagues at the University of Wisconsin have heavily influenced the development of curricula for the most severely impaired exceptional subgroups. The "criterion of ultimate functioning" was introduced in an early publication (Brown, Nietupski, & Hamre-Nietupski, 1976) and continues as a standard against which to measure the adequacy and appropriateness of instructional planning. Implicit in the criterion of ultimate functioning are six questions for teachers, related services personnel, and parents to consider *before* initiating instructional activities:

1. Why should this instructional activity be provided?
2. Will this activity prepare the student for functioning in complex heterogeneous community environments?
3. Could the student function as an adult *without* these skills?
4. Is there a different activity that will allow the student to realize the criterion of ultimate functioning more quickly and efficiently?
5. Will this activity in any way impede, reduce, or restrict the probability of ultimate functioning in community environments?
6. Are the skills, materials, tasks, and criteria of concern similar to those encountered in adult life?

These strategies for generating curricula rely basically on an ecological approach in providing direction and rationale for teaching the functional, chronological-age-related skills necessary for successful interactions in domestic, community, and vocational settings.

> Strategies for generating functional, age-appropriate curricula are presented in Chapter Six.

When applied to handicapped preschool children the criterion of ultimate functioning translates into "criterion of the next school environment"—kindergarten or first grade. The logic of this principle dictates preschool curricula focusing on teaching the skills necessary for successful transition to and maintenance in regular education kindergarten and primary level classrooms.

INTERDEPENDENT SKILL CLUSTERS

A series of articles by Doug Guess and colleagues at the University of Kansas (Mulligan, Guess, Holvoet, & Brown, 1980; Holvoet, Guess, Mulligan, & Brown, 1980; Brown, Holvoet, Guess, & Mulligan, 1980; Guess & Noonan, 1982; Sailor & Guess, 1983) describe the individualized curriculum sequencing model (ICS) for teaching clusters of skills that cut across the traditional developmental domains. This approach avoids the tendency to teach skill areas as isolated units and shifts the focus to identifying and teaching age-appropriate and functional tasks. For example, a young child might be taught to raise his head (gross motor), look at an object (visual orientation), produce a sound or sign (communication), reach for and grasp the object (fine motor), and then use the object in a functional manner (cognitive/fine motor). Contained in this cluster are five age-

> Skill clusters are described at length in Chapter Nine.

appropriate and functional skills that have been identified as critical to independent functioning. Rather than being taught separately, with repeated trials, the skills are clustered in a holistic manner so the child practices the entire sequence on every instructional occasion.

FUNCTIONAL COMMUNICATION SKILLS

Emphasis should be upon environmental interaction and control.

The majority of children, even nonverbal children, are already communicators. They communicate in a variety of ways, some subtle, some not. The problem is that we frequently fail to acknowledge certain primitive devices as communications. Such behaviors as tantrums, pushing away, persistent eye gaze, throwing a toy for attention, and crying may be answered or ignored; they may not be recognized as communication. Sometimes practitioners even deliberately intervene to extinguish these behaviors, instead of using them as a base for developing more conventional and appropriate communication devices.

Augmentative communication systems are discussed in Chapter Ten.

Some nonverbal children lack the motivation to attempt control of their environment; they have learned to be passive and helpless. When a child is not able to establish a relationship between her own behavior and what occurs in her environment, she stops trying to assert herself. "Learned helplessness," a construct introduced by Seligman (1975), refers to the state of passivity that results when there is no predictable way to control the environment. Whether this lack of control is an effect of an unresponsive or unpredictable environment *or* of the child's physical limitations is unimportant. The result is the same. Our task with these youngsters is to arrange the environment in such a way that the child can affect and control it. We must assure that each child is provided with the most effective system she can master—the one that will permit the greatest interaction with and control over the greatest number of people in the most settings.

EMPIRICALLY VALIDATED METHODOLOGY

Much remains to be learned about the concepts and procedures involved in language intervention, but we can state with some assurance that there is a validated scientific methodology. The movement from a preoccupation with language form to consideration of the minimal skills required for environmental control has lead to new training emphases. One consequence of looking at the critical effects of communication in everyday life, instead of focusing exclusively on response forms, has been the development of a wide range of augmentative and alternative communication systems. Focusing on what we want language to be able to accomplish for the student (what language should *do,* rather than how it is produced) has led to widespread adoption of manual signing and communication boards. The results of these efforts have been gratifying.

A technology for language intervention has been developed, and its application demonstrated with many populations. This technology is thoroughly described in subsequent chapters. The conditions necessary for language learning and communication have been identified and successfully manipulated. This is not to say that we have all the answers (e.g., the study of generalization of treatment effects in the natural environment is just beginning), but we are saying that certain conditions and contexts for acquisition have been established well enough that they can be applied with an expectation of success.

That some children have not acquired language or are acquiring it at a rate significantly below expectations may be evidence that they are not processing stimuli in the same manner as their peers. But it is not necessarily a reason for assuming that they cannot learn from many of the same natural interactions. It is not a sufficient rationale for rigorously controlling learning conditions, restricting the range of available stimuli, and limiting the range of acceptable responses. In fact, if learning *does* occur under these unnatural circumstances, with massed trials and repetitive stimuli, we can hold little hope of generalization. Much effort was wasted in the past because we were not sensitive to the importance of simulating natural language learning conditions.

There was a time, not so long ago, when a clinic room was considered the ideal language intervention setting. It seemed to meet all the criteria for an optimal learning environment or, at least, what we thought was an optimal learning environment: quiet, isolated from interruptions, and free from distracting stimuli. What we created instead was an unnatural and counterproductive training environment; it is difficult to talk when there is nothing interesting to talk about.

Design of the optimal language learning environment is discussed in Chapters Six, Seven, and Eight.

TRANSDISCIPLINARY PROCESSES

Statutory, judicial, fiscal, and policy developments on a national level in the mid-seventies have required interagency collaboration and collaboration across disciplines. Among other developments, the "single agency responsibility" and "related services" requirements of Public Law 94-142 have made joint planning and collaborative service arrangements mandatory. Collaboration and mutual exchange of knowledge, skills, and information across discipline boundaries are key tenets of the transdisciplinary model, which is considered to be the most desirable type of service delivery organization for severely handicapped students (e.g., McCormick & Goldman, 1979). The transdisciplinary approach is a process through which professionals from different related disciplines share information, skills, and decision-making responsibilities. A transdisciplinary team is substantially more than a group of human service providers; it is a team of professionals who consider efficient and effective service management more important than discipline boundaries.

Transdisciplinary term processes and parent involvement are discussed in Chapter Eleven.

SUMMARY

1. Etiological category labels convey little information relevant to language and communication intervention because children sharing the same label often exhibit markedly different abilities and difficulties. However, we can make some broad generalizations:
   a. Speech, language, and communication disorders occur with high frequency among children with cerebral palsy.
   b. Children with spina bifida typically display normal intelligence, but it is not unusual to find a language pattern called the "cocktail party" syndrome.
   c. Muscular disabilities and health impairments affect language development only to the extent that they restrict mobility and social interactions.
   d. The severity of a hearing-impaired child's language difficulties is determined by age of onset and degree of hearing loss.
   e. Visually impaired children often demonstrate language delays because of restricted mobility and an inability to engage in sustained search behavior.
   f. Children termed learning disabled demonstrate a range and variety of complex language-related difficulties.
   g. Whether autistic deficits are primarily linguistic, social, or cognitive is unclear; however, language and communication impairments are the most striking characteristic of autistic children.
   h. Mentally retarded children appear to develop language skills in the same sequence as nonhandicapped children, but at a slower rate.
2. In order to design proper intervention procedures, language specialists and teachers need to be able to make finer discriminations within the gross category of "language disorders," of which most handicapped children are members. Children who exhibit problems conceptualizing ideas about objects, events, and relations can be designated as having a content disorder. Those exhibiting problems with the structural aspects of language are differentiated as having a form disorder. Those who have trouble expressing communicative intent with socially appropriate and correct forms can be identified as having a language use problem.
3. Major advances in special education include:
   a. Public policy mandating an appropriate education for all handicapped children.
   b. Functional and age-appropriate curriculum objectives (particularly for the severely and profoundly handicapped).
   c. Skill clustering so that the child practices a range and variety of skills in their natural sequence.

d. Recognition of the potential usefulness of augmentative communication systems to facilitate and/or supplement vocal language.

e. Development of a technology and sufficient empirically validated information to permit simulation of optimal language learning conditions.

f. Application of transdisciplinary team processes with all types of services.

REFERENCES

BARTAK, L., & RUTTER, M. Differences between mentally retarded and normally intelligent autistic children. *Journal of Autism and Childhood Schizophrenia,* 1976, *6,* 109–120.

BLOOM, L., & LAHEY, M. *Language development and language disorders.* New York: John Wiley & Sons, 1978.

BROWN, L., NIETUPSKI, J., & HAMRE-NIETUPSKI, S. The criterion of ultimate functioning and public school services for severely handicapped students. In M.A. Thomas (Ed.), *Hey, don't forget about me!* Reston, Va.: The Council for Exceptional Children, 1976.

BROWN, F., HOLVOET, J., GUESS, D., & MULLIGAN, M. The individualized curriculum sequencing model (III): Small group instruction. *Journal of the Association for the Severely Handicapped,* 1980, *5,* 351–361.

BRYAN, T., DONAHUE, M., & PEARL, R. Studies of learning disabled children's pragmatic competence. *Topics in Learning and Language Disabilities,* 1981, *1,* 29–39.

CROMER, R. The development of language and cognition: The cognition hypothesis. In B. Foss (Ed.), *New perspectives in child development.* New York: Penguin Education, 1974.

CRUICKSHANK, W., BICE, H., & WALLEN, N. *Perception and cerebral palsy.* Syracuse: Syracuse University Press, 1957.

CUNNINGHAM, M. A comparison of the language of psychotic and non-psychotic children who are mentally retarded. *Journal of Child Psychology and Psychiatry,* 1968, *9,* 229–244.

DAVIS, H., & SILVERMAN, S.R. *Hearing and deafness.* New York: Holt, Rinehart & Winston, 1970.

DUCHAN, J.F., & ERICKSON, J.G. Normal and retarded children's understanding of semantic relations in different verbal contexts. *Journal of Speech and Hearing Research,* 1976, *19,* 767–776.

DUNCAN, D., SBARDELLATI, E., MAHEADY, L., & SAINTO, D. Nondiscriminatory assessment of severely physically handicapped individuals. *JASH,* 1981, *6,* 17–22.

EISENSON, J. *Aphasia in children.* New York: Harper & Row, 1972.

EISENSON, J., & INGRAM, D. Childhood aphasia—an updated concept based on recent research. *Acta Symbolica,* 1972, *3,* 108–116.

EVANS, D., & HAMPSON, M. The language of mongols. *British Journal of Disorders of Communication,* 1968, *3,* 171–181.

FRAIBERG, S. Parallel and divergent patterns in blind and sighted infants. *Psychoanalytic Study of the Child,* 1968, *23,* 264–300.

FRAIBERG, S. *Insights from the blind.* New York: Basic Books, 1977.

GUESS, D., & NOONAN, M.J. Curricula and instructional procedures for severely handicapped students. *Focus on Exceptional Children,* 1982, *14* (5), 1–12.

HARE, B.A., & HARE, J.M. *Teaching young handicapped children: A guide for preschool and elementary grades.* New York: Grune and Stratton, 1977.

HERMELIN, B., & O'CONNOR, N. *Psychological experiments with autistic children.* London: Pergamon Press, 1970.

HICKS, J. Language disabilities of emotionally disturbed children. In J. Irwin & M. Marge (Eds.), *Principles of childhood language disabilities.* Englewood, N.J.: Prentice-Hall, 1972.

HINGTGEN, J., & BRYSON, C. Recent developments in the study of early childhood psychoses: Infantile autism, schizophrenia and retarded disorders. *Schizophrenia Bulletin,* 1972, *5,* 8–55.

HOBBS, N. *The futures of children.* San Francisco: Jossey-Bass, 1975.

HOBBS, N. Classification options: A conversation with Nicholas Hobbs on exceptional child education. *Exceptional Children,* 1978, *44,* 494–497.

HOLVOET, J., GUESS, D., MULLIGAN, M., & BROWN, F. The individualized curriculum sequencing model (II): A teaching strategy for severely handicapped students. *Journal of the Association for the Severely Handicapped,* 1980, *5,* 337–351.

HUTCHISON, D. A model for transdisciplinary staff development (A nationally organized collaborative project to provide comprehensive services for atypical infants and their families). A monograph: *Technical Report,* 1974, *8.*

KAUFFMAN, J.M. *Characteristics of children's behavior disorders.* Columbus, Ohio: Charles E. Merrill, 1977.

LACKNER, J. A developmental study of language behavior in retarded children. *Neuropsychologia,* 1968, *6,* 301–320.

LARSON, A.D., & MILLER, J.B. The hearing impaired. In E. L. Meyen (Ed.), *Exceptional children and youth: An introduction.* Denver: Love Publishing Company, 1978.

LAWRENCE, E.R. Spina Bifida children in school: Preliminary report. *Developmental Medicine and Child Neurology,* 1971, *25,* 44–46.

LERNER, J.W. *Learning disabilities: Theories, diagnosis, and teaching strategies.* (3rd ed.). Boston: Houghton Mifflin, 1981.

LONGHURST, T.M. Assessing and increasing descriptive communication skills in retarded children. *Mental Retardation,* 1972, *19,* 42–45.

LOVAAS, O., KOEGEL, R., SIMMONS, J., & LONG, J. Some generalizations and follow-up measures on autistic children in behavior therapy. *Journal of Applied Behavior Analysis,* 1973, *6,* 131–165.

LYON, S., & LYON, G. Team functioning and staff development: A role release approach to providing integrated educational services for severely handicapped students. *JASH,* 1980, *5*(3), 250–263.

MARGE, M. The general problem of language disabilities in children. In J.V. Irwin & M. Marge (Eds.), *Principles of childhood language disabilities.* Englewood Cliffs, N.J.: Prentice-Hall, 1972.

McCORMICK, L., & GOLDMAN, R. The transdisciplinary model: Implications for service delivery and personnel preparation for the severely and profoundly handicapped. *AAESPH Review,* 1979, *4,* 152–161.

MILISEN, R. The incidence of speech disorders. In L. Travis (Ed.), *Handbook of speech pathology and audiology.* Englewood Cliffs, N.J.: Prentice-Hall, Inc., 1971.

MOORES, D.F. Nonvocal systems of verbal behavior. In R.L. Schiefelbusch & L.L. Lloyd (Eds.), *Language Perspectives: Acquisition retardation and intervention.* Baltimore: University Park Press, 1974.

MOORES, D.F. *Educating the deaf: Psychology, principles and practices.* Boston: Houghton-Mifflin, 1977.

MOREHEAD, D., & INGRAM, D. The development of base syntax in normal and linguistically deviant children. *Journal of Speech and Hearing Research,* 1973, *16*, 330–352.

MULLIGAN, M., GUESS, D., HOLVOET, J., & BROWN, F. The individualized curriculum sequencing model (I): Implications from research on massed, distributed, or spaced trial learning. *Journal of the Association for the Severely Handicapped,* 1980, *5*, 325–336.

MYERS, P.I., & HAMMILL, D.D. *Methods of learning disorders* (2nd ed.), New York: John Wiley and Sons, 1976.

National Advisory Committee on the Handicapped. *The unfinished revolution: Education for the handicapped* (1976 Annual Report). Washington, D.C.: Department of Health, Education, and Welfare, USOE, 1976.

NOBER, L. *Topics in Language Disorders,* 1982, *2,* ix–x.

NORTHERN, J.L., & LEMME, M. Hearing and Auditory Disorders. In G. H. Shames and E. H. Wiig (Eds.), *Human Communication Disorders.* Columbus, Ohio: Charles E. Merrill, 1982.

ORNITZ, E.M., & RITVO, E.R. Medical assessment. In E.R. Ritvo (Ed.), *Autism: Diagnosis, curriculum, research and management.* New York: Spectrum, 1976.

REES, N. Pragmatics of language: Applications to normal and disordered language development. In R. L. Schiefelbusch (Ed.), *Bases of language intervention.* Baltimore: University Park Press, 1978.

RICKS, D.M., & WING, L. Language, communication and the use of symbols. In L. Wing (Ed.), *Early childhood autism: Clinical, educational, and social aspects* (2nd ed.). New York: Pergamon Press, 1976.

RUTTER, M. Behavioral and cognitive characteristics. In J.K. Wing (Ed.), *Early childhood autism: Clinical, educational and social aspects.* New York: Pergamon Press, 1966.

RUTTER, M. Concepts of autism: A review of research. *Journal of Child Psychology and Psychiatry,* 1968, *9,* 1–25.

RUTTER, M. Diagnosis and definition of childhood autism. *Journal of Autism and Childhood Schizophrenia,* 1978, *8,* 139–161.

RUTTER, M., & SCHOPLER, E. (Eds.), *Autism: A reappraisal of concepts and treatment.* New York: Plenum, 1978.

RYAN, J. Mental subnormality and language development. In E. Lenneberg and E. Lenneberg (Eds.), *Foundations of language development.* New York: Academic Press, 1975.

SAILOR, W., & GUESS, D. *Severely handicapped students: An instructional design.* Boston: Houghton Mifflin Company, 1983.

SAVAGE, V. Childhood autism: A review of the literature with particular reference to the speech and language structure of the autistic child. *British Journal of Disorders of Communication,* 1968, *3,* 75–87.

SCHULER, A.L. Aspects of communication. In W.H. Fay & A.L. Schuler (Eds.), *Emerging Language in Autistic Children*. Baltimore: University Park Press, 1980, 87–112.

SELIGMAN, M.E.P. *Helplessness: On depression, development, and death.* San Francisco: W.H. Freeman, 1975.

SIMMONS, J.Q., & TYMCHUK, A. The learning deficits in childhood psychosis. *Pediatric Clinics of North America,* 1973, *20,* 665–675.

SPAIN, B. Verbal and performance ability in preschool spina bifida. *Developmental Medicine and Child Neurology,* 1972, 155.

SWISHER, L.P., & PINKSER, E.J. The language characteristics of hyperverbal hydrocephalic children. *Developmental Medical Child Neurology,* 1971, *13,* 746–755.

VAN RIPER, C. *Speech correction: Principles and methods* (6th ed.). Englewood Cliffs, N. J.: Prentice-Hall, 1978.

VERHAAREN, P., & CONNOR, F.P. Physical disabilities. In J.M. Kauffman and D. P. Hallahan (Eds.), *Handbook of Special Education.* Englewood Cliffs, N.J.: Prentice-Hall, Inc., 1981.

VITTER, D.K. Language disorders and schooling. *Topics in Language Disorders,* 1982, *2,* 13–21.

VOGEL, S.A. Morphological ability in normal and dyslexic children. *Journal of Learning Disabilities,* 1977, *10,* 35–43.

WARD, T., & HODDINOTT, B. The development of speech in an autistic child. *Acta Paedopsychiatrica,* 1968, *35,* 199–215.

WARREN, D.H. *Blindness and early childhood development.* New York: American Foundation for the Blind, 1977.

WARREN, D.H. Visual impairments. In J.M. Kauffman & D.P. Hallahan (Eds.), *Handbook of Special Education.* Englewood Cliffs, N.J.: Prentice-Hall, Inc., 1981, 195–221.

WEILAND, M., & LEGG, D. Formal speech characteristics as a diagnostic aid in childhood psychosis. *American Journal of Orthopsychiatry,* 1964, *34,* 91–94.

WIIG, E.H., & SEMEL, E.M. *Language assessment and intervention for the learning disabled.* Columbus, Ohio: Charles E. Merrill, 1980.

WILBUR, R. The linguistics of manual languages and manual systems. In L. Lloyd (Ed.), *Communication assessment and intervention strategies.* Baltimore: University Park Press, 1976.

WING, L. The handicaps of autistic children—A comparative study. *Journal of Child Psychology and Psychiatry,* 1969, *10,* 1–40.

WING, L. What is an autistic child? *Communication,* 1972, *6,* 5–10.

CHAPTER FOUR

INITIAL AND ONGOING ASSESSMENT

Richard L. Schiefelbusch and Linda McCormick

T here is no single, all-purpose format for language assessment. The lack of generality is because of children's individual differences, such as variables relating to age, environment, nature of impairment, educational status, and probable learning rates. This chapter will help the reader develop a sound approach to this difficult set of language assessment procedures. Numerous references provide options for additional readings to extend the perspectives and the procedures.

> Describing a child's language behavior for the purpose of identifying a problem or for planning intervention is referred to as assessment. [The first stages of] assessment are carried out before intervention is begun, so that the educational program begins immediately with the most appropriate and reasonable goals and procedures for facilitating language learning. [However,] assessment continues during intervention in order to chart progress, establish new goals, and make necessary changes in procedures. (Bloom & Lahey, 1978, p. 307)

In addition, the plan for assessment is interwoven with information in the other chapters to integrate assessment with the larger picture of language acquisition and intervention. For instance, the content, form, and use (interactionist) design presented in Chapters One, Two and Three is considered in selecting assessment strategies. Chapter Three provides a perspective on individual differences and suggests an approach to organizing assessment information for intervention planning. Chapter Five deals with the Individualized Educational Program (IEP) and provides the educational picture into which the language assessment and training activities are to be set. The roles of parents, specialists, teachers, and therapists are discussed in relation to the establishment of the plan. This chapter refers to and integrates with development of the IEP. Chapter Five also discusses the procedures for planning the intervention program. As such, it extends the assessment system and adds to its functions.

Finally, Chapter Six deals with the instructional process that relies on information derived from assessment and planning. The range of decision making necessary to reach a functional instruction plan is indicated in this series of chapters. Chapter Six also details designs for maintenance and generalization. Continuing assessment, together with initial or preprogram assessment, provides a functional information system to guide the teacher and specialist in identifying problems, selecting procedures for training, and adjusting the training plan, according to the child's progress.

Later chapters provide examples of how procedures for assessment, planning, and instruction are applied in different programs. Refinements are necessary to adapt the procedures for infants at-risk, preschool children, and severely and multiply handicapped children. The procedures sections in Chapters Seven, Eight, Nine and Ten amplify this discussion on assessment. This chapter covers the designs for initial and continuing assessment, and later chapters illustrate how the procedures are applied.

Successful intervention depends on thorough and careful assessment and planning.

WHO SHOULD ASSESS LANGUAGE?

Chapter Six asks, "Who should teach language?" The question is answered in two parts. The communication specialist has responsibilities for design, implementation and consultation. However, there we state that the "orchestration and follow-through of activities to promote language learning and communication are usually teacher responsibilities (with continuous consultation from the language/communication specialist)."

This rationale places the primary responsibilities for initial and ongoing assessment and planning for program implementation and evaluation on the communication specialist. Responsibility for day-to-day programming and monitoring of progress toward language objectives usually rests with the teacher. However, distribution of role functions may vary from one setting to another. Allocation of resources and negotiations about role functions are among the decisions to be considered when the service delivery team is organized. In any case, a language specialist is responsible for the initial pre-IEP assessment, and usually the preprogramming assessment.

Chapter Eleven discusses service delivery team organization and role negotiations.

The language specialist and the teacher should together seek information from, and share information with, parents, and other teachers and specialists (e.g., physical therapist). The more the specialist knows about the ecology and requirements of the classroom, and the more the teacher knows about assessing and teaching language, the more effective their collaboration will be. If communication specialists and teachers, along with parents and other relevant members, are to be an effective team they must be trainers and trainees to one another. They must share information and skills and also learn new competencies themselves.

120

ASSESSMENT STRATEGIES

Miller (1978) suggests three initial questions to ask when planning assessment procedures:

1. *Why* are we assessing the child?
2. *What* are we going to assess?
3. *How* are we going to assess the child?

An effective assessment procedure is one that provides the most useful data in the least time.

There are only three valid reasons for assessment.

An effective assessment strategy is one that provides the maximum amount of useful information in the shortest time. Table 4-1, developed by Miller, provides a basic outline of the components necessary to comprehensive assessment.

Information in each of the three columns is an elaboration of the *why, what, how* system. The *why* question is strategic because it requires clarification of the purpose for which assessment is undertaken.

The *what* strategy describes components of the language system somewhat differently than the content-form-use format described in Chapters One and Two, but the relationship of the two should be clear. In addition, Miller suggests that comprehension and production should be carefully assessed. Comprehension data is important in determining the developmental status of the child and in planning for functional language instruction, especially in regard to receptive language skills. *How* strategies involve assessment options for studying individual impairments of language forms and functions. Each of the *how* strategies of assessment is developed in subsequent pages.

WHY ASSESS LANGUAGE BEHAVIOR?

Why are we assessing this child?

One way to answer the *why* question is to say that there are as many reasons as there are individual differences in children and concerns of parents and teachers. However, for the purposes of the educational intervention system, the primary reasons for assessment are (Miller, 1978):

1. To identify children with potential language problems.
2. To establish baseline functioning.
3. To measure behavior change within a teaching program.

The first of these, screening and determining eligibility for special services, is in many ways the most difficult. It can be challenging to determine whether a child's language is developmentally abnormal. Siegel (1975) makes this point emphatically: "The question of whether or not a youngster ought to be provided speech services, ultimately is based on the considered judgment of a professionally educated and experienced clinician, and not by the application of some set of norms" (p. 214). The competent decision maker effectively uses normative and other developmental information to reach this considered judgment.

TABLE 4-1 Outline of the basic components of the assessment process

Why?	What?	How?
1. Identify potential problems	1. Components of language system	1. Procedures
A. Screening	A. Phonology	A. Standardized tests
(1) Problem/no problem	(1) Articulatory proficiency	B. Nonstandardized tests
(2) Further evaluation	(2) Phonological system	C. Developmental scales
(3) Referral to other	B. Syntax	D. Behavioral observation
professionals	(1) Sentence form/grammar	
2. Establish baseline functioning	(2) Order relationships of	
A. Determine developmental	constituents	
level	C. Semantic	
B. Describe nature of behavioral	(1) Sentence function;	
difference	meaning	
C. Specify behavior needing	(2) Case relationships	
remediation	(3) Lexicon; concepts	
3. Measure behavioral change within	2. Processes	
a teaching program	A. Comprehension	
A. Establish the nature of	(1) Hearing acuity	
behavioral change resulting	(2) Auditory processing of	
from program	linguistic units	
(1) Within context of	B. Production	
teaching situation	(1) Mechanism functioning	
(2) Within natural	(2) Production of linguistic	
environment	units	
	C. Pragmatics	
	(1) Communication	
	functions	
	(2) Conversational	
	competence	
	D. Cognitive development	

Source: Jon Miller, "Assessing Children's Language Behavior." In Richard L. Schiefelbusch (Ed.), *Bases of Language Intervention.* Baltimore: University Park Press, 1978.

Identification and screening   Screening is the use of systematic procedures to identify *provisionally* those children from a population that require further assessment. The intent is to identify those children for whom a more complete assessment is warranted. What is needed for screening is some small set of items that is critically related to language development and can be administered and scored quickly and easily by any one of a number of persons. Unfortunately no such set of discriminating items presently exists.[1]

The question is: Does the child have a problem that warrants closer examination and special services?

The most relevant screening information will come from parents, physicians, nurses, counselors, social workers, teachers and others who have frequent contact with the children. Siegel (1976) recommends establishing a referral system in which teachers and other professionals form the front line in the initial identification of communication disorders. He further suggests that "the first step in such a referral system is for the clinician to define *language disorder* in terms that are explicit and can be shared with colleagues" (p. 93). (The content-form-use definitions introduced in Chapters One, Two, and Three do this.)

---

[1]That does not mean, however, that there are not a number of norm-referenced screening tests available. Bloom and Lahey (1978) provide a carefully selected list of such tests (pp. 362–63). Several tests for identification and screening are described in Appendix A at the end of this chapter.

122

In schools the goal of screening is to determine if the child meets the eligibility criteria for special services.

In schools the goal of screening is to determine eligibility for special services as defined in a state plan, which is based on P.L. 94-142. Following is an example of criteria for eligibility for programs for the severely language impaired in one state.[2]

1. Criteria for eligibility include:
   a. Language delay of two or more years.
   b. Evidence that the language deficit is affecting or has the potential to affect academic progress.
2. Language deficits must be evident in one or more of the following areas:
   a. *Phonological disorder:* the student demonstrates a disorder in the competencies required to perceive or produce the speech sounds of the sound system in a manner in which the fully competent user of the native language perceives or produces them. (A student who demonstrates no evidence of disorder other than phonology may not be considered eligible.)
   b. *Morphological disorder:* the student demonstrates a disorder in the competencies required to perceive or produce the 14 commonly accepted morphemes (roots or affixes [Brown, 1973]) in a manner in which the fully competent user of the native language uses them.
   c. *Semantic disorder:* the student demonstrates a disorder in the competencies required to comprehend words, grammatical forms or structures imposed by time (temporal ordering of logical production), meaning or context underlying the logical grammatical structure of the native language.
   d. *Syntactic disorder:* the student demonstrates a disorder in the competencies required to understand and use phrases or sentences consistent with grammatical rules.
   e. *Functional use (pragmatic disorder):* the student demonstrates a disorder in the competencies required to utilize language appropriate to the social context of the given situation, i.e., cannot interact in conversation, says the "wrong thing at the wrong time," or uses offensive language.
   f. *Language processing:* the student demonstrates a disorder in the act of receiving, perceiving and interpreting spoken or written language within the structure of his/her native language.

Entry requirements for the severely language-impaired (in some states) also specify that the child must have average intellectual potential, normal hearing, vision, and emotional adjustment, or there must be evidence that any deficits in these areas are not problems. Other programs may specify eligibility in terms of specific handicaps.

---

[2]Document prepared under the auspices of the Bureau of Education for Exceptional Students, Division of Public Schools, Department of Education, Tallahassee, Florida.

In some states the state plan also suggests specific screening and assessment procedures. The most frequently cited language tests in Florida (listed by 50% or more of the school districts in one county) include

1. BTBC - Boehm Test of Basic Concepts
2. CELI - Carrow Elicited Language Inventory
3. DTLA - Detroit Test of Learning Aptitude
4. ITPA - Illinois Test of Psycholinguistic Abilities
5. PPVT - Peabody Picture Vocabulary Test
6. TACL - Test of Auditory Comprehension of Language
7. ZPLS - Zimmerman Preschool Language Scale

The Florida program illustrates how screening procedures may be designed. There is close agreement between these eligibility criteria and the components of language performance presented in Chapters Two and Three.

Establishing baseline functioning   The second purpose of language assessment is to establish baseline functioning. There are at least three reasons why this should be done. The most apparent reason is to determine a present level of performance. This information can be used as a reference base for planning and for subsequent comparisons. A second reason is to establish the extent of the language delay and/or disorder. A third reason is to describe the exact nature of the developmental problem. Each of these reasons will be considered briefly.

> There are three reasons for establishing a baseline functioning level.

Developmental tests provide information about the child's performance level compared to a same-age peer group. Snyder (1981) suggests three formal measures to aid in establishing levels of early communicative development.[3] These are the Receptive-Expressive Emergent Language Scale (REEL), The Sequenced Inventory of Communicative Development (SICD), and the Initial Communication Processes Scale (ICP). The REEL (Bzoch & League, 1971) uses a parental interview to sample communicative behaviors between birth and age 3. The SICD (Hedrick, Prather & Tobin, 1975) begins with parental reports and then uses performance items that tap communicative development from birth to approximately age 4. The ICP (Schery & Glover, 1982) uses examiner observation and task elicitation to sample the communicatively relevant behaviors of the sensorimotor period.

The REEL samples developments in the child's early word comprehension and ability to initiate routines (e.g., "pat-a-cake"). However, it does not sample prelinguistic gestural performatives. The SICD focuses more heavily on auditory processing at the prelinguistic and early linguistic levels and asks some discriminating questions about the content of early lexical development, sampling a wide variety of lexical categories that are consistent with data from recent research (e.g., Benedict, 1979; Snyder,

---

[3]See section on developmental scales (page 131) for a wider range of developmental issues.

Bates & Bretherton, in press). SICD items also generate information about the child's productive routines and declarative gestural behaviors. The more recently designed ICP taps all levels and types of prelinguistic and early linguistic performatives. In addition, it examines those cognitive skills that directly relate to communicative development. The assessment potential of the ICP is especially useful for young multiply handicapped and mentally retarded children. These standardized measures can provide important information about the child's prelinguistic and early linguistic development. Other procedures for determining the child's developmental level are considered in the *How* section of this chapter.

Once the child's developmental level has been determined, it is possible to specify more precisely the extent of delay and/or the nature of the disorder. The child's language performance is compared with developmental data to determine whether the child has a language delay (is performing at an earlier stage developmentally) or a language disorder (is performing differently within a particular stage of development) and profile the delay or disorder relative to content, form, and use domains. Language delays are more common. Generally, the primary difference between atypical and "normal" communicators is in rate of acquisition; otherwise, their developmental patterns may be very similar.

Information about the precise nature and extent of the child's language problems combines with other information (as described in Chapter Five) to form the basis for planning an age-appropriate and functional educational plan.

The question is: Is what we are doing having the desired impact?

Measuring behavior changes within a teaching program   The third reason for language assessment is to determine the short and long term effects of the teaching program. This form of assessment includes program evaluation, maintenance evaluation, or formative assessment. The program is judged effective if the child is progressing at an expected rate as shown by a record of his progress. These data are then used in planning adjustments in the intervention program, including methods, curricula, scheduling, and environmental arrangements. Procedures for ongoing assessments are presented in the section on behavioral evaluation on page 133.

WHAT ARE WE GOING TO ASSESS?

The determination of *what* to assess is guided by referral information, initial observations, screening information and by a working knowledge of the language system (the content-form-use system described in Chapters One, Two and Three). The assessment plan must be individually determined for each child. Assessment time, like instructional time, is a valuable commodity. Careful analysis of available information narrows the focus as described in the next section.

In the previous chapter we discussed content, form, and use difficulties, content-form-use association difficulties, and parallel content-form-use delays. This section discusses the content-form-use components of the language system as they relate to selection of assessment procedures. An understanding of these components can guide in planning the "what" of language assessment.

As Bloom and Lahey (1978) suggest, the purpose of assessment is to collect information about

> ... how the child uses the conventional system of signals to represent what the child knows and communicates about the world (content); what aspects of the language system the child understands and expresses (form); and the purposes for which the child uses the system and how the child chooses among alternative means in different contexts (use). p. 309.

In addition to information about the child's language behavior, we also need information about the conditions that will help the child learn. We need to ask a series of functional questions. These questions concern factors in the child's environment that accelerate or impede language learning, and the child's knowledge, interests, and special response preferences. The first question is the nature of the child's language problems: Is the child experiencing difficulties of content (formulating and conceptualizing ideas about objects, events, and relations), form (learning the code and rules for expressing and understanding ideas about the world), use (functional communication), the lack of associations between content, form, and use, or general language delay?

Information about how the child learns is as important as a present level of performance profile.

The following questions are intended as a guide, not a checklist. They will not generate sufficient information to determine the child's strengths and deficits, but they will guide selection of appropriate instruments or other systematic observation procedures.

Content can be assessed at two levels: general or universal knowledge and topic knowledge. General knowledge could include (a) knowledge about objects, (b) knowledge about object relations, and (c) knowledge about event relations (see Chapters One and Two). *Object knowledge* includes both classes of objects and particular objects. *Object relations* knowledge includes concepts about how objects relate to themselves or to other objects in the same class, concepts about the properties and attributes that distinguish one object from another, and concepts about relations between objects. *Event relations* knowledge includes concepts about how different events relate to each other and relations within an event.

Topic knowledge is the particular idea coded in a message—a particular object, a particular action or a particular relation. Thus, one can talk about the *family* car, eating *ice cream* or walking to school with *specific* friends.

The following questions can help determine if the child's language problems are content-related (Schiefelbusch & McCormick, 1981). The purpose of these questions is to determine the child's status relative to the sensorimotor constructs thought to be precursive to language content.

If the child's language problems appear related to content deficits, select and administer instruments referenced against concept development.

1. Does the child give evidence of remembering absent objects and/or people?
2. Does the child engage in pretend play?
3. Does the child search for a desired object if the object is not in its customary location?
4. Does the child cry or fuss when a desired object is out of reach or figure out a way to get it?
5. Does the child use or play with objects in a way that indicates understanding of function (e.g., hat to head, cup to mouth)?
6. Is the child able to match identical objects?
7. Is the child able to match nonidentical objects that have a similar function?
8. Does the child use some means (nonverbal or verbal) to indicate the desire for recurrence (continuation) of an activity or an additional amount of a substance (e.g., holding cup out for more milk)?
9. Does the child give evidence of recognizing ownership (his own versus another's possessions)?
10. Does the child act upon two objects in relation to each other?

If the child's language problems appear related to form deficits, select and administer instruments which assess phonology, morphology and syntax.

Form difficulties are problems related to the shape or surface structure of language symbol-meaning (form-content) connections. Three descriptors of form are: (a) *phonology,* the sounds of oral language; (b) *morphology,* meaning units and the internal structure of words, i.e. roots, prefixes and suffixes; and (c) *syntax,* sentence organization including word order and relationships between words. Form is somewhat easier to assess than content and use functions because it is overt and more easily recorded. The following questions can aid determination of whether the child's problems are form-related.

1. Will the child imitate vocal and/or verbal models?
2. Will the child look at or pick up a familiar toy/object when asked "Where is _____?"
3. Will the child act upon objects as directed (e.g., point, shake, etc.)?
4. Does the child make sounds as if to comment on the focus of his and another's attention?
5. Does the child use different sounds to reject objects or attention?
6. Is the child's MLU commensurate with mental age?

If the child's language problems appear related to use deficits, select and administer instruments that assess communication strategies and devices.

Use difficulties are most apparent in natural social contexts. Use of the expressive, directive and referential functions (Moerk, 1977) or perlocutionary, illocutionary and locutionary devices (Bates, 1976) indicates that the child has acquired at least an early stage of communicative competence. The following questions can help you decide if the child's problems are use-related.

1. Does the child look at an adult's face/eyes during joint interaction?
2. Does the child take turns in reciprocal games (e.g., peekaboo)?
3. Does the child follow the gaze of a familiar adult and attend to their focal point?
4. Does the child direct the behavior of adults to secure desired objects or services?
5. Does the child persist with and/or modify a signal (gesture, sound or word) when the adult does not respond as desired?
6. Does the child use vocalizations to attract an adult's attention?
7. Does the child show objects to adults for attention?
8. Does the child produce related utterances following the utterance of others?

Keep in mind that where there are severe deficits and/or delays in achievement in one dimension (e.g., content) they will usually be accompanied by deficits/delays in other dimensions because of the interdependence of form, content and use. The interdependence of the three dimensions will have an effect at the measurement level and at the child performance level. At the measurement level, deficits/delays in one dimension preclude or, at least, hamper valid assessment of other dimensions. For example, a form deficit (e.g., delayed phonological development) complicates the assessment of content and use. You must rely on estimates from nonverbal assessment devices to establish functioning in these areas. At the child knowledge level, the interdependency of achievements between and across linguistic dimensions must be considered. Learning to use language may depend on achievements in form and content and vice versa.

> Where there are *severe* deficits or delays in one dimension, expect some accompanying problems in other areas.

You should try to establish a developmental level of performance for each of the three dimensions of language. Compare whatever data are available on acquisition of form and form-content linkages (vocabulary, inflectional morphemes, and syntax) with the normal development pinpointed in Table 2-3. Compare information about the child's perceptual-cognitive skills with the developmental information in Table 2-1. Compare the child's use of language with developmental research data on the development of communication skills in Table 2-6. When these questions have been answered, the focus of assessment narrows from language in general to a particular aspect (or aspects) of language. Now consider assessment techniques to collect data on specific strengths and weaknesses in the problem area and information about the child's learning strategies (described in Chapter Five).

128

HOW ARE WE GOING TO ASSESS THE CHILD?

The major *how* options of assessment include standardized tests, developmental scales, nonstandardized tests, and behavioral observations procedures. Each option has special advantages and disadvantages. Remember that no one procedure will fit all children equally well or be applicable across all settings and all problems, and no one procedure will provide all of the information you need to plan the program.

Seek information about child's response preferences and control style and, most importantly, stay alert to all potential clues.

A few practical recommendations will help the specialist and/or teacher with initial assessment. First, *children respond differently to different people.* The child may respond very differently in a testing situation, with a stranger, than with peers or familiar adults. Parents can usually help you gain perspective about the child's novel response tendencies, e.g., with whom and at what levels does the child use language? Parents, specialists, and teachers will arrive at a more reliable estimate of the child's level of performance if they share information.

Second, children use language differently to achieve different ends. Some children use silence to control a context while others speak volubly to achieve their intentions. The volume and range of language may be misleading if it is not examined in light of the context and the child's apparent intentions. This issue is also considered in the previous section on how to assess language use.

Third, language is a complex, integrated system. Assessment of any aspect or combination of aspects will evoke responses relative to other parameters of language. Consequently, any sample of the child's language is likely to include information beyond the specific task or task category under assessment. It is important not to overlook these data.

DuBose (1981) provides a detailed form to assist the clinician in observing behaviors during the assessment process. (See Appendix E). The specialist and/or teacher can prepare a version of this form to assist in securing information during the assessment process.

ASSESSMENT PROCEDURES

Miller (1978) divides assessment procedures into four basic categories:

1. Standardized tests
2. Developmental scales
3. Nonstandardized tests
4. Behavioral observation

These procedures can provide different or similar information depending on how they are used. Standardized testing is the most structured form of assessment and observations in the natural environment are the least structured; nonstandard elicitations fall between these assessment forms. A brief analysis of each procedural category provides some perspective on the advantages and disadvantages of each.

Standardized tests   A test is said to be "standardized" if validity and reliability data are available. Skillful use of standardized tests can provide useful information *if* you are careful to select a test (or tests) that fits the purposes of the assessment. However, it is important not to lose sight of their limitations. There is growing disenchantment with total reliance on standardized, commercially produced tests for language assessment. One argument, put forth by Berry (1980) is that objective tests do not "evaluate oral language as children comprehend it and use it." They only provide information about the child's mastery of "syntactic, phonologic, and morphologic forms in unrelated tidbits of language," without taking into account the pragmatic aspect or the context in which language is used (p. xiii). Danowitz (1981) similarly believes that "formal tests of language have serious limitations for assessing the form and content of expressive language and are entirely unsatisfactory for assessing the use and comprehension of spoken language" (p. 103).

A standardized test is one that meets certain validity and reliability criteria.

  These criticisms seem to be based on the unlikely assumption that a formal test may be the primary or the only assessment procedure used. Perhaps the indictments are directed more at single instrument procedures rather than at standardized procedures. As Siegel (1979) points out, "language is simply too vast and too multifaceted to be completely represented in any single test" (p. 2).

Many criticisms of standardized tests appear to be based on the assumption of a single instrument procedure.

  The main argument advanced in support of standardized tests is their validity, reliability, and precision in comparing a child's functioning with that of other children of the same age (Bloom & Lahey, 1978). However, even this appears to be a misconception, since 28 widely used tests of language development recently reviewed by Darley (1979) were found without exception to be unacceptable in all three essential areas of validity, reliability and normative data.

  The limitations of standardized tests become even more significant when we consider that few provide the inventory of language skills needed to plan an intervention program. What is critically absent is the context which can be used to show the child's abilities to use language for the exchange of information with other persons—the social uses of language.

  Selection of effective tests for severely handicapped children is particularly difficult. No one has identified formal measures that can be used reliably and validly for general and/or specific purposes with this population. DuBose (1981) suggests that in the absence of consistent, generalizable data, examiners must continue to make decisions on an individual basis.

> A first consideration is to select the test instrument that will yield the most useful information about a particular handicapped child's development and learning. When a condition must be changed to permit a child to perform, one must identify the concept being examined, how the child's sensory or physical impairment will interfere with related task performance, and how the task can be modified. (p. 13)

  The wide range of variables with the potential to influence the results of standardized tests is another disadvantage. The most obvious variable,

There are three sets of variables with the potential to influence test results.

of course, is the child. Many children have attentional, perceptual, motivational, or memory problems. Others require special arrangements because of sensory or motor problems. Still other children have had limited experience and may not be ready to take the test. Because the child is "nonstandard," the standardized ways of administering the tasks of the test must be altered. These alterations change the test score and, likely, the reliability in any test-retest comparison. Situational variables also influence the test results. Small children, especially handicapped small children, perform variably according to the setting and the test arrangement. The time of day and the person doing the testing may also affect test results. Finally, task variables influence the child's effectiveness in test performance. As noted above, most tests are designed to fit children who can hear, see and use standard response modes.

Carrow-Woolfolk and Lynch (1982) suggest presentation of selected items of standardized tests in naturalistic settings. Just because items occur in a standardized test does not preclude modifying the items in order to further explore a child's linguistic skill. "If a child's performance improves with modification of the test item, this indicates what the child *can* do, and such information could contribute to planning the intervention program. Obviously, once the procedure has been modified, the norms may not be applied" (p. 237).

One important method for checking the validity of formal test results is to compare them to those derived from informant-interview scales. These scales are especially useful when administered to parents of children who are severely impaired. One such instrument is the Verbal Language Development Scale (VLDS) (Mecham, 1971), an extension of the communication portion of the Vineland Social Maturity Scale. When administered to the child's caregiver, the VLDS provides a rough language-age-equivalent for the child below 3 years. Bzoch and League's (1971) Receptive-Expressive-Emergent-Language (REEL) Scale is another informant-interview scale. This scale is nothing more than a series of questions about expressive and receptive language acquisition over the language age period from birth to 36 months. It yields a receptive quotient, an expressive quotient, and a composite or combined quotient. The REEL is especially useful in guiding the choice of questions in a parent case history interview.

The following guidelines, proposed by Linder (1983) for developing formal and informal assessments, summarize this section and introduce the next.

1. Use normative data to provide inter-individual comparisons (skill level of child compared with age peers).
2. Use a comprehensive normative test to provide an overview of the child's strengths and weaknesses.
3. Use normative assessment to provide direction for further testing.
4. Keep the assessment plan flexible, so that assessments can be added or deleted as necessary.

5. Use [informal assessments] to supplement normative data and to provide intra-individual comparison (skill levels of an individual child).

6. Develop new [informal assessments] as needed for individual children.

7. Consider any biases the test may have when given under standardized conditions, and supplement the assessment with instruments designed to show maximum performance levels.

Developmental scales Developmental scales are based on the concept that speech and language emerge along predictable paths. Application of the developmental concept to instruction assumes that learning can be specified in terms of behavioral characteristics and that it is possible to locate a child on a developmental sequence.

Developmental scales are based on the premise that development is orderly and predictable.

Developmental scales are used to compare handicapped children with same age nonhandicapped peers. There are two principal types of developmental scales. One type, the informant-interview scales described above, depends on a third person, often a parent, to answer questions about items on the scale. Items are checked to determine positive and negative items as in a checklist. The second type attempts to elicit specific behaviors from the child. Thus, developmental scaling divides into two types: (a) indirect reporting of developmental milestones and (b) direct observation and objective reporting. (See Appendix C for some examples of developmental scales.)

Three scales of the indirect reporting type were discussed earlier. One of the few such scales specifically developed for use with handicapped children is the Scales of Early Communication Skills for Hearing Impaired Children (Moog & Geers, 1975). It evaluates the speech and language development of hearing-impaired children between the ages of 2 and 8. Tests for developmental assessment of young handicapped children include the Environmental Pre-language Battery (Horstmeier & MacDonald, 1978), the Environmental Language Inventory (MacDonald, 1978), the Preschool Language Scale (Zimmerman, Steiner & Evatt, 1969), and the Vane Evaluation of Language Scale (Vane, 1975).

You have probably perceived that there is often little difference between standardized developmental tests and developmental scales. The major difference is that scales are more informally applied and rely somewhat more on specialist and/or teacher judgments for scoring.

Nonstandard tests Because there are few instruments that can be used with severely handicapped children, it is often necessary for teachers or clinicians to devise informal testing procedures. As previously suggested by Linder, informal tests can extend the results of standardized tests and generate additional information about some important aspect of the child's language performance. The tasks may be derived from formal tests with stimuli and directions largely worked out in advance, or they may be informally devised and revised during the assessment session according to the responses of the child.

Nonstandard tests are teacher-made procedures.

132

A great advantage of nonstandardized tests is the potential for flexibility.

One of the greatest advantages of informal, or nonstandardized, testing is the potential for flexibility both in design and in application. The test can be designed to conform to the child, rather than forcing the child to conform to the test (Miller, 1978). The four categories of nonstandard tests found to be helpful in evaluating children's language behavior are: (a) free speech analysis, (b) elicited production, (c) comprehension, and (d) elicited imitation.

The idea in recording a free speech sample is to collect representative evidence of the child's usual productive language. If the sample is indeed representative, then repeated samples will be similar in content. Miller (1978, p. 293) provides a list of person, setting and stimulus variables to consider in establishing the context for free speech samples:

1. Person
   a. Adult-child, including parent-child and clinician-child interactions
   b. Child-child, including playmates or siblings
2. Setting
   a. Home in various activities: eating, dressing, playing, etc.
   b. School: classroom, therapy room or playground
   c. Residential facility: day room, ward, school room, therapy room
   d. Clinic: waiting room, therapy room
3. Materials
   a. Stories
   b. Pictures
   c. Toys

The goal of free speech samples is recording spontaneous utterances.

The method of recording free speech samples also has a bearing on whether the data are representative and useful. Audio or videotape recordings are preferred, but it is possible to record in writing if the child's production rate is low. It is important to get an accurate record of the child's productions, as well as the activities that accompany the verbal behavior. A recent manual edited by Miller (1981) presents techniques for eliciting language samples and describes procedures for analysis.

Elicited production procedures can provide more specific information in less time.

The goal in collecting free speech samples is to record spontaneous productions. In contrast, *elicited production* procedures provide samples that do not occur frequently in natural arrangements. To secure a detailed analysis of specific features within a short time, the teacher and/or specialist can ask questions or make statements to evoke particular responses. Most procedures for sampling articulation, instruction following, problem solving, or information giving require elicited production procedures.

Elicited production, in addition to being a short cut for sampling of important aspects of content, form and use, also provides for contextual design that may be useful in planning intervention. Person, setting and materials variables can be explored in elicitation activities to determine which is most facilitative in subsequent sessions with the child.

Contextual variables are particularly important when assessing *comprehension*. The comprehension assessment process poses unique validity problems because it is often difficult to differentiate responses indicating understanding of linguistic input from those based on contextual cues. There is always a possibility that the child is attending to cues other than linguistic cues in determining the meaning of an utterance. In a sense, the child inadvertently "fudges," and the consequence is an inaccurate "picture" of his knowledge.

Elicited imitation can reveal a great deal about the child's language understanding and expression. Imitation samples provide clues about the child's memory functions and rule knowledge. Generally, a child reproduces a sentence using the grammatical rules she knows, so rule knowledge is easy to assess.

> Use elicited imitation strategies to assess form skills.

The informality of nonstandardized assessments can be both an advantage and a disadvantage in assessing language. The advantages are time saving, individualization, and high validity features. The limitation is best stated by Slobin and Welsh (1971), who caution that information obtained in this way should be supplemented by other data.

Behavioral evaluation A behavioral evaluation can be as simple as observing and listening to a child while making informal notations, but more often specialists and teachers use more careful, systematic procedures to collect baseline data and monitor subsequent behavior change. The behavioral information can be used also as a basis for planning, for indications of progress, or for a means of comparison with the reports given by others who talk with the child in other settings. Behavioral recording is especially useful when assessing communication functions, e.g. requesting, greeting, responding, and conversational devices such as taking turns. (These functions are described in Chapter Six.)

> The advantage of *behavioral observations* is that they can be continuous across tasks, settings, and people.

The first step in selecting a behavioral observation strategy is to clarify the purpose of the observation and the precise behavior to be observed. Most often the purpose is related to intervention objectives; the child will be observed to determine his placement in, and/or progress through, the program. Then select a recording system appropriate to the purpose and the target behavior.

> Collecting and graphing behavioral observation data.

Narrative recording is probably the oldest and best known method for collecting behavioral information. Narrative recordings are called anecdotal records. They are most commonly used for preliminary definition of categories preceding identification of precise observational strategies. Narrative information may be written or recorded by audio or video tapes for later transcription.

Interpreting narrative data can be simplified by providing time notes and organizing the descriptions into three columns. In the first column record (a) events that occur before the communicative utterance (antecedent events); in the second column, (b) the child's verbal or nonverbal

> Once recorded, narrative records are analyzed to identify specific program targets.

behavior; in the third column, (c) the effect (consequence) of the communication. The description should include everything the child says and does and to/with whom, as well as what is said and done to/with the child.

Nonnarrative recording simplifies the data collection process because only occurrences of a limited set of preselected behaviors are recorded. Target behaviors must be identified and defined before observation.

Practical considerations and what behavioral dimension (e.g., rate, duration) is of concern determines the choice of a particular recording procedure. The following discussion provides several strategic procedures for recording observations and for reporting the data. Implementing these procedures is usually the responsibility of the teacher, with planning and analysis assistance from the specialist.

Event or frequency recording involves counting the number of times the target behavior occurs during a specified time period. This method is appropriate for recording discrete behavior units of short duration with easily discernable beginnings and endings. Sentences, phrases, words, syllables, and phonemes are examples of discrete verbal units which, if they are not delivered at a high rate, can be easily counted. When the behavior occurs at a high rate or lasts for variable or extended periods of time (e.g., participation in ritualized games, interactive play), there is a loss of precision with event recording. Other methods such as duration recording, interval recording, or time sampling (discussed below) will provide a more accurate picture of the child's behavior.

Frequency recording is realistic for classroom data collection because it can be easily incorporated into daily routines. Data collection devices are simple, usually just a pen or pencil and paper or a counter. Here are some ideas for recording frequency data:

1. Keep tallies on a 3 x 5 index card premarked as the samples in Figure 4-1. The first teacher-made data card in Figure 4-1 was designed to record demonstration of tool use behavior. The criterion was 8 correct responses in 10 trials over two consecutive sessions. When no trials were presented for a stimulus on that day, it is indicated. Otherwise, 10 trials per stimulus are presented. The second data card permits scoring of data for three children. Use of intentional nonverbal symbols to regulate the behavior of others, a prelinguistic goal of language use, is being monitored. The third card was designed to record verbal imitations. Slashes indicate presentation of the stimulus model. If the model is imitated, the slash is crossed through to become a plus sign (+). Once completed, the cards are filed and the data later transferred to IEP records or graphed.

2. A layout (similar to that on the cards or expanded to cover more days, more children, or more stimuli) may be printed on 8½ x 11 paper and attached to student clipboards or kept in program notebooks. The larger paper has space for more program information and recording instructions.

Event or frequency recording yields a count of how many times the behavior occurred.

Objective: Tool use Trials — 10 per stimulus		Child's Name: Susannah Week of: 4/21/83				
	Car	Clown	Necklace	Telephone	Apple
Monday	//	Not Presented	Not Presented	Not Presented	Not Presented
Tuesday	ЖҬ //	/	Not Presented	Not Presented	Not Presented
Wednesday	ЖҬ ///	//	Not Presented	Not Presented	Not Presented
Thursday	ЖҬ ////	///	Not Presented	Not Presented	Not Presented
Friday	Not Presented	////	/	Not Presented	Not Presented

Objective: Use of intentional nonverbal symbols to regulate the behavior of others Time: 8:40 - 9:00			Week of: 2/14/83		
Names Date	2/14/83	2/15/83	2/16/83	2/17/83	2/18/83
Kelli	///	ЖҬ			
Mark	///	//			
Cami	//	///			

Objective: Verbal imitation		Child's Name: Mark Week of: 12/16/83			
Model	Monday	Tuesday	Wednesday	Thursday	Friday
play	/ ++	// +++			
Hi	//	// +			
juice	++ /	+ +			
up	// +	+ +			
go	+	/ +			
yes	+++	+			
bye-bye	+ ///	+ +			
coat	/// +	/ + +			

FIGURE 4-1 Teacher-made data card

3. Hand-held or wrist worn counters help you count higher rate behaviors. Different types can be purchased in sporting goods departments (golf counter) and needlework departments (knitting stitch counter). Behavior counts can be recorded on a data sheet/card after the session, at convenient breaks, or at the end of the day. Another useful device is a piece of white bandage tape around the left wrist or a sleeveband. Behavior occurrences are tallied with a pencil or ball-point pen.

In addition to recording frequency of occurrences, it is critical to record the number of trials (opportunities for the response) if performance is based on opportunity. For example, on the first card (Figure 4-1) each toy (stimulus) was made available 10 times; there was a fixed number of opportunities (10 per stimulus) to retrieve the toy. In this case the resultant data may be graphed as a percentage (e.g., retrieved the toy car Monday, 20%; Tuesday, 70%; Wednesday, 80%; etc.). Because training/observation time is not held constant, we cannot compute rate from these data.

When opportunities to respond vary, it is important to maintain a constant observation period.

When the number of opportunities for a response varies from one time period to the next, as is the case with the behavior monitored on the second data card, then a constant observation period is critical. Note that in this case it was 20 minutes. This permits computation of rate (frequency ÷ time) or simple frequency (e.g., "used three intentional nonverbal symbols to regulate the behavior of others in the 20 minute observation period").

The data recorded on the third data card could present a problem. We have no idea of the length of the training/observation sessions, and so rate calculations are precluded. The number of opportunities (trials) per day apparently has not been held constant, and so expression of percentages would have no meaning. There is an answer to the dilemma, however. The back of the card reads, "Provide 18 to 20 trials per stimulus over a weekly period." Attention and fatigue factors were a concern with this particular child, and so a decision was made to maintain opportunities constant over a weekly rather than a daily, period.

Interval recording allows fairly accurate measurement of low and medium rates of responding.

Interval recording permits fairly sensitive measurement of both duration and frequency simultaneously. The observation period is divided into equal time intervals (usually from 5 to 50 seconds) depending on the average frequency and duration of the behavior. Regardless of the number of times the target behavior occurs during an interval, the interval is scored only once. When more than one behavior is being observed or recorded, or when more than one child is to be observed and recorded, there may be separate rows for each behavior or child, or a single row where a symbol for the behavior occurring or child responding in that unit is recorded (Figure 4-2).

One limitation of the interval recording method is lack of precision. Repp, Roberts, Slack, Repp and Berkler (1976), in a comparison of observation recording methods, found that low and medium rates of responding can be measured with some accuracy (with 10-second intervals), but that high rates of responding are significantly underestimated with interval measurements (as compared to frequency recording). Behaviors emitted at a high rate should be measured with a frequency method, or very short intervals (less than 10 seconds) should be used. Another limitation of this method is that it requires the observer's undivided attention.

When using an interval system, it is important to specify the proportion of the interval in which the behavior must occur to be scored prior to observation. Does it have to occur for the entire interval? If it occurs during part of the interval, is that sufficient to be scored as an occurrence?

SECONDS	10	20	30	40	50	60
CUP	/	/				
BALL						
COMB			/	/	/	/

Functional use (3 toys/objects available)

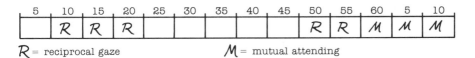

R = reciprocal gaze   *M* = mutual attending

Reciprocal gaze and mutual attending during free play.

FIGURE 4-2 Interval Recording Examples

When a "whole interval method" is used, there is the potential for losing some information. If, for example, the behavior "reciprocal gaze" is noted to begin during the 3rd second of the 10-second interval and continue until the 8th second (see Figure 4-2), there would be no count. However, if prior to beginning the observations, you decided that the target behavior is to be scored if it exists for 3 consecutive seconds during the 5-second interval, then "reciprocal gaze" would be scored in the 2nd interval, but not in the 1st. This method helps, but does not completely solve the problem of information loss. What actually occurred in this session was that the severely handicapped child established eye contact ("reciprocal gaze") during the 3rd second, maintained it until the 8th second (5 seconds), then looked away for 3 seconds before reestablishing "reciprocal gaze" in the 12th second. He then maintained contact until the 19th second. The fact that there was a break and actually two eye contact episodes is not reflected in the data. In this case, shorter intervals are required.

Interval recording requires some type of timing device. A watch or a clock with a second hand or a portable recorder with taped prerecorded interval signals (and an ear plug attachment) are most common. For classroom purposes such devices as egg timers and kitchen timers (with a muffled bell) can be used for recording when the intervals are as long as 3 to 5 minutes.

Duration recording is used when the length of time a behavior occurs is of interest. The number of seconds or minutes from initiation to termination of the target behavior is recorded. Duration recording is most

When the temporal dimension of the behavior is of concern, duration recording is the best system.

appropriate for (a) behaviors that occur at rates too high to count, (b) behaviors that occur for extended time periods, and (c) behaviors that are variable in length (e.g., attention, play, crying). Duration data may be reported in total seconds or total minutes or percentage of time relative to the observation period.

One way of recording duration is the time accumulation method. The stopwatch is started as the behavior begins, stopped when the child moves to another activity, restarted when the target behavior is begun again, etc. Since the watch is never returned to zero, it shows total accumulated duration at the end of the observation period. Here again, however, it is important to be aware of some information loss. Although the stopwatch reading shows the total number of seconds or minutes the target behavior occurs, one does not know how many separate behavioral episodes there were or when they occurred.

The *time sampling* recording method is more suited to use in applied settings than is interval or duration recording because it does not require the observer's undivided attention. Similar to interval recording, time sample data can be converted to and reported as percentages. The observation period is divided into equal intervals, as in interval recording; but instead of scoring the target behavior(s) during the interval, observation and recording take place at the end of each interval. Hall, Hawkins and Axelrod (1975) describe this method as "analogous to taking a snapshot of the subject . . . capturing the subject's behavior at a given moment in time" (p. 210). The "snapshots" need not be taken at regular intervals but number of samples per observation session should be predetermined. Hall et al. (1975) suggest setting a timer randomly, then recording when the bell sounds, resetting, and continuing the process for the predetermined number of samples.

A wide range and variety of behaviors lend themselves to the time sampling method. Information about one or several behaviors of a single child or a group can be recorded concurrently. Data is recorded for a number of children by rotating from one child to another (attending to and recording the behavior of each sequentially). The sequential observation process is continued until each child has been observed the prespecified number of times.

Time sampling has many of the advantages of interval recording, without the undivided attention requirement. The only precaution is that behaviors that occur at a low frequency or have a very short duration must be sampled on a frequent interval basis or they will be missed.

In addition to the four major types of observation measurement methods, there are two variations which may be applicable to some language behaviors: latency recording, which is a type of duration measure, and trials-to-criterion recording, which entails event recording.

Instead of recording the length of time a behavior is performed, *latency recording* focuses on the time that elapses between stimulus and response initiation. There are any number of situations when promptness or immediacy of the response is as significant as accuracy and independ-

Time sampling is similar to interval recording except that recording takes place at the end of the interval.

In latency recording, the amount of time lapse between stimulus and response is recorded.

ence. The most common examples are situations where the child is asked a question or expected to respond to a request. When establishing a rein-forcement hierarchy, response latency may be considered an indication of the child's relative preferences for various objects and activities. The amount of time that elapses between when the stimulus is presented (e.g., displaying a toy, offering a play activity) and when the child begins to act on the object or actively participate in the play activity may be recorded as a measure of stimulus attractiveness and desirability.

Trials-to-criterion recording is a variation of event recording that has proven particularly useful in programming for the severely handicapped (Haring, 1978). Once a desired performance level has been established, the instructor simply counts the number of trials the child requires to at-tain that performance level. This method is not sensitive and does not pro-vide meaningful data unless skills are broken down into discrete subtasks and appropriately sequenced. Ideally, practice of each subskill is inherent in performance of subsequent subskills. An example of a skill sequence that lends itself to this type of analysis and recording is the development of sound localization (Robinson & Robinson, 1978):

Some training sequences lend themselves well to trials-to-criterion recording.

1. Child hears a sound outside visual field
2. Child visually searches for sound source
3. Child turns head in direction of sound and visually searches for sound source
4. Child turns head in horizontal direction and then looks down to visually locate sound source
5. Child turns head and directs gaze downward simultaneously to visually locate sound source

At each stage in the sound localization sequence, the number of trials required before the child demonstrates the desired behavior is re-corded. The child may be required to demonstrate the subskill a number of times as criterion for moving on to the next subtask. Each subskill is es-sentially "checked off" as attained, a procedure which makes this method similar to a checklist.

Once data have been collected, the next decision is how to report and display the information so that it will be functional (visible and easily interpretable) for program decision making. The data collection methods discussed in the previous section will generate information about whether the selected program is indeed affecting child behavior. In addition to pro-viding a basis for decisions related to modification of instructional strate-gies, these data are important for documenting progress toward attain-ment of IEP goals and objectives. The question is how to report the information: Should you use proportional concepts, such as percentage and ratio, or frequency and rate? How should you display it? The first part of this question is already answered if you have correctly formulated the in-structional objectives.

Data reporting methods.

The type of data collected will dictate the reporting method.

If appropriately stated, each of the child's language instruction objectives includes specific criteria. These criteria provide a basis for determining when the objective is achieved. Just as the nature of the desired behavior dictates the observation methods and criteria, the data dictate reporting methods. For example, consider this objective: During interpersonal exchanges, child will maintain eye contact for at least 1 minute. The word "maintain" indicates a duration recording method because we are interested in the length of time the behavior occurs. The accumulation duration method is not appropriate because we are concerned with the length of each episode—not total time. The duration criterion for this objective may be based on (a) a measure of baseline functioning, (b) normal development findings (that normal learners typically maintain eye contact for a specified period of time in reciprocal play), or (c) the entry requirements of subsequent tasks. A 1-minute duration was determined to be an appropriate criterion for this objective in our example. Mastery required demonstration of the response over 5 consecutive days. Thus, the criteria are properly stated "for a minimum of 1 minute over 5 consecutive days." The two types of observation procedures dictated by these criteria are duration (of eye contact) and frequency (of 1-minute eye contact episodes). Because any interpersonal exchange provides an occasion for this behavior, the number of opportunities will vary, but time is held constant (the length of the school day). If you think that the use of a stopwatch could interfere with your interaction with the child during this type of exchange, you may simply count seconds to yourself (*one-thousand-one, one-thousand-two, etc.*) and note only the 1-minute episodes. Such an imprecise procedure would be unacceptable in research, but it is sufficiently precise for classroom monitoring purposes. Report the number of 1-minute eye contact occurrences per day on a data card or program sheet. When the criterion is reached, note the date the objective was completed on the child's IEP form or in some other convenient record. Latency data are reported in the same manner as you would report the occurrence of behavior units because there is no ceiling on the time requirement.

Data are usually reported as frequency, rate, percentage or ratio.

All data are not as easily collected or reported as the example just cited. Some objectives include several skills and require more careful documentation to monitor progress. Data may be reported as frequency, rate, percentage, or ratio, and displayed graphically. An advantage of graphs is the potential for depicting small changes in behavior and rate of change that may otherwise go unnoticed. Before considering simple graphing conventions, however, review these general guidelines for reporting data.

Frequency and rate The number of times the behavior occurs may be reported as simple frequency if the time is held constant (e.g., the total number of initiated verbal interactions each day during the 10-minute recess period). If time is not held constant, convert the frequency into rate per standard unit of time. If, for example, the child initiated verbal requests six times over two hours one day and four times over three hours the next day, calculate rate per hour by dividing the number of behaviors by the number of hours. The resultant rates are 3 and 1.3 per hour respectively.

Percentage and ratio   Percentages may be used to report many different types of data—frequency data, if the number of response opportunities (trials) per observation period is fixed, duration data, and interval data. Percentage is an effective reporting procedure for duration and interval data, even if observation periods are not constant. Compute percentage by dividing total correct responses by number of opportunities (in the case of frequency data), total amount of time by total length of the observation period (for duration data), or total intervals in which the behavior occurred by total intervals in the observation period (for interval data). In each case multiply the results by 100. Ratio reports are similar to percentage reports, except the number of opportunities or trials is noted (e.g., 8 of 10).

Graphing conventions   The basic graph employs two axes, a vertical axis called the ordinate and a horizontal axis called the abscissa. Units of behavior (frequency, rate, percentage, duration) are usually recorded on the ordinate and time units (e.g., sessions, days, weeks) on the abscissa (Figure 4-3).

> The most common type of graph is a simple line graph with two axes.

Squared graph paper simplifies the plotting of data. Plot the data point at the intersection of the axes, then connect them with a line. Figure 4-4 is an example of a graph displaying event data.

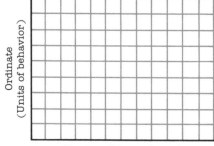

Abscissa (Units of time)

FIGURE 4-3

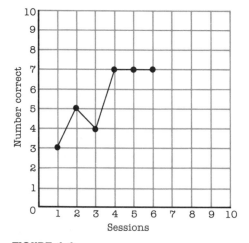

FIGURE 4-4

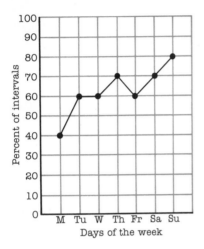

FIGURE 4-5

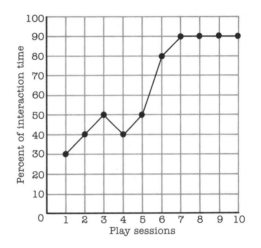

FIGURE 4-6

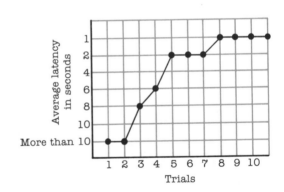

FIGURE 4-7

Figure 4-5 is an example of a graph displaying interval data reported as percentage. A similar display method is used for reporting time sample data.

Figure 4-6 shows duration data expressed as percentage.

Latency data are displayed in Figure 4–7. Note that trials are depicted on the abscissa. An alternative to reporting response latency for each trial, which takes considerable space, is to report average latency per session.

THE LINKAGES BETWEEN ASSESSMENT AND TEACHING

In reality the most difficult and critical part of assessment and evaluation is using the resulting information to develop and/or modify programs. If assessment data do not contribute to the promotion of effective language and communication experiences, they are useless. Assessment and evaluation data should guide decision making, initially and continually, and should provide the focal point for team meetings and decisions on subsequent reassessments.

Most importantly, assessment and evaluation information must guide the process of language instruction. It should contain specific information about the child as a communicator and learner, about attainments and usages, and about variability in different contexts. Teaching begins during the initial screening assessment, and assessment continues throughout the intervention process. After the child has learned to perform the skill consistently in the instructional setting, data should be collected on performance in natural settings. (Facilitating and evaluating generalization will be discussed in Chapter Six.)

We should now return to the content-form-use design that was discussed in the section, *What are we going to assess?* The information we have considered in the various assessment strategies should be collated based on this language design. The questions that were asked in the content-form-use sections can now be posed using the aggregated information. To facilitate this process the language specialist and/or teacher may develop a schematic chart which lists the various assessment sources, along with the relevant developmental information and the child's charted language data. The important thing is to have a design for integrating the data and setting training priorities.

There are two general strategies for such planning. One is a *deficit* strategy: identifying the low points on the child's language profile and then developing arrangements to train these areas to criteria. A second strategy is to begin with positive indicators, the child's strengths, so that the training can provide for immediately successful experiences. In either approach the purpose of assessment data is to guide and assist planning of an individualized curriculum and teaching strategies. The integrated assessment information should guide both the *what* and the *how* of intervention planning. Further information about linkages between assessment and teaching are presented in Chapters Five and Six.

ADDITIONAL ISSUES: THE ASSESSMENT TEAM AND PARENTS AS PARTICIPANTS IN ASSESSMENT

A discussion of assessment that does not consider the assessment team composition and the involvement of parents as active assessment participants is incomplete. Although each of these issues is discussed further in Chapter Eleven, they are considered briefly here because of their relevance to assessment.

A major test of the evaluation team's effectiveness is sharing all information so that a complete and comprehensive functional plan can be developed. Creating and maintaining this plan requires the team to collect and collate information so that there is consensus for planning. Most importantly, each member must clearly understand his or her role. The child's parents or guardians must be notified of any assessment plans and results. Their role in assessment is as important as their role in training.

Parents should actively participate in the assessment of their child at the early stages of planning and throughout the course of intervention. Parent involvement is also discussed in the section on IEP committee activities in Chapters Five and Eleven. In reality parents may play different roles (see Chapter Eleven) that reflect varying degrees of involvement. One of their important functions is to exchange information with specialists and teaching staff. Through the process of giving and receiving information, the parents become functional members of both assessment and service teams.

SUMMARY

1. Language/communication specialists typically assume major responsibility for initial, and ongoing assessment and planning the program evaluation; teaching staff responsibilities include orchestration and implementation of these activities.

2. The primary reasons for assessment are (a) to determine whether language intervention is indicated, (b) to specify the goals and objectives of that intervention, and (c) to monitor its effectiveness.

3. The purpose of screening is to identify those children for whom more complete and comprehensive assessment is warranted and/or to determine if a child meets the eligibility criteria for special services.

4. When the purpose of assessment is to determine baseline functioning levels, sufficient information must be collected to pinpoint the precise level of the target behavior across all relevant domains as a basis for planning and, subsequently, evaluating intervention goals and objectives.

5. There are four basic types of assessment and evaluation procedures: (a) standardized tests, (b) developmental scales, (c) nonstandardized tests, and (d) behavioral observation procedures.

6. There are two types of behavioral observation strategies: narrative recording and nonnarrative recording. The latter category includes event recording, interval recording, duration recording, time sampling, latency recording, and trials to criterion recording.

7. The type of behavioral observation data collected determines the reporting methods; data are usually reported as frequency, rate, percentage, or ratio.

8. The most difficult and critical aspect of child assessment and program evaluation is interpreting and analyzing the information they generate to develop and/or improve programming.

9. Parent involvement is a critical element in the success of both assessment and intervention.

REFERENCES

ALLEN, K.E., HOLM, V., & SCHIEFELBUSCH, R.L. *Early intervention: A team approach.* Baltimore: University Park Press, 1978.

ANDERSON, R., MILES, M., & MATHENY, P. *Communication evaluation chart from infancy to five years.* Cambridge, Mass.: Educators Publishing Service, Inc., 1963.

BATES, E. *Language and context: The acquisition of pragmatics.* New York: Academic Press, 1976.

BENEDICT, R. Early lexical development: Comprehension and production. *Journal of Child Language,* 1979, *6,* 183-200.

BERRY, M. *Teaching linguistically handicapped children.* Englewood Cliffs, N.J.: Prentice Hall, 1980.

BLOOM, L., & LAHEY, M. *Language development and language disorders.* New York: Wiley and Sons, 1978.

BROWN, R. *A first language: The early stages.* Cambridge, Mass.: Harvard University Press, 1973.

BZOCH, K., & LEAGUE, R. *The receptive-expressive emergent language scale.* Gainesville, Fla.: Computer Management Corporation, 1971.

CARROW-WOOLFOLK, E., & LYNCH, J.I. *An integrative approach to language disorders in children.* New York: Grune and Stratton, 1982.

CARTWRIGHT, C. Effective programs for parents of young handicapped children. *Families of Handicapped Children, Topics in Early Childhood Special Education,* 1:3, October, 1981.

CHAPMAN, R., & MILLER, J. Analyzing language and communication in the child. In R.L. Schiefelbusch (Ed.), *Nonspeech language and communication: Analysis and intervention.* Baltimore: University Park Press, 1980.

COOPER, J.O. *Measurement and analysis of behavior techniques.* Columbus, Ohio: Charles E. Merrill, 1974.

DANOWITZ, SISTER M.W. Formal versus informal assessment: Fragmentation versus holism. *Topics in Language Disorders,* 1981, *1*(3).

DARLEY, F. *Evaluation and appraisal techniques in speech and language pathology.* Reading, Mass.: Addison-Wesley Publishing Co., 1979.

DuBOSE, R. Assessment of severely impaired young children. *Assessing the handicapped preschooler, Topics in Early Childhood Special Education,* 1981, *1*(2).

DUNN, L. Expanded manual: Peabody Picture Vocabulary *List.* Circle Pines, Minn.: American Guidance Service, 1965.

GERBER, A., & BRYEN, D. *Language and learning disabilities.* Baltimore: University Park Press, 1981.

HALL, R.V., HAWKINS, R.P., & AXELROD, S. Measuring and recording student behavior: A behavior analysis approach. In R.A. Weinberg & F.H. Wood (Eds.), *Observation of pupils and teachers in mainstream and special education settings: Alternate strategies.* Minneapolis, Minn.: Leadership Training Institute, University of Minnesota, 1975.

HANNAH, E. *Applied Linguistic Analyses II.* Pacific Palisades, Calif.: Sincom Associates, 1977.

HARING, N.G. (Ed.) *Behavior of exceptional children.* (2nd ed.). Columbus, Ohio: Charles E. Merrill, 1978.

HEDRICK, D., PRATHER, E., & TOBIN, A. *Sequenced inventory of communication development (SICD).* Seattle: University of Washington Press, 1976.

HILL, J. *Models for screening.* Paper presented at the annual meeting of the American Education Research Association, 1970.

HORSTMEIER, D., & MacDONALD, J. *Environmental prelanguage battery.* Columbus, Ohio: Charles E. Merrill, 1978.

KIRK, S., McCARTHY, J., & KIRK, W. *The Illinois test of psycholinguistic abilities* (Rev. ed.). Urbana, Ill.: University of Illinois Press, 1968.

LEE, L. *Northwestern syntax screening test (NSST).* Evanston, Ill.: Northwestern University Press, 1971.

LEE, L. *Developmental sentence analysis.* Evanston, Ill.: Northwestern University Press, 1974.

LINDER, T.W. *Early childhood special education: Program development and administration.* Baltimore: Paul H. Brookes Publishing Co., 1983.

MacDONALD, J. *Environmental language inventory.* Columbus, Ohio: Charles E. Merrill, 1978.

McLEAN, J. Language structure and communication disorders. In N.G. Haring (Ed.), *Behavior of exceptional children* (2nd ed.). Columbus, Ohio: Charles E. Merrill, 1978.

McREYNOLDS, L. Contingencies and consequences in speech therapy. *Journal of Speech and Hearing Disorders,* 1970, *35,* 12-24.

MECHAM, M. *Verbal language development scale (VLDS).* American Guidance Service, 1971.

MILLER, J. Assessing children's language behavior: A developmental process approach. In R.L. Schiefelbusch (Ed.), *Bases of language intervention.* Baltimore: University Park Press, 1978.

MILLER, J. *Assessing language production in children: Experimental procedures.* Baltimore: University Park Press, 1981.

MOERK, E. *Pragmatic and semantic aspects of early language development.* Baltimore: University Park Press, 1977.

MOOG, J., & GEERS, A. *Scales of early communication skills for hearing impaired children.* Central Institute for the Deaf, 1975.

PRUTTING, C. Process /pra/, ses/n: the action of moving forward progressively from one point to another on the way to completion. *Journal of Speech and Hearing Disorders,* 1979, *44,* 3-30.

REPP, A.C., ROBERTS, D.M., SLACK, D.J., REPP, C.F., & BERKLER, M.S. A comparison of frequency, interval, and time sampling methods of data collection. *Journal of Applied Behavior Analysis,* 1976, *9,* 501-508.

ROBINSON, C., & ROBINSON, J.H. Sensorimotor functions and cognitive development. In M. Snell (Ed.), *Systematic instruction of the moderately and severely handicapped.* Columbus, Ohio: Charles E. Merrill, 1978.

SCHERY, T., & GLOVER, A. *The initial communication processes scale.* Monterey, Calif.: Publishers Test Service, 1982.

SCHIEFELBUSCH, R.L., & McCORMICK, L. Language and speech disorders. In J.M. Kaufman & D.P. Hallahan (Eds.), *Handbook of special education.* Englewood Cliffs, N.J.: Prentice-Hall, 1980.

SIEGEL, G. Appraisal of language development. In F.L. Darley (Ed.), *Evaluation of appraisal techniques in speech and language pathology.* Reading, Mass.: Addison-Wesley Publishing Co., 1979.

SIEGEL, G. The use of language tests. *Language Speech-Hearing Service Schools,* 1975, VI(4), 211-217.

SIEGEL, G., & BROEN, P.A. Language assessment. In L.L. Lloyd (Ed.), *Communication assessment and intervention strategies.* Baltimore: University Park Press, 1976.

SLOBIN, D.I., & WELSH, C.A. Elicited imitation as a research tool in developmental psycho-linguistics. In C.S. Lavatelli (Ed.), *Language training in early childhood education.* Urbana, Ill.: University of Illinois Press, 1971.

SMITH, D.D., & SNELL, M.E. Intervention strategies. In M.E. Snell (Ed.), *Systematic instruction of the moderately and severely handicapped.* Columbus, Ohio: Charles E. Merrill, 1978.

SNYDER, L. Assessing communicative abilities in the sensorimotor period: Content and context. *Topics in Language Disorders,* 1981, *1*(3), 31-46.

SNYDER, L., BATES, E., & BRETHERTON, I. Content and context in early lexical development. *Journal of Child Language,* in press.

VANE, J. *Vane evaluation of language scale.* Clinical Psychology Publishing Company, Inc., 1975.

WARYAS, C., & STREMEL-CAMPBELL, K. Grammatical training for the language-delayed child: A new perspective. In R.L. Schiefelbusch (Ed.), *Language intervention strategies.* Baltimore: University Park Press, 1978.

ZIMMERMAN, I., STEINER, V., & EVATT, R. *Preschool language scale.* Columbus, Ohio: Charles E. Merrill, 1969.

APPENDIX A

Prices given in appendixes are subject to change.

IDENTIFICATION AND SCREENING

Boehm Test of Basic Concepts (BTBC)

Grades K–2; 1967–71; a picture test based on concepts (e.g., below, more, last) "commonly found in preschool and primary instructional materials"; BTBC; Forms A ('69, 16 pages in two booklets), B ('70, 16 pages in two booklets); revised manual ('71, 30 pages); instructional materials on concepts available; $7 per 30 tests; 75¢ per manual; $1.50 per specimen set; postage extra; Spanish directions ('70) available; (30-40) minutes in two sessions; Ann E. Boehm; Psychological Corporation.*

Carrow Elicited Language Inventory (CELI)

Ages 3–7; 1974; CELI; 18 scores: grammar (articles, adjectives, nouns, noun plurals, pronouns, verbs, negatives, contractions, adverbs, prepositions, demonstratives, conjunctions), type (substitutions, omissions, additions, transpositions, reversals), total; individual; no reading by examinees; I form; scoring/analysis form (4 pages); manual (49 pages); verb protocol (6 pages); training guide (51 pages); training tape, 5 inch reel or cassette; audio-tape equipment necessary for administration; $44.95 per set of testing materials including 25 scoring/analysis forms and 10 protocols; $4.50 per 25 tests; $4.50 per 25 protocols; cash orders postpaid; specimen set not available; (10-15) minutes; Elizabeth Carrow; Learning Concepts.*

Detroit Tests of Learning Aptitude (DTLA)

Ages 3 and over; 1935–75; DTLA; 20 scores; pictorial absurdities, verbal absurdities, pictorial opposites, verbal opposites, motor speed and precision, auditory attention span (for unrelated words, for related syllables), oral commissions, social adjustment A, visual attention span (for objects, for letters), orientation, free association, memory for designs, number ability, social adjustment B, broken pictures, oral directions, likenesses and differences, total; no data on reliability of part scores; individual; 1 form; revised examiner's handbook ('67, 143 pages, with 1955 norms); supplement ('68, 15 pages); pictorial material ('58, 97 pages); revised record booklet ('59, 16 pages); descriptive and interpretive brochure ('75, 26 pages); $3.95 per pictorial material; $6.95 per 35 record booklets; 60¢ per single copy; $2 per descriptive brochure; $5.30 per handbook; $1.95 per supplement; postage extra; (60–95) minutes; Harry J. Baker and Bernice Leland (except descriptive brochure); Bobbs-Merrill Co., Inc.*

Illinois Test of Psycholinguistic Abilities Revised Edition (ITPA)

Ages 2–10; 1961–68; ITPA; 11–13 scores; auditory reception, visual reception, visual sequential memory, auditory association, auditory sequential memory, visual association, visual closure, verbal expression, grammatic closure, manual expression, auditory closure (optional), sound blending (optional), total; individual; 1 form ('68); Manual ('68, 134 pages); record form ('68, 16 pages); visual closure picture strips ('68, 5 pages); $58 per set of testing materials, 25 record forms, and 25 sets of picture strips; $6.50 per manual; cash orders postpaid; (45–60) minutes; Samuel A. Kirk, James J. McCarthy, and Winifred D. Kirk; University of Illinois Press.*

Peabody Picture Vocabulary Test (PPVT)

Ages 2.5–18; 1959–65; PPVT; individual; Forms A, B, ('59, 154 pages, picture booklet used with both forms); plastic edition of pictures also available; expanded manual ('65, 51 pages); individual record ('59, 4 pages) for each form; $14 per set of testing materials including 25 individual records for each form ($19.50 with set of plastic plates); $3.65 per 50 individual records; postage extra; (10–15) minutes; Lloyd M. Dunn; American Guidance Service, Inc.*

Test of Auditory Comprehension Language (TACL)

Ages 3–6; 1973; 2 tests which may be administered in English or Spanish; no norms for Spanish edition; cash orders postpaid; Elizabeth Carrow; Learning Concepts. (a) Screening Test for Auditory Comprehension of Language. STACL; short form for identifying children who need further testing with long form; 1 form (31 pages); manual (24 pages); 80¢ per test; $3.95 per manual; (5–10) minutes. (b) Test for Auditory Comprehension of Language Fifth Edition. TACL; long form; individual; 1 form (210 pages in manual); manual (37 pages plus test); scoring form (4 pages) for each language; $39.95 per manual and 25 English or Spanish scoring forms; $3.75 per 25 English or Spanish scoring forms; specimen set not available; (20) minutes.*

*Reprinted by permission of the Buros Institute of Mental Measurements. Copyright 1978 by The University of Nebraska.

150

APPENDIX B

STANDARDIZED TESTS

Northwestern Syntax Screening Test (NSST)

Ages 3–7; 1969–71; NSST; 2 scores: receptive, expressive; no data on reliability; individual; 1 form ('69, 42 cards in manual); manual ('71, 13 pages plus cards and record form); record form ('69, 1 page); $10.30 per kit including 50 record forms; $2.71 per 50 record forms; cash orders only; (15) minutes; Laura Lee; Northwestern University Press.*

Verbal Language Development Scale (VLDS)

Ages 0–14. 1971; Provides an indirect method of assessing the language of children who "cannot or will not respond to direct testing methods" (Manual, p. 2). Manual, 16 pages, $.75; 25 3-page score sheets, $2.00; Merlin J. Mecham; American Guidance Service, 1971.

Communication Evaluation Chart (CEC)

Is divided into 9 age levels ranging from 3 months to 5 years. Useful as a survey instrument to determine if the child is below normal limits. R. Anderson, M. Miles and Metheny, P., Golden, Colorado: Golden Colorado Business Forms, Inc., 1964.

APPENDIX C

DEVELOPMENTAL SCALES

Scales of Early Communication Skills for Hearing Impaired

2–8 year olds; 1975; 4 scales: Receptive Language Skills, Expressive Language Skills, Nonverbal Receptive Skills, and Nonverbal Expressive Skills. Manual with 1 scale, $7.50; 25 scales $3.00 per package; Examiner's Manual, 42 pages; test blank, 4 pages. Jean S. Moog and Ann V. Geers, Central Institute for the Deaf.

Environmental Language Inventory (ELI)

1978, "a diagnostic strategy for assessment and training of children with severe delay in expressive language." Manual, $7.95, spiral-bound, soft-cover manual. James D. MacDonald, Charles E. Merrill.

---

*Reprinted by permission of the Buros Institute of Mental Measurements. Copyright 1978 by The University of Nebraska.

Environmental Pre-Language Battery (EPB)

1978, "a diagnostic and training instrument designed for use with nonverbal or minimally verbal individuals who are functioning below or at the single-word level. Manual, $7.95 for spiral-bound soft cover. DeAnna Horstmeier and James D. MacDonald, Charles E. Merrill.

Preschool Language Scale (PLS)

Ages 2–6; 1969; PLS; 3 scores: auditory comprehension, verbal ability, total, plus an articulation section; no data on reliability and validity; individual; 1 form; picture book (36 pages); record booklet (18 pages); manual (88 pages); $9.50 per set of picture book, record booklet, and manual; $7.50 per 10 record booklets; postage extra; (30) minutes; Irla Lee Zimmerman, Violette G. Steiner, and Roberta L. Evatt; Charles E. Merrill Publishing Co.*

Vane Evaluation of Language Scale (VELS)

Ages 2.5 to 6.5; 1975; VELS, also called VANE-L; language acquisition; 3 scores: receptive language, expressive language, memory; no data on reliability and validity; individual; 1 form; record booklet (2 pages); manual (32 pages); class record sheet (2 pages); $15 per set of test objects, 50 record booklets, and manual; $3.50 per 50 record booklets; $8 per set of test objects; $5 per manual; cash orders postpaid; (10) minutes; Julia R. Vane; Clinical Psychology Publishing Co.*

APPENDIX D

BASELINE FUNCTIONING

The Bzoch-League Receptive-Expressive Emergent Language Scale.

For the Measurement of Language Skills in Infancy. Birth to age 3; 1970–1971; also called REEL Scale; 3 scores: receptive, expressive, combined; no data on reliability of part scores; 1 form ('70, 8 pages): manual ('71, 46 pages plus scale) entitled *Assessing Language Skills in Infancy;* $15.50 per 25 scales and manual; $6.75 per 25 scales; $9.75 per manual; postage extra; (10) minutes; Kenneth R. Bzoch and Richard League; Anhinga Press.*

Initial Communication Process Scale (ICP)

Ages 0–3; 1982; language acquisition; 3 domains: perceptual, motor, and functional integrations (non-social and social); reliability and

---

validity checked; ten scales (1 and 2, perceptual capacities; 3 and 4, motor capacities; and 5-10, functional integrations); manual (35 pages); Objectives Bank Progress Monitoring Log; Publishers Test Service, A service of CTB/McGraw-Hill, 2500 Garden Road, Monterey, California 93940.

Sequenced Inventory of Communication Development (SICD)
For children under two, 30 minutes, administration; 10 minutes, scoring. For children over two, up to one hour, administration; 10 minutes, scoring. Kit, $95.50; separate manual, $8.50; packages of 50 response booklets, $7.50. Test Kit contains Examiner's Manual, 100 pages; Expressive Communication Age Scale Response Booklet (packages of 50); Receptive Communication Age Scale Response Booklet (packages of 50); *Photo Articulation Test* Stimulus Cards (large and small); Collection of stimulus items. D.L. Hedrick, E.M. Prather, and A.R. Tobin, University of Washington Press, 1975.

APPENDIX E

GUIDELINES FOR OBSERVING BEHAVIORS DURING THE ASSESSMENT PROCESS

Child's Name: _____ Observer: _____

I. Screening, adaptive or informal assessment

A. What *did* the child do?

B. Which tasks were the most difficult for the child?

C. Which materials evoked optimal responses from the child?

D. What was the average length of time the child attended to each task? Did any specific tasks hold his/her attention longer?

E. How quickly did the child learn new tasks? Could s/he generalize new skills to other materials? Could s/he remember new skills over time?

F. Through what means did the child approach the majority of tasks?

G. What questions would you pursue based on the child's performance? What type of tasks will answer your questions?

H. How did the child respond to the evaluator? Was rapport established and how was this accomplished?

I. What type of behavioral management techniques were successful?

J. What appears to be the origin of the child's cognitive/adaptive delay?

K. What informal assessment instruments or subtests would you use to further investigate this child's skills?
Cognitive _____
Language _____
Motor _____
Social/Self-care _____

L. What is the approximate level of this child's functioning?

0–6 mos. _____	36–42 mos. _____
6–12 mos. _____	42–48 mos. _____
12–18 mos. _____	48–54 mos. _____
18–24 mos. _____	54–60 mos. _____
24–30 mos. _____	60–66 mos. _____
30–36 mos. _____	66–72 mos. _____

Comments:

M. What appears to be the most handicapping condition? Based on the screening information, how would you rate this child's auditory, visual, physical, and intellectual systems?
Rating Key: 0 = no or very minimal impairment; 1 = impairment that interferes with performance but not significantly; 2 = severe impairment, system is nonfunctional or extremely damaged.

Auditory _____ Visual _____ Physical _____ Intellectual _____

II. Fine Motor Skills

A. Did the child approach materials with one hand more than the other? Which?

B. Did the child: reach _____ grasp _____ release voluntarily _____?

C. Did the child hold objects in both hands? _____

D. Did the child use two hands together? In the same direction? In opposing directions?

E. Did the child cross his/her midline? _____

F. How did the child hold (grasp) pegs, blocks, beads, rings, cups, scissors, writing implements?

G. Could the child rotate wrists to: RH?   LH?
turn the handle on a jack-in-the-box _____ open a door _____

twist off tops and lids _____ operate an eggbeater _____ wind a mechanical toy _____

H. How would you describe his/her eye-hand coordination?

Accuracy _____ Control _____ Rhythm _____ Speed _____

I. Could s/he plan motorically?

Paper and markers _____ Beads _____ Blocks _____ Cutting _____ Paper folding _____ Washers and rings _____

J. What is the primary origin of this motor delay?

K. What other motor instruments or subtests would you use?

_____

What is approximate developmental level? _____

III. Gross Motor

A. What is the primary origin of the gross motor delay?

B. Does the child have basic movement patterns?

Head control _____ Trunk control _____ Sitting balance _____ Cutting _____

C. Describe the child's highest level of movement: *How* did the child do it?

D. Did the child maintain balance?

From a sitting position _____ While walking _____

While standing on one foot _____ While walking beams _____

E. Did the child run?   jump?   climb stairs?   HOW?

F. Did the child interact with balls? Did the child track projectory? *RH, LH,* Catch _____ Throw _____ Kick _____

G. Did the child follow a series of movements?

H. What formal gross motor instrument or subtests would you use to further evaluate these skills?

I. What is the child's approximate developmental motor level?

IV. Language

A. What is the origin of the child's language delay?

B. Does the child's hearing appear to be intact? What responses support your answer?

C. Does the child use hearing functionally, i.e., for language and communication?

D. What cues are used by the child for comprehension?

Physical guidance _____ Tactual _____ Contextual
situation _____
Gestures and signs _____ Visual and tactual _____
Tactual and verbal _____ Verbal and visual _____ Verbal
only _____
Other _____

E. Was the child responsive to the evaluator's verbal cues or "tuned out"?

F. Does the child vocalize?
cries and laughs _____ vocal play _____ words _____
screams _____ babbling _____ phrases _____ phonemes
(speech sounds) _____ jargon _____ echolalic _____

G. Can the child name objects, pictures presented either verbally or manually?

H. Describe the sounds, words, signs, etc. the child used.

I. Does the child use his/her voice for communication, i.e., as opposed to self-stimulation?

J. Does the child communicate verbally?

Touch the evaluator _____

Place the evaluator's hand on an object _____

Return the object to the evaluator _____

Points _____ Pulls the evaluator to the desired effect _____

Gestures _____ Signs _____

K. Does the child know what objects are for and how to use them?

L. Does the child possess the prerequisites for language?

M. If the child communicates in phrases or sentences, try to list 10 examples.

N. What other formal instruments or subtests would you use to gather further information about this child's language? _____

O. What is the child's approximate developmental language level?

V. Socialization Self-Care Skills

A. Did the child separate easily from the parent(s)?

B. Was rapport established easily?

C. Was eye contact established with the evaluator(s)?

D. Did the child cooperate with the evaluators? Enthusiastically or passively?

E. Did the child resist performing tasks?

F. Did the child exibit any unusual behaviors, i.e., self-stimulation?

G. Was the child abusive or aggressive?

H. Did the child interact with people and toys appropriately?

I. To what extent could the child toilet self?

J. To what extent could the child wash hands?

K. To what extent could the child undress and dress?

L. What other instruments would you use to gather more information?

M. What was the approximate developmental level?

VI. Other Observations/Impressions

Reprinted from *Topics in Early Childhood Special Education* 1:2, "Assessment of Severely Impaired Young Children: Problems and Recommendations" by Rebecca Fewell DuBose, by permission of Aspen Systems Corporation, © 1981.

CHAPTER FIVE

INTERVENTION PLANNING

Linda McCormick

Intervention planning should be approached in much the same way as you would approach a research project. All educational planning is necessarily experimental because we cannot specify with any assurance precisely what will be successful with different children. One reason for this tentativeness is that programming effectiveness depends on the complex interaction of numerous variables. Not all of these are under the control of educational personnel.

The proper attitude for teachers and language specialists planning for children with language problems should be that of a scientist or detective. Form hypotheses about what will be effective (the assessment and planning process), operate in accordance with these hypotheses (the intervention process), continually monitor effects of the operations (the evaluation process), and then revise, modify, expand, or form new hypotheses as indicated (assessment and planning, again). Planning is a continuous and circular activity which does not stop when the child's Individualized Educational Program (IEP) has been developed. It is important to remember that at least the child's first IEP represents only "a set of hypotheses about what might work in teaching a youngster" (Ysseldyke & Algozzine, 1982). Teaching staff and appropriate ancillary personnel must follow through with the hypothesis testing process, or this planning document will have little validity and usefulness.

This chapter and the next are intended to guide the hypothesis formulation and testing processes.

The notion that instructional decision making and design must be viewed as a hypothesis testing process guided development and organization of this chapter and the next chapter. This chapter presents a brief discussion of the IEP planning process because most agree that even if the economic and political incentives for compliance with P.L. 94-142 should be removed (and this is always a possibility), the program planning requirements of this legislation are not likely to be discontinued. Effective interventionists were advocating and formulating individualized programs long before P.L. 94-142 became a reality, and it is highly unlikely that this practice will end.

The remainder of this chapter suggests procedures for identifying the conditions under which a child can learn and respond most effectively. Applying this information to design and application of instructional practices and arrangements, particularly related to language, is the subject of Chapter Six.

THE IEP PROCESS

Discussion of the broad purposes and processes mandated by Public Law 94-142 is beyond the scope of this book. There are many excellent books (e.g., Lerner, Dawson, & Horvath, 1980; Shrag, 1977; Torres, 1977; Turnbull, Strickland, & Brantley, 1978) and numerous articles and chapters that cover the subject comprehensively. This discussion is limited to that section of the law which provides for development of an Individualized Education Program (IEP) and briefly outlines the requirements and procedures of the IEP process. Child and environmental variables to consider when formulating hypotheses about language and communication training and methods goals are discussed at length.

THE IEP COMMITTEE

The odds are overwhelming that by the end of your first year of professional employment you will have formulated or participated in the formulation of a number of IEPs. This function is one for which neither teachers nor specialists can be too well prepared. P.L. 94-142 lays out clear guidelines on when and how the IEP process is to proceed, but it is up to school personnel to assure proper implementation.

An IEP must be developed within 30 calendar days of the determination of eligibility for special education services. P.L. 94-142 establishes both the composition and functions of the committee charged with formulating this services plan. At least the following persons must be included in the planning process: The child's teacher (who will implement the IEP), a representative from special education administration (often a coordinator or consultant level staff member), the child's parent(s) or guardian(s), the person conducting the assessment (or a person knowledgeable in interpretation of the results), and where appropriate, the child. Participation of the prospective teacher is not required by law unless the child is not presently in school. However, this professional is a most desirable addition to the committee because he or she will be responsible for implementing the plan, selecting procedures and materials to accomplish the goals and objectives, evaluating progress, and monitoring the delivery of related services.

If the law has been followed, the parents have been provided with a report prior to the IEP meeting. The procedural safeguards of P.L. 94-142, the action that is being proposed for their child, and a description of the evaluation procedures that led to the decision should have been explained

If at all possible, the receiving teacher should be a member of the IEP committee.

to them prior to the meeting. As noted in Chapter Four, one reason the active involvement of parents or guardians is so critical is their unique ability to contribute pertinent information concerning their child's behavior in nonschool settings. Presumably, the greater the parental involvement at the point of determining programming directions, the greater degree of cooperation can be expected from them later. Parents indicate their approval of the plan by signing it. If, at some future time, they are not satisfied with any aspect of their child's services, they may request a revision or a hearing by an impartial hearing officer.

Parent involvement is discussed at length in Chapter Eleven.

DEVELOPMENT OF THE PLAN

The IEP committee is charged with the responsibility of developing the IEP and is told by the law precisely what this plan must include. It must include (a) a statement of present performance levels, (b) annual goals and short-term objectives, (c) a statement of the specific special education and related services to be provided, (d) the projected date of initiation of services and anticipated duration of these services, (e) objective criteria, evaluation procedures, and schedules for determining at least once a year whether the anticipated objectives are being met.

Sometimes a rough draft of all, or some portion, of the IEP is outlined prior to the committee meeting. Some systems justify this procedure as necessary for efficient use of committee time. At or before the meeting, committee members are provided with this tentative draft that has been developed by one or more of the involved professionals. Another approach is to assign different segments to various members according to their area of expertise and then assemble the segments at the meeting. In either case, the total plan is discussed and modified or amended at the IEP meeting.

Whether the plan is being developed by the committee as a whole or by some of its members, the first task is to review information provided by the multidisciplinary team responsible for the assessment process. At this point, if there is any doubt at all about the adequacy of the available data, additional information needs should be specified with a request that supplementary data be collected. Ideally, the assessment team's report should

As discussed in Chapter Four, the more specific and comprehensive the products of the assessment process are, the more valid the planning process.

1. Be organized according to developmental and/or functional domains, rather than by the administered tests
2. Describe specific areas of strength as well as skill deficits in clear, behavioral terms
3. Note conditions (setting, materials, reinforcers, cues, task variables) which evoke optimal performance
4. Indicate, based on natural environmental observations and/or interviews with significant others, whether identified skills are performed across tasks, persons, and settings
5. Present findings in a manner that can be easily translated into goals and objectives
6. Identify physical, medical, and sensory limitations

The next step in the process is drafting annual goals and short-term objectives. There should be two or three annual goals addressing each of the child's special needs. Goals may, of course, also describe achievements in other than academic areas, e.g., physical education, vocational training, social development or self-help areas. Most importantly, each should be broad enough to encompass a range of specific short-term or intermediary objectives.

Annual goals may be in development or functional domains.

Objectives should be sequential (ordered developmentally, functionally, or logically), specific, realistically manageable and, most importantly, measurable. Mager's (1975) "behavior-conditions-criteria" format is by far the most popular method to operationalize these "means" statements. The *behavior component* of the objective describes precisely what the learner is expected to do (the behavior that will be accepted as evidence that the objective has been achieved). In stating this desired behavior, verbs such as "understand," "know," and "learn" should be avoided in favor of observable actions like "point to," "initiate," "state," "sign," "verbalize" and "label."

An objective has three components—behavior, conditions and criteria.

The context in which the learner is to perform (the "givens" under which the behavior should occur) is specified in the *conditions component.* Commonly included in this component are setting variables (structured, unstructured), materials (pictures of familiar objects), equipment (typewriter, walker) body position (side-lying, supine) and time (after lunch, at snack time). The conditions component aids the teacher in designing specific aspects of the instructional program and also assists the individualization of instruction.

The *criterion component* is in many ways the most difficult because it assumes understanding of the child's learning characteristics *and* the nature of the desired behavior. Types of criteria include timed procedures, percentage or number of responses correct, and percentage of time or intervals. Guard against the tendency to indiscriminately rely on a single "standard" criterion (e.g., 9 of 10, 80%) for all children, all behaviors, and all programs. This is a deplorable, but all too prevalent, practice which assumes that all children learn in the same way and that all skills and concepts are mastered at the same level when, in fact, the case is quite the opposite. The same child may master one skill (as demonstrated by accurate performance in subsequent maintenance probes and generalization to the natural environment) if trained to seven (or 70%) consecutive correct responses on that skill, and require nine (or 90%) correct trials for three days in a row before mastering another skill. Likewise, different children master the same skill at different criterion levels.

Do not rely on a single criterion for all objectives.

Analyze all available information about the child and try to agree on a valid standard for mastery. Remember that if the criterion is set too high, there is a risk of the child becoming bored with the task or satiated on the reinforcer; training may continue interminably without meeting the predetermined "success" standard. Neither you nor the child can afford to waste valuable instructional time in this manner.

When there is reason to suspect that a criterion has been set too high, terminate instruction prior to attainment of the criterion and observe whether the concept is demonstrated in the natural environment (or administer probes at some future time to see if the desired behavior has been mastered.) If it *has* been retained and generalized (without reaching the original criterion), then the criterion was, indeed, too high. If not, of course, training must be reinstated. The same type of classroom experimentation can establish whether a criterion has been set too low.

The criterion is a "best guess" as to the response level a particular child must demonstrate before the target concept or skill has been mastered.

Formulate a child's first IEP with the understanding that the criteria are tentative and revisions may be necessary before the end of the school year. Development of criteria for objectives on subsequent IEPs will be easier because the child's special learning characteristics will have been identified.

The third task facing the IEP committee is delineation of special education and related services needs (e.g., speech and/or language therapy, physical therapy, psychological services, transportation, etc.). The IEP must list all of the special services that will be required to provide an appropriate education.

The next consideration is the "least restrictive environment" (LRE). This provision of P.L. 94-142 states that handicapped children are to be educated with nonhandicapped children "to the maximum extent appropriate." The LRE is not easy to interpret and it is even more difficult to operationally define because the meaning of "appropriate" depends on the child. Identification of LRE for a particular child requires substantial information about the child's skills relative to the demands of various placement options. Because the IEP committee rarely has sufficient data to assure an appropriate match between the child's performance capabilities and environmental characteristics, this decision is another in the "best guess" category. It should be noted that the need for a means of collecting empirical data for objective decision making in this area is recognized, but still unmet (McCormick & Kawate, 1982). What is needed are (a) standard procedures to determine and justify the extent to which children should receive regular and/or special education services and (b) training models which focus on preparation for integration with same age peers.

The term "less restrictive" can only be defined in relation to a child's present circumstances. Logically, the more restrictive the child's present environments, the greater the range and variety of future environments that qualify as "less restrictive." Less restrictive subsequent school environments for preschoolers will be those instructional arrangements where there are opportunities for maximum exposure to and interaction with more competent children. Less restrictive nonschool environments will be home settings (e.g., kitchen, backyard) and community settings (e.g., playground, grocery store), where "normal" 4, 5, and 6-year-old children routinely participate (Vincent, Brown, & Gatz-Sheftel, 1981).

Projected timelines serve a useful purpose because they affirm the temporary status of special services.

The next topic for IEP committee consideration is timelines (projected dates for initiation of services and the anticipated duration of each of these services). These dates are not binding; they are merely projections, but they focus attention on possible termination of the special services and the ultimate goal of full support in the regular education system.

One purpose of these timelines is to affirm the temporary status of the special services.

In addition to procedures for evaluating individual objectives, the IEP must establish in writing the system for periodic review and evaluation by the state education agency. The state educational agency is required to develop and implement monitoring procedures to insure, at least on an annual basis, that the child is making progress. When the anticipated progress is not evident, steps must be taken to identify and eliminate barriers.

Each of the five mandated IEP components has a purpose. In addition to providing teachers and other professionals with instructional direction, they promote accountability, communication, and cooperation. Each component plays an important role in assuring the intent of the IEP—individualized instruction to meet the special needs of the special child.

To summarize, the functions of the IEP committee are:

1. identification of the problem areas where special instruction is indicated
2. quantification of present performance levels in the problem areas
3. determination of goals and objectives which, when obtained, will ameliorate the problem areas
4. selection of the environment(s) and persons to achieve the goals and objectives
5. determination of precise quantitative methods to monitor and evaluate achievement of the goals and objectives

The IEP committee has five major *responsibilities.*

ASKING INSTRUCTIONALLY RELEVANT QUESTIONS

Formulating a meaningful individualized educational plan involves substantially more than coming up with a list of target behaviors. Design of appropriate and effective procedures requires systematic investigation of the child's learning strengths and weaknesses, and analysis of environmental demands and consequences. Some questions that are particularly relevant to development of procedures for language and communication programming are

In actual practice, decisions on *how* to teach are usually left to the service delivery team (see Chapter Eleven).

1. What are the child's preferred and/or intact sensory modalities?
2. Does the child have learning strategy problems?
3. What are the child's functional output capabilities?
4. What are the environmental events most likely to motivate some form of controlling response?

These broad questions raise many issues. Some are dealt with in this chapter. Others, including the basis for sequencing of instruction, curricula adaptation, arranging the instructional environment to maximize

The remainder of this chapter focuses upon asking instructionally relevant questions about: 1. sensory acuity, 2. learning strategies, 3. output capabilities, and 4. motivational variables.

learning, basic components of instruction and developing "age-appropriate" objectives are addressed in Chapter Six.

The considerations and strategies suggested in this chapter will assist you to formulate appropriate and functional (operationally defined as "enhancing positive effects for the child") communication goals and objectives, and identify and implement individualized intervention strategies. The objective of this chapter is to prepare you to make informed decisions about (a) sensory acuity, (b) learning strategies (limitations and preferences), (c) output capabilities, and (d) motivational variables. Table 5-1 presents an overview of the factors relevant to planning intervention strategies.

Before discussing these variables that have a profound effect on the likelihood of generating functional and effective intervention strategies, we must make an important point about interpreting assessment data. It is not unusual to find, upon close examination of a child's language assessment data (or data in any domain) that there are many inconsistencies and even, sometimes, what appear to be contradictions among scores and reports. Too often the initial reaction to such inconsistencies is to view them as negating the quality or reliability of the test, the observations or the observers. This is a mistake.

Data inconsistencies may be evidence of the situation specificity of the child's language behavior, *not* an effect of imprecise observations or unreliable testing procedures. The interactionist position, which views behavior as the result of an interaction between prevailing stimulus condi-

TABLE 5-1 Factors to consider for functional and effective intervention

Instructionally Relevant Questions	Focus of Observations and Data Collection	Instructional Unit to Modify/adapt
1. What are the child's preferred and/or intact sensory modalities?	auditory acuity visual acuity tactile acuity gustatory acuity olfactory acuity	Stimulus
2. Does the child have learning strategy problems?	selective attention concept formation storage and retrieval	Stimulus
3. What are the child's functional output capabilities?	speech manual signing pointing directed gaze body movement gesture writing	Response
4. What are the environmental events most likely to motivate some form of controlling response?	desired/needed objects and events desired services	Consequences

tions and child characteristics, would, in fact, predict such inconsistencies. Evidence of differences in language performance across stimulus conditions is important data, and should be thoughtfully analyzed. If the stimulus variables contributing to the child's behavior inconsistencies can be isolated, this provides some insight as to the saliency of different stimuli (objects, settings, and persons), and the child's response preferences.

We return to those organismic and environmental variables which, because they control and/or influence language learning, affect the formulation of appropriate goals and objectives, and the selection of teaching strategies. Our emphasis is on the role each plays with respect to language learning and use, and on the relevancy of information concerning the respective roles for planning. The purpose of asking questions about the child's sensory acuity, learning strategies, output capabilities, and motivational characteristics is to generate information that will aid selection of antecedent conditions, functional output modes, and consequent events.

SENSORY ACUITY

If one or more of the avenues of learning (auditory, visual, tactile, olfactory and gustatory) is impaired or limited, the ease with which language can be acquired will be affected. In addition to providing some explanation for language difficulties, information about sensory efficiency and discrimination abilities is critical to intervention decision making. The following discussion draws heavily from Hollis and Carrier (1978), Riechle and Yoder (1979), Sailor et al. (1980), and Guess, Sailor and Baer (1977). All emphasize the importance of identifying and subsequently exploiting the child's most accessible and functional sensory modality or modalities.

The question is: What are the child's preferred and/or most intact sensory modalities?

Auditory acuity   Impaired hearing deprives the child of critical data about his physical, social, and linguistic environment. A young child who demonstrates any of the following physical or behavioral signs may have hearing difficulties and should be referred for audiometric assessment (Best, 1978; DuBose, 1979). Physical signs include

1. frequent colds and complaints of earaches
2. signs of discharge from the ears
3. breathing through the mouth
4. reported buzzing or ringing in the ears
5. frequent tonsil problems

Behavioral signs include

1. failure to respond when spoken to
2. failure to understand directions or simple questions
3. looking puzzled and/or asking for words of sentences to be repeated
4. avoidance of contact and extreme shyness with peers
5. cocking head to one side and studying a speaker's face

6. articulation problems
7. voice problems
8. a preference for high or low pitched sounds

Not surprisingly, hearing impairment affects performance on stand-ardized intelligence tests (Sullivan & Vernon, 1979). An alternative for hearing impaired infants is *Uzgiris and Hunt Ordinal Scales of Psycho-logical Development* (Uzgiris & Hunt, 1975) or, for 2 to 4 year olds, the *Smith-Johnson Nonverbal Performance Scale* (Smith & Johnson, 1977). Whatever tests are administered, it is important to interpret the re-sults in light of the interaction between the child's auditory capabilities and her test performance (Brackett, 1982). Distinguish between errors re-sulting from deficiencies in language knowledge and knowledge of the world, and those resulting from difficulty with the reception of auditory stimuli.

A variety of special assessment techniques has been developed for difficult-to-test infants and severely handicapped children (e.g., Bricker & Bricker, 1969; Lloyd, Spradlin & Reid, 1968; Fulton, 1974). However, even with the high success rate these techniques report (Fulton reports 92% success rate), most are not suitable for use with young and/or severely handicapped children. The conditioned play technique developed by Lloyd, Reid, and McManis (1968) also has limited usefulness because it re-quires motor responses that are beyond the capabilities of many children with severe neuromotor impairment. Likewise, the tangible reinforcement techniques suggested by Bricker and Bricker and others are inappropriate for severely developmentally delayed children who do not demonstrate the necessary awareness of cause-effect relationships (Bricker & Campbell, 1980). Light reinforcement techniques (Miller, Rabinowitz, Frost, & Sea-ger, 1969) are somewhat more promising except, of course, with the visu-ally impaired.

> It is extremely difficult to find assessment techniques appropriate for very young and/or severely handicapped children.

A group at San Francisco State University has recently addressed the problem of difficult-to-test children (Sailor, Guess, Goetz, Schuler, Utley & Baldwin, 1980). Suitable for classroom implementation, these screening procedures yield some data about accessibility of the auditory channel and prepare the child for more intensive assessment by an audi-ologist. They are relatively simple to implement, with or without amplifica-tion.

> There are some promising new techniques for as-sessing the auditory acuity of severely handicapped children.

If the child is imitative, the specialist or teacher should provide a vo-cal model of sounds in the child's repertoire and compare the child's vocal imitations when she can see the model's face versus trials without a visual cue. If the child is nonimitative, the specialist or teacher should record re-sponses to different sounds such as speech, environmental noises, and noisemakers (e.g., small bells, squeak toys). One sound at a time should be presented (no more than 12 inches from the child's head), with alterna-tive presentations of the stimuli 3 to 4 inches on either side of the posterior midline. Hold each stimulus in position for 10 seconds or so before activating the sound for 2 to 3 seconds. Any differences in response, even the most subtle, when signals are sounded on the right or the left side should be recorded.

Cohen and Gross (1979) provide a list of infant auditory development pinpoints that provide categories for scoring of the child's responses to the recorded sounds. Roughly three developmental response stages can be delineated:

Look for evidence that will allow you to identify the child's responses stage.

Stage 1 Attention responses:
1. stops or lessens movement
2. tightens eyelids, blinks or shifts eyes
3. startles-stiffens, quivers, extends limbs

Stage 2 Localization responses:
1. turns head and visually searches on either side of stimulus
2. turns head and localizes below and above the stimulus
3. locates sound stimulus immediately at all angles

Stage 3 Discrimination responses:
1. vocalizes more in response to animate than to inanimate sounds
2. smiles when talked to
3. stops ongoing activity in response to "no-no"
4. quiets and attends to mother's voice more than to a stranger's voice

Responses at any of the three levels indicate receipt of auditory signals, but Stage 3 responses are most sophisticated. Higher level responses may suggest greater auditory acuity and/or a somewhat more advanced cognitive ability.

Visual acuity   The educational implications of poor conjugate eye movements (when the child's eyes do not work together) are pervasive. The child's field of vision is limited, there is no compensation for the blind spot in each eye, and depth perception is impaired (Sailor et al., 1980).

As in the area of auditory acuity, procedures to assess the visual acuity of very young and/or severely handicapped children have been limited by the restricted response capabilities of these populations. Until recently, what procedures were available were difficult to implement in classroom settings. The following strategies, like those suggested in the previous section, were generated by Sailor et al. Data from these observations should be reported to a pediatric ophthalmologist experienced in dealing with the severely handicapped. Very often, corrective lens, patches, and/or training exercises can be prescribed.

Conjugate eye movements can be assessed by following these steps in a darkened room. (a) Seat the child approximately 12-18 inches in front of you. If the child is unable to maintain a sitting position, place her supine with flexion at neck, hips and knees. Position yourself so that the child's face is on the same plane as yours and look directly into her eyes.

Assess the child's conjugate eye movements, visual field, and central vision.

Introduce a brightly colored (yellow or green) object such as a penlight inside a "pop" bead or a finger puppet and note whether the object is reflected exactly in the center of each pupil. Practice this procedure with an adult before implementation with children to assure that the observation can be made as quickly and accurately as necessary. (b) Conjugate tracking can be assessed with the same object and with you and the child in the same position. After she has fixated on the object, move it on a horizontal plane to both sides and note (1) if tracking occurs, and (2) whether both eyes follow the object smoothly. If one eye wanders, that eye is probably not providing the child with meaningful input. (c) Now, using the same object again and the same positioning, obtain fixation on the object at a distance of 18 inches in front of the child. Move it quickly toward the tip of her nose, and note whether the object is reflected evenly in both pupils up to 4-6 inches from the tip of her nose.

Evaluation of the child's *visual field* requires the manipulation of two penlights in a darkened room. Position yourself and the child in the same manner as before with your faces on the same plane. One of the child's eyes should be "occluded" with an eye patch. Hold one penlight at nose level approximately 18 inches from midline, and the second penlight at arm's length in eight different positions, one at a time. You will eventually want to make a complete circle around the child's head with the penlight at arm's length.

These tests do not replace thorough assessment by an ophthalmologist.

Begin the test with both lights off. Switch on the penlight that is held at nose level (repeated flicking on/off may be required initially to get the child's attention) until the child fixates. Then, simultaneously, switch this midline light off and switch the light that is held at arm's length on. Note whether the child shifts fixation to the second light source. Then, turn the second light off and, in the darkness, position your outstretched arm up and repeat the procedure. Record the child's shift or lack of shifting in fixation to up, down, right, and left and midway points for two complete circles. Repeat this procedure for a smaller circle 10-12 inches from the child's nose.

Failures to respond to the light in outer or inner circle positions is reason for immediate referral to an ophthalmologist because it may indicate a degenerative condition of the retina requiring medical intervention. The learning implication of a restricted visual field is inefficient visual scanning.

Central vision is the third class of visual behavior that you should consider. If the child is reasonably cooperative, central vision can be measured by an ophthalmologist with the use of drops to dilate the pupils and an ophthalmoscope. If the child is not cooperative enough for this procedure, you can experiment with stimuli at different measured distances to determine the distance appropriate for presentation of training stimuli.

The findings from these visual tests, like those from auditory assessment, should be considered when making decisions about antecedent stimuli for language training. They also contribute to understanding the child's language problems. Severely impaired or totally nonfunctional vision (even if the child demonstrates no other handicaps) can partially account for language delay because the reduction or absence of visual input affects the child's exploration of her environment which, in turn, affects language development. The visually impaired child is also at a disadvantage in social interactions. The development of social interactions, through which the normal child learns interactive communication devices, is hampered because facial expressions, body postures, and other avenues of nonverbal communication are largely unavailable to the vision-impaired child. Visual impairment also interferes with the acquisition of basic self-help skills like dressing, eating, and personal hygiene which children with vision acquire to some extent through modeling.

Language delay in the visually impaired child can be attributed to lack of mobility and socialization opportunities as well as reduced visual input.

Tactile acuity   Impairment in tactile perception modifies and distorts the detail of a child's cognitive map of the environment in much the same way, though to a lesser extent, as visual or auditory impairments (Hollis & Schiefelbusch, 1979). Unfortunately there is practically no research on tactile acuity and preferences of severely handicapped children. The primary source of information in this area is limited developmental data on the tactile preferences of infants and the tactile discrimination abilities of nonhandicapped children.

Wolff (1963) observed that 7-week old infants smile in response to tactile-kinesthetic stimulation (patting and gentle rubbing). At 4 months, they smile when tickled (Washburn, 1929). Later, 2-year-olds demonstrate maximum enjoyment in contact with water (splashing, hand washing, and water play with containers), sand, and sand/water combinations (Gesell, Ilg, Ames, & Rodell, 1974). At 2½, their sense of touch is well developed as demonstrated by preferences for such textures as silk, fur, and angora. However, they continue to revel in water and water-based substances like mud. Discrimination of textures continues to improve until a child is about 8 or 10 years old and then levels off (Warren, 1977). Most studies that have compared the tactile discrimination abilities of visually impaired children with those of sighted children have failed to support the notion that the former group are somehow endowed with superior capabilities.

Assess tactile responsiveness by experimenting with different types of physical contact, and different textures and sensations.

It is not unusual to find severely handicapped children who demonstrate *tactile defensiveness* (an adverse reaction to being touched). The child has to be desensitized to touching and holding. Meals are a good time to begin gradually increasing the degree and duration of tactile contact. When the child readily accepts contact during caregiving, different types and degrees of tactile stimulation can be systematically programmed.

Gustatory and olfactory acuity   Except for some tertiary attention from educators of the blind, the senses of taste and smell have been virtually ignored as learning modalities. These senses are very primitive compared to the visual, auditory and tactile senses, but they are sometimes extremely important when dealing with severely multiply handicapped children.

The usual approach to assessing smell is to note differential responses to the various common spices (e.g., ginger, cloves, cinnamon) and types of perfume (Cohen & Gross, 1979). Considering that infants even as young as 32–68 hours respond differently to a variety of olfactory stimuli (Engen & Lipsett, 1965), it is highly probable that even the most severely impaired children are able to discriminate some smells.

Assess responses to substances in each of the major taste categories.

Normally, five major taste categories—sweet, sour, bitter, salty, and metallic—are discriminable by the gustatory sense. With one exception, taste preferences appear to be learned. The exception is sweetness which is excluded because of evidence that even newborns can differentiate among different concentrations of sugar as well as different kinds of sugar like glucose and lactose (Scott, 1969; Caplan, 1973). Very young infants prefer the sweetness of fruit (bananas and applesauce are first choices) over vegetables, as anyone who has been sprayed with strained spinach or some other vegetable will readily attest.

Texture should be considered along with taste when assessing gustatory preferences. A 1-year old probably rejects pureed meat because of its sticky, granular texture rather than its taste. As wide and varied a range of foods and drinks as possible, including smooth, crunchy, chewy, and dry textures as well as sour, salty, bitter, and sweet tastes, should be provided to obtain a true picture of discrimination ability and preferences.

When selecting instructional stimuli, take the child's sensory preferences and strengths into account.

In summary, it is important to identify and capitalize on a child's preferred sensory modalities and avoid instructional stimuli that rely on the less preferred and/or weaker senses. This does not mean ignoring the weaker senses when developing intervention strategies because, in many cases, the weaker senses can be significantly strengthened, either with prosthetic devices or training. The point is to arrange antecedent conditions to take advantage of the child's strengths, particularly when new and complex stimuli are being presented.

LEARNING STRATEGIES

In Farham-Diggory (1972), Bruner defines information processing as the way in which an individual achieves, transforms, and retains knowledge.

The process approach to intervention should not be confused with information processing *research*, which has generated some very useful data.

There are several reasons we prefer to use the term *learning strategies* for this phenomenon. First is the connotation of more active and deliberate control; a learning strategy is usually thought of as an activity undertaken by an individual to cope with the requirements of a task or solve a problem. In contrast, information processing suggests a passive flow of information through perceptual and cognitive systems (e.g., Waugh & Norman, 1965). There is an implication that the information is active, but the individual is not.

Another reason for preferring the term *learning strategies* is that it allows some dissociation from intervention philosophies referred to as the *process approach* or *specific abilities approach*. The lack of clearcut experimental data verifying these intervention philosophies has lead to skepticism about the validity of information processing constructs in general (Salvia & Ysseldyke, 1981).

One reason the information processing approach has fallen into disrepute is that early proponents of this approach (e.g., Frostig & Horne, 1964; Getman, 1965; Kephart, 1971; Kirk & Kirk, 1971) tended to view processing abilities as *causing* specific language and reading related diffi-culties. The implication was that processing problems, even though not directly observable, can be reliably assessed and remediated, and that remediation will have a direct effect on such critical skills as language and reading. All currently available tests and programs based on this premise have serious shortcomings.

There is no evidence that information processing dif-ficulties *cause* learning problems but they are use-ful in *describing* them.

The Illinois Test of Psycholinguistic Abilities (ITPA) (Kirk, McCarthy, & Kirk, 1968) is one example of a test based on the information processing approach. It consists of 12 subtests, each designed to measure an aspect of psycholinguistic processing ability *presumed* to be central to language learning. There are numerous remedial programs and activities, particu-larly for learning disabled children, based on the processing ability deficits this test purports to isolate. Some professionals continue to use these pro-cedures despite the lack of data demonstrating that psycholinguistic train-ing based on the ITPA is successful, at least when the ITPA is the criterion for successful training (Hammill & Larsen, 1974, 1978).

There is little scientific sup-port for the ITPA as a diag-nostic tool or as the basis for remediation.

There are at least three possible explanations for the fact that "psy-cholinguistic training" based on ITPA results has not been very successful (Bloom & Lahey, 1978):

1. The ITPA subtests do not, in fact, measure the distinct abilities underlying language knowledge and use
2. Low scores on the subtests may not be valid indicators of weak-nesses in the abilities underlying language knowledge and use
3. Remediation of the deficits identified by subtest scores simply may not transfer to general improvement in the knowledge or use of language

We must emphasize again that we are not contending that there is no relationship between information processing (or learning strategies) and language learning (or between psycholinguistic abilities and language performance). We contend that there is no clear relationship between ITPA scores, training based on these scores, and language learning. To the credit of its developers, the ITPA ushered in a new assessment perspective. At the time that it was introduced, the majority of assessment instruments were designed for identification and placement only. The ITPA was one of the first instruments developed for the express purpose of generating data useful for planning and implementing individualized instruction. As such, it was a valuable contribution to discovery of new dimensions for assessment-intervention linkages.

The basic problem with the ITPA (and other instruments and proce-dures directed towards information processing) seems to be a confusion of correlation with causation. That there are processing differences be-tween normal and atypical language learners is undeniable. The mistake is in assuming that these differences are sufficient to cause language diffi-culties. It could as easily be the other way around; language difficulties may, in some way, affect information processing. Also, there is the reality

The extent to which lan-guage problems affect in-formation processing, or vice versa, is not at all clear.

of environmental variables, the effects of which simply cannot be overlooked when considering language learning. Processing dysfunctions alone, although they may be demonstrated to *correlate* with language learning problems, are not sufficient to *cause* them. There are many other variables to take into account.

As emphasized above, the fact that information processing approaches to assessment and remediation have not been particularly successful *does not negate* the usefulness of the phenomena referred to as information processing abilities or learning strategies. That we have not been able to effectively isolate, measure, and/or train these abilities is no reason to ignore their potential contributions to language learning. Understanding the learning strategies a child lacks, or is not applying, can help you decide *how* and, to a lesser extent, *what* to program.

The selection and display of training stimuli, determination of response modalities, and other instructional decisions require knowledge of the language learning process and understanding of a child's learning strategies. Stated another way, developing the most effective intervention procedures requires us to "stack the cards in the child's favor." Arranging conditions so that the potential for success is maximized requires a thorough understanding of the game itself (language learning), as much information as possible about the cards (knowledge) the child is presently holding, and data concerning her playing strategies (skills). How well the child plays the game (and ultimately, whether she wins it) depends, in large part, on how skilled we are in stacking the deck (collecting and using relevant information).

The next section considers the learning activities thought to occur between sensation and response in normal learners. We summarize what is known about these learning strategies and present some programming suggestions based on these findings. If information about the learning strategies of a handicapped child is not available at the time the IEP is developed, place a high priority on collecting information about the child's selective attention, concept formation, and memory strategies during the initial phases of instruction.

To get an idea of what learning strategies are, consider how a child comes to "know" an object, event, or relation. First she must selectively attend to its relevant features. The next step is interpreting, transforming, organizing, and comparing whatever sensory information the stimulus provides to stored memory representations (concepts) accumulated from past experiences with similar stimuli. These learning strategies (attending, interpreting, transforming, organizing, and comparing) are cognitive responses intermediary between the sensory input (seeing, hearing, touching, smelling, and tasting) and language. Every new sensation and experience represents a learning problem that calls for identification and mobilization of these essential strategies. They are the means of knowing.

Learning strategies are cognitive responses intermediary between sensory impressions and language.

The sensorimotor actions of infancy described in Chapter Two (e.g., object manipulation, imitation, play) are operations or learning experiences that stimulate and develop the child's earliest learning strategies.

From birth, the infant begins preparing for the complex perceptual and cognitive problem solving related to "knowing" at the representational level, evident around 18 to 24 months.

One of the most interesting characteristics of learning, at any age but particularly during the developmental years, is its selectivity. There are certain qualifications that appear to affect what can and will be learned at any time (when and if learning strategies will be mobilized). There are two readiness hypotheses—Hunt's "match hypothesis" (1961, 1965) and Seligman's "preparedness hypothesis" (1975)—that highlight the selectivity of learning.

Readiness theories highlight the selectivity of learning.

Seligman proposes a "preparedness" continuum with "prepared" at one extreme and "contraprepared" at the other as a way of conceptualizing readiness for learning. Two types of events or stimuli are at the prepared extreme: (a) those the child is perceptually and cognitively ready to learn and (b) those that are critical or adaptive for survival. An example of perceptual readiness would be the infant's sensitivity and responsiveness to speech sounds (preparedness to learn language). An example of learning critical for survival would be the concept *hot,* which the young child learns early and quickly, usually after only one experience with something hot.

Contraprepared learning, at the other extreme of the continuum, is learning for which the child is not motorically or cognitively prepared. For example, toddlers do not have the perceptual and cognitive sophistication to perform conservation operations; their attraction to irrelevant perceptual cues such as height, width, size, shape, and color precludes selective attention to the relevant task dimensions. This is not to say that preparedness is *essential* for learning or that contrapreparedness means that learning is impossible. It simply suggests what is learned most easily and what is most likely to be retained. Seligman's preparedness continuum, like Piagetian stages, predicts the amount of time and effort that is required to teach a given task and the extent of generalization to expect.

The "preparedness hypothesis" states that experiences and stimuli the child is perceptually and cognitively ready to learn and those that are critical for survival will be learned more easily than others.

Closely related to Seligman's preparedness hypothesis is Hunt's "match hypothesis" (Hunt, 1961, 1965) which suggests that children are intrigued by, and therefore selectively attend to, information that is moderately discrepant from what they already know. What is too similar to prior experiences (termed low discrepancy stimuli) or too complex (high discrepancy stimuli) will be discounted and generally ignored. Only stimuli halfway on the continuum of complexity (or discrepancy) relative to the child's cognitive level will be meaningful and learned. The instructional challenge is to arrange a proper relationship between environmental stimuli and preestablished concepts.

The "match hypothesis" suggests that children will more readily learn that which is moderately discrepant from what they already know.

The moderately discrepant construct applies at any level and age. Imagine yourself in a high school social studies class or an advanced anatomy class in medical school. In either case, the low complexity/discrepancy high school setting or the high complexity/discrepancy medical school setting, you will most likely tune out the instructional stimuli as too easy or too difficult. Presumably, the stimuli in your present classes are somewhere in the middle of these extremes, or moderately discrepant from what you already know.

Instructional stimuli should be difficult enough to make learning a challenge but not so complex that new concepts cannot be associated with knowledge formed through past experience. When planning and evaluating language training programs, keep both readiness hypotheses in mind. Readiness will undoubtedly affect the child's application of learning strategies. Our purpose in the next section is not to explicate the research concerned with learning processes in any detail, or to explore theoretical issues. We want to convey a sense of how some learning strategies, selective attention, concept formation, and storage and retrieval, are thought to operate.

Learning requires the identification of and attention to relevant stimuli or stimulus features.

Selective attention   Selective attention can be operationally defined as singling out and focusing upon particular stimuli or stimulus features in the vast array that is available at any time. More specifically, it is the child's ability to identify and attend to relevant sources of information and ignore the irrelevant features of a stimulus or task. The perception and localization of auditory and visual stimuli have received the most attention, but the ability to attend to relevant dimensions of other sensory information is also important. The existence of age-related changes in selective attention suggests a developmental continuum.

Historically, the most detailed and comprehensive work on attention was provided by Eleanor J. Gibson (1969). The essence of Gibson's theory is that with experience and practice children learn to isolate and attend to the specific features or feature combinations that differentiate between similar (but not too similar) stimuli. They also learn to attend with more than one sense at a time, and to coordinate input from two or more senses. The major tenets of Gibson's theory are: (a) The child's cognitive development imposes limitations on what can be attended to (among competing stimuli) and, therefore, what can be learned, and (b) the child learns to attend with increasing specificity. What this means is that learning tasks are approached with attentional biases and preferences at each stage of development; some stimulus dimensions (e.g., shape, size, color) are more or less salient at different times. To complicate matters further, different children have different preferences, and the same child may have different preferences in different settings (Flavell, 1977).

Selective attention propensities can be influenced by training and experiences.

On an optimistic note, Gibson suggests that the tendency to be distracted by irrelevant features can be reduced through training. Attentional dispositions should not discourage attempts to guide a young child's focus (e.g., highlighting relevant features). Certainly caregivers guide attention from their very earliest interactions with their infants. Research with handicapped children, as discussed in a subsequent section, has verified the assertion that selective attention can be influenced by training.

The terminology used by Piaget (Piaget and Inhelder, 1969) to talk about the selective attention process is different from Gibson's, but the conclusions are virtually the same. Piaget uses the term "decentration" to describe the child's increasing ability to selectively attend. He contends that children in the preoperational period (roughly the ages 2 to 4) focus or "centrate" on only one feature or property of a stimulus or one dimension of a task, and exclude all others. The inability of children at this age to conserve is attributed to this propensity for overselective attention. The preoperational child centrates either on the height of the taller container or the width of the wider container but seems incapable of attending to both. The fact that one dimension compensates for the other escapes the child's notice because they are not attended to simultaneously.

The ability to sustain attention focus, referred to as attention span or, more behaviorally, as "on task" behavior, is equally important for learning. Like selective attention, attention span varies among children, depending on the task and the child's age. When there are no distractions, attention span provides a rough measure of task or stimulus complexity and the intensity of whatever learning strategies are being brought to bear on the task. However, this measure must be interpreted with some caution. Differences in the duration of attention to a task may also indicate different cognitive styles. Children who display a tendency to respond quickly to task demands (with a high error rate) may have learned an impulsive cognitive style. Those who devote more attention to the task before responding (with a low error rate) may have learned to respond in this manner.

> Attention span is a rough measure of task complexity and the intensity of learning strategies that are being applied to the task.

Concept formation   Whether we favor the semantic position described in Chapter One (that language learning is learning to map preexisting nonlinguistic concepts) or the interactionist position (that language learning is a two-way street with preexisting concepts influencing the acquisition of linguistic skills and language influencing cognition), there is significant mental activity involved. It is difficult to functionally separate thinking from talking. The form of selected sensory information must be changed (without altering its meaning) and organized in some efficient manner, or it will not be useful for future reference. Concepts are the products of cognitive development; they are presumably measured by cognitive assessment instruments.

Recall from Chapter Two that we used the analogy of getting the kitchen in order to illustrate the classification or categorization task that faces the young child. At one point the kitchen analogy breaks down. We do not need to change the form of the kitchen items prior to organizing and storing them, but sensory input must be transformed before, or in the process of, classification. As Flavell (1977) says: "meaningful, structured inputs are not just copied or printed into memory at storage time . . . the act of comprehending and encoding into memory is a Piagetian assimilation-type process of *construction* of an internal conceptual representation of the input" (p. 192).

> Sensory input is not just copied or printed into memory; its form must be changed prior to organization and storage.

The young child is faced with the enormous task of constructing nonlinguistic categories (knowledge about objects and object relations) and linguistic categories (knowledge about words and relations between words). Construction of nonlinguistic categories begins at birth or shortly

You may want to review Chapter Two to refresh your memory of the details of early cognitive and linguistic development.

after. The child begins working on the second set of constructions at about the time of her first birthday. With experience and maturation of the central nervous system, she becomes more adept at recognizing linguistic and nonlinguistic constants among different events and stimuli and can deal with increasingly more numerous and varied sensory inputs.

Both linguistic and nonlinguistic concepts are necessary for language. As noted above, linguistic categories include knowledge about words (vocabulary) and relations between words (how words are combined to generate meaning). Construction of these categories entails substantially more than the mental representation of the sound sequence, so that the word can be spoken or recognized when it is heard. Each word concept must include sufficient information to "know" the word on five levels: (a) referential, (b) extended, (c) relational, (d) categorical, and (e) metalinguistic (Bloom & Lahey, 1978).

A word concept includes referential, extended, relational, categorical, and metalinguistic information about that word.

To know a word in the *referential* sense means knowing the object or event to which it refers. Knowing a word in its *extended* sense is knowing something about the range of objects and events to which it can be extended. The word "ball," for example, can be extended to many different round, bounceable, throwable objects (and to one type of not-so-round object which is as often kicked as thrown). Knowing a word in its *relational* sense means knowing the meanings it assumes when used with different words. For example, knowing "throw" in relation to "ball" is understanding the relational meaning between words that refer to an action and an affected object. Knowing a word in its *categorical* sense is knowing the different categories the word may belong to, knowing what semantic, perceptual, and functional categories this particular word shares with other words. "Ball" shares its throwable aspect of meaning with a number of other objects with otherwise different meanings. Likewise, its roundness property could lead to different categorization based on this perceptual attribute. The fifth sense in which a word must be known is termed *metalinguistic,* knowing about the word itself—that it is a word composed of sounds, etc.

Nonlinguistic categories are of two types, object concepts and concepts about object relations. Constructing a concept about a particular object requires sufficient knowledge of its physical structure (how it looks, sounds, feels, smells, tastes, what it is made of, etc.), so that the object can be recognized on subsequent encounters. Piaget (1954, 1970) calls the mental representation of this type of information "figurative knowing."

Additional questions to quantify concept formation are provided in Chapter Four.

Concepts about object relations, or "operative knowing," on the other hand, are mental representations of how the object relates to other objects (including the child) through movements or actions. This second category of concepts has to do with understanding what the object can do and/or what can be done with it. Together, these two broad categories of nonlinguistic concepts, object concepts and relational concepts, give the child something to talk about.

For prelinguistic children and children at the single-word stage, your observations and data collection to quantify concept formation strategies should focus on

1. Functional and symbolic play skills

   Does the child repeat various learned actions and combine them in a meaningful manner during object play?

   Does she demonstrate familiar actions and routines (without the objects to which they are usually applied) during play?

2. Means-end relationships and causality

   Does the child use objects as tools and apply foresight in solving simple problems?

3. Matching, sorting, and sequencing skills

   Can the child match similar objects? Can she sort objects by perceptual features (color, shape, etc.)?

   Can she sequence by size?

Other questions to guide observations of concept formation strategies for the child *functioning* cognitively below age 2 are presented in Chapter Four in the discussion on identifying *content* deficits.

Storage and retrieval   As the terms suggest, storage refers to putting information into memory; retrieval refers to recovery or recall of that information. There is no need to belabor the considerable importance of these abilities. If the conceptual products of experience are to be useful in the future, they must be retained and recoverable. Differentiation between what is called "memory" and what is called "knowledge" is difficult, and perhaps not too important; the two terms are almost synonymous as commonly applied.

> Information must be retained and recoverable if it is to be of future use.

Research generally differentiates three levels of memory: (a) sensory or immediate memory, (b) short-term memory, and (c) long-term memory. *Sensory or immediate memory* (also called iconic memory) is assumed to have a relatively large capacity, but an extremely brief duration. For approximately ¼ of a second, a trace of sensory stimuli is recorded and then, as quickly, lost or transferred on in the memory system. *Short-term memory* is also transitory; information is forgotten in a very short time.

> There are three levels of memory.

To be remembered, related information must be somehow organized in memory. The process of organizing related pieces of information together is called *chunking*. Chunking increases short-term memory capacity. Although there are numerous ways to chunk bits of information, chunking based on meaning has received the most attention. Ceci and Howe (1978) identify the competent "memorizer" as a child who is able to recall items by reference to meaning—e.g., "Is there something to eat on the list?". Nonsemantic chunking strategies, such as thinking of an item's color or location, are noticeably inferior to the semantic method (Geis & Hall, 1977).

> Two strategies to increase short-term memory are chunking and rehearsal.

The major syntactic breaks between clauses in sentences are an example of linguistic chunking. Without chunking of words into clauses, it would be difficult to remember a lengthy utterance long enough to comprehend the meaning and respond. Sentences, particularly complex ones, are not entered into and subsequently retrieved from short-term memory as lists of independent words. They are stored and retrieved as chunks or phrases. Likewise, the chunking of sounds into words makes it possible to retain far more than if sounds were unrelated and not separated by brief pauses.

A second short-term memory strategy is *rehearsal,* covert practice or repeating of bits or units to be remembered. In addition to reducing the time limitation on short-term memory, this strategy serves to strengthen the chained associations between units. Research by numerous investigators demonstrates enormous variability in when, what, and how people rehearse (e.g., Butterfield, Wambold, & Belmont, 1973; Flavell, 1970). Rehearsal strategies also vary considerably in complexity and sophistication.

Theoretically, the storage capacity of long-term memory is unlimited. Storage duration varies from minutes to a lifetime. The content of long-term memory (what is stored, retained, and retrieved) depends on what fits readily into existing knowledge structures. It remains an open question whether linguistic concepts are stored in a manner similar to nonlinguistic concepts but separately, or whether the two are part of a general mental capability (Bloom & Lahey, 1978). What is clear, however, is that there is a mental plan for language. This plan includes stored information about linkages between linguistic and nonlinguistic categories and basic principles guiding use and expansion of language knowledge. No matter how this plan is organized (by feature collections, semantic categories, and/or associative labyrinths), one thing is certain—the storage system is exceedingly complex and constantly changing.

Information can be stored in long-term memory by rehearsal, chunking, imagery, and associations.

Strategies for putting information into *long-term memory* include (a) rehearsal, (b) chunking, (c) imagery, and (d) association. Because rehearsal and chunking are also short-term memory strategies they have already been described. *Imagery* involves visualizing (imagining a picture of) either the event or events to be remembered or something that symbolizes the event(s). One imagery technique is to deliberately generate an absurd situation linking two or more objects or events that you want to remember. This imagery strategy works best with concrete concepts and for people with good visualization skills. A new event may be given significance by deliberate *association* with existing linguistic or nonlinguistic categories, or new information may be associated (pre-grouped) according to semantic commonalities. The greater the number and strength of meaningful associations with existing knowledge, and the better new items or events cluster by semantic category (e.g., food, utensils, emotions), the greater the likelihood for retention.

Retrieval strategies include the use of specific cues, use of general knowledge, and inference.

Retrieval strategies are as important as storage strategies. *Perseverance* (continuing to search for a sought after item which does not come to mind immediately) is one retrieval strategy. More elaborate retrieval strategies involve the use of specific cues (e.g., "I remember she was wearing shorts..."), use of general knowledge about the world, and inference or logic ("so it must have been last summer sometime"). Research considering retrieval strategies shows the same age-by-treatment effects encountered in other memory research. The strategic use of retrieval cues seems to involve a complex interaction of knowledge and skill (Kobashigawa, 1974, 1976). Relatively little is known about deficiencies in this area, but Flavell (1977) suggests that they may be a consequence of lack of foresight in storing, application of the wrong retrieval strategy, or lack of knowledge about retrieval strategies.

In summary, while learning strategies are not observable, their effects on a child's performance certainly are. As Sidman (1980, p. 286) has noted "...all responses are controlled, if not by stimuli the experimenter has specified, then by others." The teacher's and/or communication specialist's task is to analyze the elements of stimuli or tasks to which the child gives a correct response, those to which she gives an incorrect response, *and* the nature of the response. Etzel, Bickel, Stella, and LeBlanc (1982, p. 197) caution that "it is not enough to know that a child makes an error. It is necessary to know the specific dimensions that are related to the occurrence of that error." Information generated by this type of error analysis can guide selection of effective procedures and materials.

There is one additional set of learning strategies—the selection and initiation of responses. These strategies are discussed in the next section because they relate to output capabilities. We state now that humans "can react with only a relatively small variety of behaviors to an immensely large number of distinct stimuli" (Moerk, 1977, p. 69). Response limitations are most evident when dealing with infants, young children, and the severely multiply handicapped.

ATYPICAL LEARNING STRATEGIES

There are still many unanswered questions about how the various aspects of learning develop and interact, and the relationship of certain learning strategies (or lack of them) to observable performance. However, there has been a significant amount of research demonstrating that handicapped and nonhandicapped children differ in how and when they apply certain learning strategies. Further, there are some data, summarized below, that suggest differences across disability subgroups. We emphasize, however, that these differences are not sufficient to require qualitatively different instructional programming. The recommendations for arranging antecedent conditions presented at the end of this section will benefit any child who gives evidence of having the identified learning strategy problem.

Handicapped and nonhandicapped children differ in how and when they apply certain learning strategies.

Learning strategy problems associated with mental retardation   At least some of the problems of mentally retarded children summarized in Table 5-2 may derive from the fact that they have not developed the learning strategies that will enable them to benefit maximally from their experiences. They frequently overlook the cues that could help them solve problems and generally fail to take outcomes of previous trials into account (Robinson & Robinson, 1976). However, once cues are perceived as relevant to problem solving and attended to, learning may proceed in much the same manner as for normal learners.

TABLE 5-2 Learning strategy problems associated with mental retardation

Selective attention problems

1. Failure to differentiate relevant from irrelevant stimuli (Robinson & Robinson, 1976)
2. Taking longer to attend to relevant task dimensions (Zeaman & House, 1963). This finding may only apply to the more severely retarded
3. Overselective attention to only a few stimuli dimensions to the exclusion of other information (Wolfe & Cuvo, 1978)

Concept formation problems

1. Atypical pattern of development of object permanence (Wohlheuter & Sindberg, 1975)
2. Inefficient use of verbal mediation to learn associations (MacMillan, 1977)
3. Difficulty grouping sensory impressions into appropriate semantic categories (Roaden, McCauley, & Sperber, 1980)

Storage and retrieval problems

1. Failure to spontaneously apply mnemonic strategies such as rehearsal, chunking, and association (McDade & Adler, 1980)

Selective attention can be enhanced by careful selection, arrangement and presentation of training stimuli.

There are a variety of methods to enhance and maximize selective attention. Most require careful attention to the selection, arrangement and presentation of antecedent training stimuli. (Applying systematic reinforcement procedures for orientation and focus on the learning task and extending attention span are discussed in Chapter Six.) Training stimuli should vary only on critical dimensions. For example, if you are teaching color, initially it should be the only dimension on which the training stimuli differ, and target colors should be significantly brighter than distractor colors. Linguistic signals can be varied by intensity, frequency, rate, and prosody (pitch, intonation, stress, pause, and duration). The salience of a sound, word, or phrase can be increased by exaggerating one or several of these dimensions. Caregivers and effective preschool teachers are skilled in application of highlighting devices to direct the attention of infants and young children. They use higher pitch, special intonations and rhythm structures, rhymes and repetitions to exaggerate relevant linguistic stimuli. Emphasizing important sounds, words, and phrases with these input features cues the child to pay attention and assists mental organization of units.

One way to reduce the potential of irrelevant visual stimuli in the acquisition stage of learning is to darken the room and spotlight relevant stimuli with a flashlight. Noisemakers, such as bells or a buzzer, can be used to attract the child's attention to a linguistic signal. It is possible to take advantage of natural attentional predispositions by selecting antecedent stimuli with the properties of novelty, movement and change. The key is to simplify the child's learning task and compensate for selective attention deficiencies by exaggerating and highlighting to maximize saliency.

There is also evidence that construction of the object permanence concept, which is problematic for many retarded children, can be affected by training (Brassell & Dunst, 1978; Bricker, Macke, Levin & Campbell, 1981; Robinson, 1975). Most training programs derive from Piaget's (1926) descriptions of his own children's progress toward attainment of object permanence or from the Uzgiris-Hunt scales that are based on Piaget's work. Programming should proceed through an ordered series of activities: (a) basic sensory organization responses (e.g., visual orientation, fixation, tracking), (b) multisensory coordinations (e.g., looking-sucking, looking-reaching, looking-grasping, looking-listening), (c) recognition of partly hidden objects, (d) search for objects seen disappearing, and (e) search for objects when the hiding place is unknown.

> Programming for object permanence should proceed through an orderly sequence of steps.

Another deficiency demonstrated by some retarded children is difficulty clustering or grouping their sensory impressions into the appropriate semantic categories. They do not seem to approach the task in the same way as normal learners or arrive at the same basic classifications (Roaden, McCauley, and Sperber, 1980). Instead of basing construction of semantic classes on relevant thematic or semantic bits of information, retarded children are likely to rely on such irrelevant cues as spatial arrangement (Baumeister and Smith, 1979). It is easy to see how inappropriate organizational strategies of this nature could be interrelated with and, in part, responsible for the semantic (content) difficulties demonstrated by mentally retarded children (Bartel, Bryan, & Keehn, 1973; Semmel, Barritt, Bennett & Perfetti, 1968; Strichart & Gottlieb, 1982) and for their general delay in language development.

> Retarded children often demonstrate problems related to categorization of sensory information.

Any type of instructional method that reduces the information load (by making the particular invariant properties more salient) will assist the child to abstract, transform and classify information. The intrinsic-action properties of inanimate objects and the static properties of animate objects need to be particularly stressed because retarded children tend to overlook these less salient characteristics. Concept formation can be aided by presenting instructional stimuli, linguistic and nonlinguistic, in blocks. Linguistic stimuli can be grouped by repetition and/or pauses. Nonlinguistic stimuli can be placed in close physical proximity and you can remind the learner to organize by requesting recall by category (e.g., "Tell me about the animals you saw").

In addition to strategies for forming nonlinguistic (content) categories and linguistic (form) categories, children must learn strategies for linking content and form. To assist this learning, it is important to make certain that the linguistic form (either word, sign, or graphic symbol) or forms that express a concept and the concept itself co-occur. Arrange for the child to experience the nonlinguistic concept (what is being referred to) and the symbol(s) simultaneously. For example, stress and repeat the word "ride" while the child is engaging in that activity (e.g., on a tricycle, in the car), and always label objects that the child demonstrates an interest in.

Retarded individuals are less apt to spontaneously apply mnemonic strategies such as rehearsal, chunking and association to cope with task

> Retarded children often fail to apply appropriate memory strategies.

demands and solve problems (McDade & Adler, 1980). They generally fail to adopt a mnemonic strategy, even when a strategy is clearly indicated and would be beneficial and adaptive (Brown, 1974; Ellis, 1970). Data pointing to a rehearsal deficit are particularly persuasive. However, the researchers who have investigated this phenomenon have found that retarded subjects can, with systematic instruction, be taught rehearsal strategies (Belmont & Butterfield, 1971), and there is also evidence of maintenance and generalization of the trained strategies to later tasks (Brown, Campione, & Murphy, 1974; Kellas, Ashcroft, & Johnson, 1973). Research on rehearsal strategy training suggests the value of labeling and verbal associations. Continuous repetition and practice of acquired skills (overlearning) in the training setting and in other contexts is desirable. In the acquisition stage of training, select tasks that are meaningful to the child, analyze the tasks into sequential steps, and incorporate multisensory stimuli.

Learning strategy problems associated with learning disabilities Although some authorities continue to maintain that a processing deficiency is at the core of the learning problems of learning disabled children (e.g., Cruickshank, 1976), others attach more significance to lack of understanding of when and how to apply particular learning strategies (e.g., Hallahan & Reeve, 1980). Learning disabled children do seem to approach learning differently. There appears to be little generalization of learned strategies across problems, even very similar ones. Table 5-3 provides a summary of the learning strategy problems of learning disabled children.

TABLE 5-3   Learning strategy problems associated with learning disabilities

---

Selective attention problems
1. Two to three year developmental lag in the ability to selectively attend (Hallahan & Reeve, 1980)
2. Failure to apply verbal rehearsal strategies to tasks requiring selective attention (Hallahan & Reeve, 1980)
3. Poor performance when there are proximal distractors (Hallahan & Bryan, 1981)

Concept formation problems
1. Failure to generalize problem-solving strategies across contexts
2. Deficiencies in reasoning and visualization (Hill, 1980)
3. Semantic or syntactic deficit in the processing of rapidly presented auditory material (McNutt & Chia-Yen Li, 1980)

Storage and retrieval problems
1. Greater likelihood of experiencing memory problems with linguistic than with nonlinguistic information (Hallahan and Bryan, 1981)
2. Failure to spontaneously apply affective strategies on memory tasks
   · (Haines & Torgesen, 1979)

Learning-disabled children are often characterized as having an impulsive cognitive style. When the correct response to a task is ambiguous, they respond hastily without thinking, and make many errors because they do not take the time to consider available alternatives. Attempts to modify impulsive responding, in the hope that altering response style will improve academic performance, have generally met with limited success (e.g., Zelniker & Jeffrey, 1976). It may be, as McKinney and Haskins (1980) argue, that impulsivity is not a response style problem at all but rather a learning strategy problem. Impulsive children can be taught to slow down; when they do, they make significantly fewer mistakes.

> Impulsivity may be less a response style problem than a learning strategy problem.

In an extensive review of research dealing with the learning strategies of learning disabled children, Hallahan and Bryan (1981) found that selective attention abilities and memory have been studied the most. The consensus of the selective attention research is that learning disabled children do not appear to be bothered by distal distractors but perform poorly when there are proximal (near) distractors. They perform as well, and sometimes even better, than their normal peers when an experimenter attempts to distract them with distal distractors such as a loud noise, flashing lights or balloons dropping from the ceiling. However, they have difficulty attending to relevant stimuli in the presence of proximal irrelevant stimuli (e.g., too many pictures on a worksheet). Instead of selectively attending to the central learning task, they focus on incidental and irrelevant details.

> Learning disabled children are most distracted by *proximal* irrelevant stimuli.

Recent research on the memory abilities of learning disabled children (Hallahan & Bryan, 1981) leads to the conclusion that storage and retrieval of linguistic information is a greater problem than remembering nonlinguistic information. Described as passive rather than active learners, these youngsters appear capable of performing the appropriate memory activities, but they do not apply them when application is indicated.

Instructional procedures under the broad rubric of "cognitive-behavior-modification" (CBM) may be the most promising for these youngsters. These methods, which combine behavior therapy and cognitive theory, assume that children can learn to guide themselves through a series of steps to solve a problem. The child is taught and provided with opportunities to practice a small set of problem attack subskills and rules for combining these subskills.

Learning strategy problems associated with autism   Table 5-4 summarizes the learning strategy problems demonstrated by many autistic children. A large body of experimental research shows that many children labeled as autistic have attention problems (e.g., Lovaas, Schreibman, Koegel, & Rehm, 1971; Lovaas, Koegel & Schreibman, 1979; Lovaas & Schreibman, 1971). When presented with a multimodal stimulus array, they tend to perseveratively focus on one stimulus or a particular set of cues to the exclusion of others. Instead of selectively searching for relevant cues to facilitate learning, as normal learners do, their behavior is often controlled by irrelevant stimuli; they attend to a narrowed range of the available stimuli. *Stimulus overselectivity* is the term given to this attention problem.

TABLE 5-4   Learning strategy problems associated with autism

Selective attention problems

1. Tendency to perseveratively focus on one irrelevant stimulus (or a particular set of cues) rather than search for relevant stimuli (Lovaas et al., 1971)

2. Tendency to respond to acoustic stimuli as a whole rather than separate features (Hermelin, 1971)

Concept formation problems

1. Failure to profit from the systematic and rule-governed (as opposed to random) presentation of stimuli (Hermelin, 1976)

2. Deficient coding and classification of sensory information (Hermelin, 1976)

3. Tendency to learn isolated discrimination rather than underlying rules (Bormann & Schuler, 1978)

Storage and retrieval problems

1. Tendency to recall nonsense material equally as well as meaningful information (Hermelin, 1971)

2. Severe deficits in short-term memory skills (Hermelin & O'Connor, 1970)

One of the most commonly cited learning problems associated with autism is overselectivity.

Some researchers suggest that overselectivity to both auditory and visual stimuli may be responsible for the language difficulties that characterize autistic children (Lovaas et al., 1971; Reynolds, Newsom, & Lovaas, 1974). Language learning requires attention to a range of linguistic and nonlinguistic stimuli as well as visual-auditory associations. To acquire meaningful language a child needs to hear or see a word representing a concept and experience the object or relation the concept represents simultaneously. The more experience she has with these visual-auditory associations, the greater the likelihood of inducing form/content interactions. If a child attends to only one cue or one feature of a stimulus at a time, she is not going to learn the correct associations. She may not learn any associations at all.

Stimulus overselectivity has pervasive and negative consequences for learning.

Stimulus overselectivity can also affect social interactions. The child misses nonverbal social cues if she attends to the auditory signal and vice versa. Most autistic children avoid social interactions—the primary context for language learning.

Observational learning is also severely restricted by stimulus overselectivity. Varni, Lovaas, Koegal, and Everett (1979) found that when autistic children observed a situation where a teacher gave a command and then rewarded a model for compliance, most of their autistic subjects learned only part of the response chain. Those few autistic children who did learn the complete response failed to associate it with the appropriate stimulus.

Other consequences of stimulus overselectivity include difficulty shifting from prompts to training stimuli (Koegel & Rincover, 1976) and lack of generalization. A study by Rincover and Koegel (1975) suggests that, for autistic children, the amount of generalization varies with the number of relevant cues that control the behavior in the training setting. The fewer the stimuli initially controlling the behavior, the less likely it is to generalize to other settings.

Many researchers have investigated ways to circumvent the overselectivity problem. The most effective seems to be within-stimulus prompting. Schreibman (1975) found that children could be taught to discriminate distinctive features by using a within-stimulus prompt and then fading-in less relevant stimuli. (A within-stimulus prompt is one that emphasizes or exaggerates the relevant stimulus element.) This eliminates the necessity to respond to multiple cues initially.

Rincover (1978) extended overselectivity research. He examined four treatment procedures designed to facilitate prompt fading: (a) within-stimulus distinctive feature, (b) within-stimulus nondistinctive feature, (c) extra-stimulus distinctive feature, and (d) extra-stimulus nondistinctive feature. The first was most effective. Using the within-stimulus distinctive feature plan, the child is first pretrained to respond to the feature of the target stimulus that discriminates it from the other stimulus. This feature is exaggerated and presented alone. Then the target stimulus and distractor stimulus are presented together, with the pretrained exaggerated feature superimposed on the target stimulus. The exaggerated feature is gradually faded until the target stimulus takes its normal form and the child consistently discriminates it from the distractor.

Evidence of cross-modal association deficits and severe deficits in short-term memory skills further complicates learning for autistic children (Hermelin & O'Connor, 1970). It has been suggested that spatial, as opposed to temporal, arrangement of stimuli may facilitate the language learning of autistic children because a spatial arrangement does not place the same memory requirements on the child. Speech and manual signals are temporal stimuli (because they are essentially lost as soon as they have been produced), as opposed to graphic representations or concrete symbols such as the plywood or plastic form used by Premack (1970), and McLean (McCormick) and McLean (1974). Pictures, written words, and Blissymbols are others that also remain available as a relatively permanent reference.

Programming suggestions for children with learning strategy problems
There are two basic approaches to dealing with atypical learning strategies. Both require an understanding of the acquisition process and how it affects performance, and a clarification of the child's strategy deficit/deviation. The first question to ask is whether the problem is a selective attention deficit, a concept formation problem, or a memory difficulty. Once the child's problem has been pinpointed as precisely as possible, the next decision is procedural. Should the problem be dealt with by attending to the construction of antecedent conditions that compensate for and counteract the deficit? Or, should the programming focus be on teaching the

Use of within-stimulus prompts can circumvent the overselectivity problems.

Spatial, as opposed to temporal, arrangement of stimuli facilitates learning.

child how and when to use the learning strategies she is not effectively applying? In other words, the decision is whether to circumvent the problem or attack it directly.

The following basic recommendations derive from research about the learning strategy deficits of atypical learners. Some are recommendations for alterations to the arrangement of antecedent conditions. Others focus on establishing or increasing the use of particular learning strategies.

1. **Vary training stimuli on critical dimensions only** For example, when size is the critical dimension, initial training stimuli should not vary along any other dimensions. The same applies to color, shape, position, etc.

2. **Emphasize critical linguistic stimuli** Vary language input features along the dimensions of intensity, frequency, rate and prosody to increase saliency. Make use of pitch, special intonations, rhythm structures, rhymes, and repetitions to gain the child's attention. Highlight relevant sounds, words and phrases. Aid organization. These cues can be systematically decreased as the child acquires the response.

3. **Reduce the distracting potential of irrelevant stimuli** Decrease the intensity and frequency of irrelevant stimuli during the acquisition learning stage to maximize the saliency of instructional cues. When the child demonstrates acquisition of the desired behavior at an acceptable level, gradually increase the intensity and frequency of the less relevant stimuli until they are at a natural level. For example, darkening the room will decrease the intensity of irrelevant stimuli (distractors). The room should gradually be returned to natural illumination when the child attains the criterion performance level.

4. **Take advantage of attentional predispositions** Select instructional stimuli from the range of objects and events the child demonstrates an interest in looking at and manipulating. Consider objects with novelty, movement, and change as well as human stimuli (voice and face)—these naturally attract attention.

5. **Consider the status of social and cognitive skills** Keep in mind that there are necessary continuities within and across social, cognitive, and language domains that influence the development of communication. If the child has not established object permanence and/or is not using any form of intentional communication, it may be premature to attempt to train the use of words symbolically (meaningfully) or socially (for communication). Target motoric, signal, and symbolic communicative behavior (in that order).

6. **Use group-related stimuli to facilitate categorization** Reduce organizational demands on the child by pregrouping those stimuli that should be categorized and stored together. Train catego-

ries such as foods, clothing, and animals together and empha-size the relevant invariant properties (e.g., foods to be eaten) of concept instances. Request recall by categories (e.g., "What foods did you have for breakfast?")

7. **Arrange for referent and reference to be experienced simultaneously**   Assist the child to establish form-content associations by providing the reference (word, sign or gesture) when the referent (the object, person, or event which the form should be associated with) is the focus of attention. Label objects and events as they are shared and attended to.

8. **Teach how and when to apply mnemonic strategies**   Rehearsal, chunking, and association should be taught and practiced across tasks and across settings.

9. **Use cognitive-behavior-modification (CBM) procedures to teach problem solving strategies**   Teach the child to guide herself through the steps in solving problems.

10. **Use within-stimulus prompts**   Enhance the differences between stimuli to be discriminated by exaggerating and intensifying some element of the instructional stimulus rather than using extrastimulus (added on) prompts that have nothing inherently to do with the discrimination.

11. **Consider spatial as opposed to temporal arrangement of stimuli**   Speech does not provide a constant auditory display, nor do manual systems provide a constant visual display. For children with attention and memory deficits, this is a problem. Communication modes with a spatial arrangement of visual stimuli, like a communication board with pictures or Blissymbols, reduce the short-term memory requirements of communication because the child does not have to remember what has been communicated.

OUTPUT CAPABILITIES

The term *mode* refers to the form of a response—the manner in which an idea or intention is conveyed. Speech is the most common communication mode. The response *modality* of speech is verbal (or vocal). Because it is the most common (the overwhelming majority of human beings use speech for communicating), speech is the preferred communication mode. In many ways, it is also the most difficult.

There are a number of terms used interchangeably for individuals being taught and using augmentative communication modes. When one or the other of these terms (nonverbal, nonvocal, nonoral, nonspeech) is used, it usually means that the individual cannot, or will not, learn speech. The individual relies on some other communication mode (e.g., pointing to pictures on a communication board, manual signing, writing) to express ideas and intentions. Keep in mind, however, that because a child does not use verbal communication does not mean she does not under-

Chapter Ten discusses augmentative communication modes in detail.

stand verbal language. The child may receive and understand information through auditory as well as through visual, tactile, gustatory and olfactory senses.

Identification, or, if necessary, training of an output mode must necessarily precede any language intervention efforts. At the most general level, the purpose of assessment of output capabilities is to decide (a) whether the child has sufficient motor control of speech mechanisms to produce intelligible speech sounds, (b) whether the child has sufficient fine motor control to produce intelligible manual signs, or whether pointing, directed gaze, and/or gross motor mechanisms are the only available output modes. (These decisions and observation guidelines are discussed in Chapter Ten.)

> It is impossible to assess and evaluate learning until a reliable response has been established.

Many of the problems encountered in assessment of severely physically impaired children are analoguous to those surrounding infant assessment. Output problems interact with the inadequacy of language assessment devices to produce enormous error potential. Arriving at even the most general estimate of what the child knows and does not know about communication is an arduous task because most language assessment devices rely heavily on motor responses (e.g., compliance to commands, vocal responses and/or pointing and handing). The severely physically handicapped child's discrimination abilities and understanding of language are difficult to assess with any reliability because of her limited output capabilities. For this reason, any assessment *must* include extensive observations of the child under a variety of setting conditions.

> Knowledge of the response propensities of normal infants aids identification of response modes for handicapped children.

One source of information to aid the search for potential response modes is the normal development literature, but these findings suggest the need for caution in interpreting young children's responses. In addition to the possibility of underestimating the child's knowledge, there is the potential for overestimation. Chapman's (1977, 1981) description of the nonlinguistic response strategies of normal infants (which follows) may be equally applicable to severely handicapped children.

Between 8 and 12 months the normal infant gives evidence of selective attention and discrimination ability by shifting gaze to objects that another is attending to, acting in some way on objects she notices, and imitating the ongoing motor behavior of another. Not until the first half of her second year does the child begin to pay close attention to and respond to vocal as well as contextual stimuli. Comprehension of people and object words (if the referents are in the immediate visual field) is signaled by looking at the named person or object. Her primary "sentence comprehension" strategy at this age is to locate the object named in the sentence and "do what you usually do" with it. For example, if blocks and a container are immediately available and a request is made that includes the word "block," the child is likely to drop the blocks in the container, because this is a typical block-container activity. If a container is not available, she may respond to the sentence differently, for example, by throwing the block.

Around 18 months, the child begins responding to two words but also continues to apply the "do what you usually do" strategy. Objects mentioned in a sentence are often acted upon according to their functional properties. When requested to "hand the hairbrush" for example, the child is just as likely to brush her hair with it as to hand it. Simple action requests are complied with appropriately toward the end of the latter half of the second year. At this age, if told to "point to the cup," the child will point rather than pretending to drink from it. Out of sight objects may be retrieved *if* they are in a familiar location.

As noted above, these findings suggest the need for caution in the interpretation of young children's responses. There is a very real possibility of crediting the child with more linguistic knowledge than she has, in fact, acquired. The child who drops blocks in a can in response to the request to "put the blocks in the can" may not have achieved the sophisticated level of morphological knowledge this response would seem to indicate. She may be responding to one word, "block," and then applying the "do what you usually do" strategy. Even at the level of gaze shifting, misinterpretation is very possible. The child may appear to demonstrate a reliable eye pointing response when, in fact, she is simply imitating the adult's shift of gaze to the appropriate visual stimulus after it has been named.

Once a reliable output mode has been identified or established, there are three types of information that can be gleaned from the child's responses: (a) data concerning what she discriminates and understands, (b) information about what she does not discriminate or understand, and (c) information about her learning and response strategies. These data can be collected by systematically manipulating antecedent conditions and carefully observing the effects of different arrangements on the child's performance.

In the first example with the blocks, the child's receptive language skills and response strategies can be assessed by presenting several familiar objects (including a block) and several different action requests with the word "block." If the child responds with the same block activity to all requests, you can assume she has the word "block" in her receptive vocabulary but does not understand the action-object function since she applies the "do what you usually do" strategy. To verify or refute the hypothesis that the child is using a gaze imitation response strategy, monitor the adult's gaze after presentation of the verbal stimulus. If correct responding depends on following the adult's gaze, she is demonstrating a response strategy typical of the normal infant between 8 and 12 months of age. Do not credit her with more sophisticated linguistic knowledge than these responses indicate.

Curricula for severely multiply handicapped children developed by Reichle and Yoder (1979), Robinson and Robinson (1978), and others provide procedures to facilitate the identification and development of a response mode (or modes). Assessment and training of an output mode (or modes) should precede like this: (a) awareness, (b) sound localization and

Often, initial training for severely physically handicapped children must focus upon developing a reliable response mode.

visual tracking, (c) line of regard following and diverted gaze, (d) imitation, (e) reach-and-grasp behavior and finally, (f) showing, giving, and pointing behaviors. The following discussion summarizes each step; however, the sources mentioned above provide more precise directions.

1. Assessing awareness Infant behaviors indicating awareness of environmental events prior to language include startling, smiling, crying, movement cessation, blinking, and visual fixation. Initially these early behaviors, called orienting behaviors, are reactions to gross stimuli (not voluntary responses), which can be evoked in a wide variety of situations by an equally wide variety of stimuli. (The sensory organs record stimuli and the child reacts reflexively.) The effect of these reactions is usually immediate feedback of a sensory nature for the infant. Assess awareness with gross environmental changes such as the slamming of a door or bright lights. These observations provide data regarding the child's sensory acuity and receipt of information from the environment. Note the type of reaction (e.g., blinking, startle, smiling) as an indication of the child's response capabilities.

2. Assessing and training sound localization and visual tracking Two behaviors provide evidence of auditory and visual acuity: (a) turning toward and visually fixating on a sound source, and (b) visually following the movement of an object. The first, sound localization, also provides evidence of auditory-visual association ability that is the beginning of cause-effect recognition. The second, visual tracking skills, are evidence that the child has taken a first step toward construction of object permanence.

Infants younger than 4 months can track slowly moving visual targets, even if they pass behind an obscuring screen and re-emerge on the other side (Bower, 1974). These responses provide evidence that the infant is orienting and beginning to learn from the environment. Equally as important as the information they provide about the child's learning progress, however, is the response potential of these behaviors. There are a variety of communication modes possible if the child is capable of directional eye movements and smooth visual scanning.

Reichle and Yoder (1979) emphasize the need to use a variety of stimuli and a variety of placements for the sound source in localization training to prevent the child from learning an immature perseverative response rather than the desired search behavior. Training should continue until the child localizes to verbal stimuli. Robinson and Robinson (1978) suggest shift of gaze (visual fixation at one point, release, and re-fixation at another point) as an alternative when motor limitations preclude head turning.

3. Training line of regard following and diverted gaze Line of regard following has been observed in normal infants as early as 4 months of age (Bruner, 1975). Though obviously related to localization and tracking, it appears to be a somewhat higher level response. Diverted gaze (looking at a named object) is even more sophisticated and should be the next step in preparing the child for an "eye pointing" response. "Eye pointing," as noted on page 190, can be a very functional response mode: the child with a reliable eye pointing response can indicate her receptive language knowledge and learn to use a simple communication board.

4. Training imitation Reichle and Yoder suggest training motor and vocal imitation simultaneously. They recommend it because (a) there is little evidence from normative findings that motor imitation *necessarily* precedes vocal imitation, and (b) at the time that imitation training is begun, there is no way to predict which of the two response modes (motor or vocal) will be most available to the child. They also recommend that motor imitation training target approximations of manual signs.

> Imitation training is discussed at length in Chapter Six.

    Vocal imitation training should begin with mutual imitation (waiting until the child vocalizes and immediately imitating the vocalization with the expectation that the child will then produce the utterance a second time) if the child is nonimitative.

5. Training reach and grasp behavior The normal infant achieves coordinated reach and grasp at approximately 5 months of age. Development of reach and grasp behaviors is one of many challenges for children who demonstrate severe neuromotor problems (e.g., abnormal persistence of the asymmetric tonic neck reflex) and/or visual impairments. The terminal objective of this training is for the child to (a) lift her hand (from outside her visual field), (b) anticipate the shape of an object in the visual field, and (c) grasp the stimulus object. When this reach and grasp objective is attained the child has acquired some limited ability to act upon objects. The ability to reach and grasp means that the child is capable of indicating a discriminated object and communicating by proffering an object, picture, or symbol card; both potentially very useful response modes.

    The sequence of training for reach and grasp skills begins with swiping behavior. To elicit swiping behavior, move an object slowly toward the child's face. When it gets close, she will usually reach up to bat it away. Over successive trials, movement is stopped at points farther from the child's face until eventually she is extending her arm to bat it away.

6. Training showing, giving, and pointing behaviors Showing, giving, and pointing behaviors require little more in the way of motor control than reach and grasp behaviors. Once these motor behaviors are an established response mode, the environment can be arranged so that the child uses these skills to respond to and initiate interactions. Pointing is particularly important because of the environmental control it affords and as a communication board response mode.

    In concluding this section, we reiterate the importance of attention to reliable and measurable response modes. With the severely multiply handicapped in particular, we are often in a position of having to circumvent concomitant conditions such as physical impairments and sensori-motor deficits that may not exist concurrently in other handicapped children. Response modes (e.g., eye pointing) that are not usually considered communicative must be identified (if available) or systematically trained (if not already in the child's repertoire) prior to attempting assessment and training of either receptive or expressive language.

MOTIVATION

The environment contains a variety of events that influence the *what, when* and *where* of language learning; it is not dependent on ability alone. Similarly, the likelihood that a language deficient child will benefit from intervention depends upon a variety of factors other than ability. The most obvious and significant of these factors is motivation. To the extent that functional relationships can be established or identified between certain stimulus events and language behaviors, the means of facilitating functional communication are available. However, these relationships are not always easy to establish, particularly with severely impaired children.

The severely handicapped child who is not consistently responsive to food, liquids, vibration, or any other easily identifiable stimuli is also likely to be the child with few communication skills: the narrower the range of desires and needs, the less reason there is to communicate. Many severely handicapped children engage in little activity of any kind, and they are not consistently responsive to the usual reinforcers. They may have a fixed and narrow range of preferences (e.g., only one type of edible, or only edibles) and situation-specific response-consequence chains (Bricker & Campbell, 1980). Sometimes a particular consequence will function as a positive reinforcer (defined relative to its effect on the preceding behavior) with one task, but not with other tasks.

With severely handicapped children we often have to commit considerable instructional effort to establishing functional relationships (changing neutral stimulus events that have no reliable influence on, or meaning to, the child into events that can effect behavior change) and identifying existing relationships. These functional relationships are enormously important to teachers and communication specialists because they are the means for teaching language.

Paying attention to and praising language are reinforcers for most less severely impaired children, but securing desired and needed objects and events is usually even more reinforcing. In fact, it is relatively safe to assume some correlation between the child's communication skills and the range and variety of functional reinforcers in her environment. You can assume that whatever communication skills she has learned have been learned because there was some type of "pay-off," very often in the form of goods and/or services (e.g., a cookie, toy, etc., and/or being picked up or swung).

Within the broad class of external reinforcers, there are contrived or artificial rewards (introduced specifically for instructional purposes), and natural rewards (objects and events in the environment which are natural

Identification or establishment of reinforcers for severely handicapped children is often extremely difficult.

Operant behaviors are influenced by their consequences; respondent behaviors are influenced by preceding events.

The most desirable reinforcers are those desired objects and events that occur naturally, contingent upon appropriate responses.

consequences for certain behaviors). Contrived reinforcers are undoubt-edly an important facilitator of learning, particularly in the initial phases of instruction, but extreme caution must be exercised in selecting and ap-plying these rewards. There is a danger of contributing to rather than ameliorating passivity and helplessness, and precluding rather than en-hancing generalization. In the application of contrived reinforcers, be par-ticularly careful not to (a) get so caught up with the idea of establishing control that the child is relegated to a passive state and the real goal of lan-guage instruction (establishing communication as a mediator of desired and needed goods and services) is forgotten, and (b) assume that "natu-ral" reinforcement will *automatically* take over.

There is one final admonition about motivation. Sometimes external objects or events may *appear* to be responsible for strengthening a de-sired language behavior when, in fact, that is not the case at all. An amus-ing example of confounding of reinforcement effects that illustrates this caveat is provided by Rumbaugh (1977). One of the chimpanzees he was working with in his computer language experiments did not consume the banana slices she earned as reinforcement for solving a problem. Instead she saved them and returned them to the experimenter on the next part of the experiment (possibly in hopes of increasing *his* future behavior of presenting interesting problem solving trials). Apparently, the banana slices were not reinforcers at all as the trainer had assumed.

> Teachers and communica-tion specialists must stay continually alert to response-consequence re-lationships.

SUMMARY

1. The completed IEP represents a set of hypotheses about what might work; it is up to the service delivery team to test, refine, and expand this tentative planning effort.

2. P.L. 94-142 specifies the process through which an IEP is formu-lated, the persons responsible for its formulation, and what the com-pleted document should contain.

3. There are at least four sets of variables to be considered in planning and developing effective and individualized curricular procedures: (a) sensory preferences and capabilities, (b) learning strategies, (c) out-put capabilities, and (d) motivational factors.

4. Impaired or limited acuity in any one or more sensory areas (audito-ry, visual, tactile, olfactory, and gustatory) will in some way affect lan-guage learning; therefore, sensory acuity information is critical to valid intervention planning.

5. Understanding the learning strategies (selective attention, concept formation, storage and retrieval) a child lacks or is not applying aids determination of *how* and, to a lesser extent, *what* to teach that child.

6. There are two readiness theories—the "preparedness hypothesis" and the "match hypothesis"—that can help professionals decide what concepts and tasks the child will learn more efficiently.

7. There are a variety of procedures available for either circumventing or attempting to remediate atypical and/or deficient learning strategies of handicapped children.

8. A reliable response mode must be identified or established before initiating language assessment and training efforts.

9. The effectiveness of language and communication training efforts depends on the ability of the teacher and specialist to identify or establish functional response-consequence relationships.

REFERENCES

AYRES, J.A. Types of sensory integrative dysfunction among disabled learners. *American Journal of Occupational Therapy,* 1972, *26,* 13–18.

BARTEL, N.R., BRYAN, D., & KEEHN, S. Language comprehension in the mentally retarded child. *Exceptional Children,* 1973, *39,* 375–382.

BAUMEISTER, A.A., & SMITH, S. Thematic elaboration and proximity in children's recall, organization and long-term retention of pictorial materials. *Journal of Experimental Child Psychology,* 1979, *28,* 132–148.

BELMONT, J.M., & BUTTERFIELD, E.C. Learning strategies as determinants of memory deficiencies. *Cognitive Psychology,* 1971, *2,* 411–420.

BEST, G.A. *Individuals with physical disabilities.* St. Louis: C.V. Mosby Co., 1978.

BLOOM, L., & LAHEY, M. *Language development and language disorders.* New York: John Wiley & Sons, 1978.

BORMANN, C., & SCHULER, A.L. Discrimination training on the basis of a single acoustic parameter in echolalic autistic adolescents. Unpublished paper, Behavior Development and Learning Center, Camarillo State Hospital, Camarillo, California, 1978.

BOWER, T.G.R. The evolution of sensory systems. In R.B. Macleod & H.L. Pick (Eds.), *Essays in honour of J.J. Gibson.* New York: Cornell University Press, 1974.

BRACKETT, D. Language assessment protocols for hearing-impaired students. *Topics in Language Disorders,* 1982, *2*(3), 46–56.

BRASSELL, W.R., & DUNST, C.J. Fostering the object construct: Large-scale intervention with handicapped infants. *American Journal of Mental Deficiency,* 1978, *82*(5), 507–510.

BRICKER, D.O., & BRICKER, W.A. A programmed approach to operant audiometry for low-functioning children. *Journal of Speech and Hearing Disorders,* 1969, *34,* 312–320.

BRICKER, W.A., & CAMPBELL, P.H. Interdisciplinary assessment and programming for multihandicapped students. In W. Sailor, B. Wilcox, & L. Brown (Eds.), *Methods of instruction for severely handicapped students.* Baltimore: Paul H. Brookes Publishing Co., 1980.

BRICKER, W.A., MACKE, P.R., LEVIN, J.A., & CAMPBELL, P.H. The modifiability of intelligent behavior. *Journal of Special Education,* 1981, *15,* 145–163.

BROWN, A.L. The role of strategic behavior in retardate memory. In N.R. Ellis (Ed.), *International review of research in mental retardation* (Vol. 7). New York: Academic Press, 1974.

BROWN, A.L., CAMPIONE, J.C., & MURPHY, M.D. Keeping track of changing variables: Long term retention of a trained rehearsal strategy by retarded adolescents. *American Journal of Mental Deficiency,* 1974, *78,* 446–453.

BRUNER, J. The ontogenesis of speech acts. *Journal of Child Language,* 1975, *2,* 1–19.

BUTTERFIELD, E.C., WAMBOLD, C., & BELMONT, J.M. On the theory and practice of improving short-term memory. *American Journal of Mental Deficiency,* 1973, *77,* 654–669.

CAPLAN, F. *The first twelve months of life.* New York: Grossett & Dunlap, Inc., 1973.

CECI, S.J., & HOWE, J.A. Semantic knowledge as a determinant of developmental differences in recall. *Journal of Experimental Child Psychology,* 1978, *26,* 230–245.

CHAPMAN, R. Comprehension strategies in children. In J. Kavanagh & P. Strange (Eds.), *Language and speech in the laboratory, school and clinic.* Cambridge, Mass.: The MIT Press, 1977.

CHAPMAN, R.S. Mother-child interaction in the second year of life: Its role in language development. In R.L. Schiefelbusch & D. Bricker (Eds.), *Early language: Acquisition and intervention.* Baltimore: University Park Press, 1981.

COHEN, M.A., & GROSS, P.J. *The developmental resource: Behavioral sequences for assessment and program planning* (Vol. 2). New York: Grune & Stratton, Inc., 1979.

CRUICKSHANK, W.M. (Ed.). *Cerebral palsy: A developmental disability* (3rd rev. ed.). Syracuse, N.Y.: Syracuse University Press, 1976.

DAVIS, H., & SILVERMAN, S.R. *Hearing and deafness.* New York: Holt, Rinehart, and Winston, 1970.

DuBOSE, R.F. Working with sensorily impaired children—Part I: Visual impairments. In S.G. Garwood (Ed.), *Educating young handicapped children: A developmental approach.* Germantown, Maryland: Aspen Systems Corporation, 1979.

ELLIS, N.R. Memory processes in retardates and normals. In N.R. Ellis (Ed.), *International review of research in mental retardation* (Vol. 4). New York: Academic Press, 1970.

ENGEN, T., & LIPSETT, L. Decrement and recovery of responses to olfactory stimuli in the human neonate. *Journal of Comparative and Physiological Psychology,* 1965, *59*(2), 312–316.

ETZEL, B.C., BICKEL, W.K., STELLA, M.E., & LeBLANC, J.M. The assessment of problem solving skills of atypical children. *Analysis and Intervention in Developmental Disabilities,* 1982, *2,* 187–206.

FARHAM-DIGGORY, S. *Cognitive processes in education: A psychological preparation for teaching and curriculum development.* New York: Harper & Row, 1972.

FLAVELL, J.H. Concept development. In P.H. Mussen (Ed.), *Carmichael's manual of child psychology* (Vol. 1). New York: John Wiley & Sons, 1970.

FLAVELL, J.H. *Cognitive development.* Englewood Cliffs, N.J.: Prentice-Hall, Inc., 1977.

FROSTIG, M., & HORNE, D. *The Frostig Program for Development of Visual Perception.* Chicago, Follett: 1964.

FULTON, R.T. *Auditory stimulus—response control.* Baltimore: University Park Press, 1974.

GEIS, M.F., & HALL, D. Encoding and incidental memory in children. *Journal of Experimental Child Psychology,* 1977, *22,* 58–66.

GESELL, A., ILG, F.L., AMES, L.B., & RODELL, J.L. *Infant and child in the culture of today: The guidance of development in home and nursery school.* New York: Harper & Row, Publishers, 1974.

GETMAN, G.N. The visual-motor complex in the acquisition of learning skills. In J. Hellmuth (Ed.), *Learning disorders* (Vol. 1). Seattle, Washington: Special Child Publications, 1965.

GIBSON, E.J. *Principles of perceptual learning and development.* New York: Appleton-Century-Crofts, 1969.

GUESS, D., SAILOR, W., & BAER, D. A behavioral remedial approach to language training for the severely handicapped. In E. Sontag (Ed.), *Educational programming for the severely handicapped.* Reston, Va.: A Special Publication of the Division on Mental Retardation, CEC, 1977.

HAINES, D.J., & TORGESEN, J.K. The effects of incentives on rehearsal and short-term memory in children with reading problems. *Learning Disability Quarterly,* 1979, *2,* 48–55.

HALLAHAN, D.P., & BRYAN, T.H. Learning disabilities. In J.M. Kauffman & D.P. Hallahan (Eds.), *Handbook of special education.* Englewood Cliffs, N.J.: Prentice-Hall, Inc., 1981.

HALLAHAN, D.P., & REEVE, R.E. Selective attention and distractibility. In B.K. Koegh (Ed.), *Advances in special education* (Vol. 1). Greenwich, Conn.: JAI Press, 1980.

HAMMILL, D.D., & LARSEN, S. The relationship of selected auditory perceptual skills and reading ability. *Journal of Learning Disabilities,* 1974, *7,* 429–435.

HAMMILL, D.D., & LARSEN, S.C. *The test of written language (TOWL).* Austin, Tex.: Pro-Ed., 1978.

HERMELIN, B. Rules and language. In M. Rutter (Ed.), *Infantile autism: Concepts, characteristics, and treatment.* London: Churchill Livingstone, 1971.

HERMELIN, B. Coding and the sense modalities. In L. Wing (Ed.), *Early childhood autism.* London: Pergamon Press, 1976.

HERMELIN, B., & O'CONNOR, N. *Psychological experiments with autistic children.* London: Pergamon Press, 1970.

HILL, D.S. A comparison of the performance of normal, learning disabled, and educable mentally retarded children on Cattell's ability constructs. *Journal of Learning Disabilities,* 1980, *13*(7), 38–41.

HOLLIS, J.H., & CARRIER, J. Intervention strategies for nonspeech children. In R.L. Schiefelbusch (Ed.), *Language intervention strategies.* Baltimore: University Park Press, 1978.

HOLLIS, J.H., & SCHIEFELBUSCH, R.L. A general system for language analysis. In R.L. Schiefelbusch & J.H. Hollis (Eds.), *Language intervention from ape to child.* Baltimore: University Park Press, 1979.

HOROWITZ, F.D. (Ed.). Visual attention, auditory stimulation, and language discrimination in young infants. *Monographs of the Society for Research in Child Development,* 1974, *39*(5), Serial No. 158.

HUNT, J.M. *Intelligence and experience.* New York: Ronald Press, 1961.

HUNT, J.M. Intrinsic motivation and its role in psychological development. In D. Levine (Ed.), *Nebraska Symposium on Motivation* (Vol. 13). Lincoln: University of Nebraska Press, 1965.

JOHNSON, D., & MYKLEBUST, H. *Learning disabilities: Educational principles and practices.* New York: Grune and Stratton, 1967.

KELLAS, G., ASHCROFT, M.H., & JOHNSON, N.S. Rehearsal processes in the short-term memory performance of mildly retarded adolescents. *American Journal of Mental Deficiency,* 1973, *77,* 670–679.

KEPHART, N.C. *The slow learner in the classroom* (2nd ed.). Columbus, Ohio: Charles E. Merrill, 1971.

KIRK, S.A., & KIRK, W. *Psycholinguistic learning disabilities: Diagnosis and remediation.* Urbana, Ill.: University of Illinois Press, 1971.

KIRK, S.A., McCARTHY, J.J., & KIRK, W.D. *The Illinois Test of Psycholinguistic Abilities.* Urbana, Ill.: University of Illinois Press, 1968.

KOBASHIGAWA, A. Utilization of retrieval cues by children in recall. *Child Development,* 1974, *45,* 127–134.

KOBASHIGAWA, A. Retrieval strategies in the development of memory. In R.V. Kail & J.W. Hagan (Eds.), *Memory in cognitive development.* Hillsdale, N.J.: Lawrence Earlbaum Associates, 1976.

KOEGEL, R.L., & RINCOVER, A. Some detrimental effects of using extra stimuli to guide learning in normal and autistic children. *Journal of Abnormal Child Psychology,* 1976, *4,* 59–71.

LERNER, J., DAWSON, D., & HORVATH, L. *Cases in learning and behavior problems: A guide to individualized education programs.* Boston: Houghton Mifflin Co., 1980.

LLOYD, L.L., REID, M.J., & McMANIS, D.L. Puretone reliability of a clinical sample of institutionalized MR children. *American Journal of Mental Deficiency,* 1968, *73,* 279–282.

LLOYD, L.L., SPRADLIN, J.E., & REID, M.J. An operant audiometric procedure for difficult-to-test patients. *Journal of Speech and Hearing Disorders,* 1968, *33,* 236–245.

LOVAAS, O.I., KOEGEL, R.L., & SCHREIBMAN, L. Stimulus overselectivity in autism: A review of research. *Psychological Bulletin,* 1979, *86,* 1236–1254.

LOVAAS, O.I., & SCHREIBMAN, L. Stimulus overselectivity of autistic children in a two stimulus situation. *Behavior Research and Therapy,* 1971, *9,* 305–310.

LOVAAS, O.I., SCHREIBMAN, L., KOEGEL, R., & REHM, R. Selective responding by autistic children to multiple sensory input. *Journal of Abnormal Psychology,* 1971, *77,* 211–222.

MacMILLAN, D.L. *Mental retardation in school and society.* Boston: Little, Brown, 1977.

MAGER, R.F. *Preparing instructional objectives* (2nd ed.). Belmont, Calif.: Fearon Publishers, 1975.

McCORMICK, L.P., & KAWATE, J. Kindergarten survival skills: New directions for preschool special education. *Education and Training of the Mentally Retarded,* 1982, *17,* 247–251.

McDADE, H.L., & ADLER, S. Down syndrome and short-term memory impairment: A storage or retrieval deficit? *American Journal of Mental Deficiency,* 1980, *84*(6), 561–567.

McKINNEY, J.D., & HASKINS, R. Cognitive training and the development of problem-solving strategies. *Exceptional Education Quarterly,* 1980, *1*(1), 41–51.

McLEAN (McCORMICK), L.P., & McLEAN, J.E. A language training program for non-verbal autistic children. *Journal of Speech and Hearing Disorders,* 1974, *39,* 186–193.

McNUTT, J.C., & CHIA-YEN LI, J. Repetition of time altered sentences by normal and learning disabled children. *Journal of Learning Disabilities,* 1980, *13*(1), 30–34.

MILLER, G.A. The magical number seven plus or minus two: Some limits in our ability for processing of information. *Psychological Review,* 1956, *63,* 81–97.

MILLER, M.H., RABINOWITZ, M., FROST, J.O., & SEAGER, G.M. Audiological problems associated with maternal rubella. *The Laryngoscope,* 1969, *79,* 417–426.

MOERK, E.L. *Pragmatic and semantic aspects of early language development.* Baltimore: University Park Press, 1977.

PIAGET, J. *The language and thought of the child.* New York: Harcourt Brace, 1926.

PIAGET, J. *The construction of reality in the child.* New York: Basic Books, 1954.

PIAGET, J. Piaget's theory. In P.H. Mussen (Ed.), *Carmichael's manual of child psychology* (Vol. 1). New York: Wiley, 1970.

PIAGET, J., & INHELDER, B. *The psychology of the child.* New York: Basic Books, 1969.

PREMACK, D. A functional analysis of language. *Journal of Experimental Analysis of Behavior,* 1970, *14,* 107–125.

REICHLE, J.E., & YODER, D.E. Assessment and early stimulation of communication in the severely and profoundly mentally retarded. In R.L. York & E. Edgar (Eds.), *Teaching the severely handicapped* (Vol. 4). Columbus, Ohio: Special Press, 1979.

REYNOLDS, G., NEWSOM, C., & LOVAAS, O. Auditory overselectivity in autistic children. *Journal of Abnormal Child Psychology,* 1974, *2,* 253–263.

RINCOVER, A. Variables affecting stimulus fading and discriminative responding in psychotic children. *Journal of Abnormal Psychology,* 1978, *87,* 541–553.

RINCOVER, A., & KOEGEL, R.L. Setting generality and stimulus control in autistic children. *Journal of Applied Behavior Analysis,* 1975, *8,* 235–246.

ROADEN, S.K., McCAULEY, C., & SPERBER, R.D. Intelligence-related differences in the relative salience of object-property relationships. *Journal of Mental Deficiency,* 1980, *84*(5), 518–525.

ROBINSON, C.C. Error patterns in Level 4 and Level 5 object permanence training. *American Journal of Mental Deficiency,* 1975, *78,* 389–396.

ROBINSON, C.C., & ROBINSON, J.H. Sensorimotor functions and cognitive development. In M.E. Snell (Ed.), *Systematic instruction of the moderately and severely handicapped.* Columbus: Charles E. Merrill, 1978.

ROBINSON, N.M., & ROBINSON, H.B. *The mentally retarded child: A psychological approach.* New York: McGraw-Hill, 1976.

RUMBAUGH, D.M. (Ed.). *Language learning by a chimpanzee: The Lana project.* New York: Academic Press, 1977.

SAILOR, W., GUESS, D., GOETZ, L., SCHULER, A., UTLEY, B., & BALDWIN, M. Language and severely handicapped persons: Deciding what to teach to whom. In W. Sailor, B. Wilcox, & L. Brown (Eds.), *Methods of instruction for severely handicapped students.* Baltimore: Paul H. Brookes Publishing Co., 1980.

SALVIA, J., & YSSELDYKE, J. *Assessment in special and remedial education* (2nd ed.). Boston: Houghton-Mifflin, 1981.

SCHREIBMAN, L. Effects of within-stimulus and extra-stimulus prompting on discrimination learning in autistic children. *Journal of Applied Behavior Analysis,* 1975, *7,* 91–112.

SCOTT, J. The process of primary socialization in canine and human infants. In J. Hellmuth (Ed.), *Exceptional Infant* (Vol. 1). Seattle, Washington: Special Child Publications, 1969.

SELIGMAN, M.E. *Helplessness: On depression, death, and development.* San Francisco: W.H. Freeman, 1975.

SEMMEL, M., BARRITT, L., BENNETT, S., & PERFETTI, C. A grammatical analysis of word associations of educable mentally retarded and normal children. *American Journal of Mental Deficiency,* 1968, *72,* 567–576.

SHRAG, J.A. *Individualized educational programming (IEP): A child study team process.* Austin, Tex.: Learning Concepts, 1977.

SIDMAN, M. A note on the measurement of conditional discrimination. *Journal of the Experimental Analysis of Behavior,* 1980, *33,* 285–289.

SMITH, A.J., & JOHNSON, R.E. *Smith-Johnson Non-Verbal Performance Scale.* Los Angeles: Western Psychological Service, 1977.

STRICHART, S.S., & GOTTLIEB, J. Characteristics of mild mental retardation. In T.L. Miller & E.E. Davis (Eds.), *The mildly handicapped student.* New York: Grune & Stratton, 1982.

SULLIVAN, P., & VERNON, M. Psychological assessment of hearing impaired children. *School Psychology Digest,* 1979, *8*(3), 271–290.

TORRES, S. (Ed.). *A primer on individualized education programs for handicapped children.* Reston, Va.: The Foundation for Exceptional Children, 1977.

TURNBULL, A.P., STRICKLAND, B.B., & BRANTLEY, J.C. *Developing and implementing individualized education programs.* Columbus: Charles E. Merrill, 1978.

UZGIRIS, I.V., & HUNT, J.McV. *Assessment in infancy: Ordinal scales of psychological development.* Urbana: University of Illinois Press, 1975.

VARNI, J., LOVAAS, O., KOEGEL, R., & EVERETT, N. An analysis of observational learning in autistic and normal children. *Journal of Abnormal Child Psychology,* 1979, *7,* 31–43.

VINCENT, L.J., BROWN, L., & GETZ-SHEFTEL, M. Integrating handicapped and typical children during the preschool years: The definition of best educational practice. *Topics in Early Childhood Special Education,* 1981, *1*(1), 17–24.

WARREN, D. *Blindness and early childhood development.* New York: American Foundation for the Blind, Inc., 1977.

WARREN, O.H. Visual impairments. In J.M. Kauffman & D.P. Hallahan (Eds.), *Handbook of Special Education.* Englewood Cliffs, New Jersey: Prentice-Hall, Inc., 1981.

WASHBURN, R.W. A study of smiling and laughing of infants in the first year of life. *Genetic Psychology Monographs,* 1929, *6,* 397–537.

WAUGH, N.C., & NORMAN, D.A. Primary memory. *Psychological Review,* 1965, *72,* 89–104.

WOHLHEUTER, M.J., & SINDBERG, R.M. Longitudinal development of object permanence in mentally retarded children: An exploratory study. *American Journal of Mental Deficiency,* 1975, *79,* 513–518.

WOLFE, V.F., & CUVO, A.J. Effects of within-stimulus and extra-stimulus prompting on letter discrimination by mentally retarded persons. *American Journal of Mental Deficiency,* 1978, *83,* 297–303.

WOLFF, P.H. Observations on the early development of smiling. In B.M. Foss (Ed.), *Determinants of infant behavior* (Vol. 2). New York: Wiley, 1963.

YSSELDYKE, J.E., & ALGOZZINE, B. *Critical issues in special and remedial education.* Boston: Houghton Mifflin Co., 1982.

ZEAMAN, D., & HOUSE, B.J. The role of attention in retardate discrimination learning. In N.R. Ellis (Ed.), *Handbook of mental deficiency.* New York: McGraw-Hill, 1963.

ZELNIKER, T., & JEFFREY, W.E. Reflective and impulsive children: Strategies of information processing underlying differences in problem solving. *Monographs of the Society for Research in Child Development,* 1976, *41,* (5, Whole No. 168).

CHAPTER SIX

DESIGNING AN OPTIMAL LEARNING PROGRAM

Linda McCormick and Ronald Goldman

T eaching is planning, organizing, and manipulating environmental conditions to promote learning; we doubt any one would argue with this definition. However, in all areas of instruction there is disagreement over *what* should be taught and precisely how to teach it.

The first two steps in the intervention process, assessment and planning, were discussed in Chapters Four and Five. The major emphasis in this chapter is on organizing and manipulating environmental conditions to promote learning. However, there are also some guidelines for curriculum content. After comparing various approaches to language intervention, we focus on the following specific teaching functions: identifying and orchestrating instructional resources, using instructional procedures and strategies, and promoting generalization and maintenance.

THE INTERVENTION TRIANGLE

To select the right intervention models you must be able to differentiate psycholinguistics, behavioral, and developmental assumptions and goals.

You probably have some notions about the disagreements over the proper content and procedures for language intervention from the previous chapters. This first section presents a brief exposition of the psycholinguistic, behavioral, and developmental approaches to language intervention.

It is valuable to understand the assumptions of these three models—psycholinguistic, behavioral, and developmental—and be able to distinguish among them when selecting and/or designing a language intervention program. However, it has become more difficult to differentiate among program models in the eighties because of (a) considerably more dialogue among applied researchers, (b) the gradual evolution toward a set of common tenets reflecting an almost universal concern for enhancing language use skills. We present assumptions and program goals for one program representing each of the three traditional intervention models. We quote the assumptions of these models, rather than paraphrase them, to avoid potential bias and illustrate differences in terminology.

A PSYCHOLINGUISTIC APPROACH

Bloom and Lahey (1978) present the following assumptions for their intervention model:

The Bloom and Lahey psycholinguistic model emphasizes training of semantic-syntactic structures.

1. "The form of utterances—words and syntactic structures—is only one of the important components of language. . .Goals of intervention must include information about the interactions among content/form/use." (p. 373)
2. "A plan for language intervention should provide information about language as the basis for evaluating and facilitating a child's progress in the development of language—information about content/form/use interactions—regardless of the cause of the disorder." (p. 373)
3. "The most reasonable and practical hypotheses on which to base intervention goals are to be derived from what is known about normal language development." (p. 374)
4. "Production rather than comprehension, should be emphasized because:. . .more is known about the development of children's production of content/form/use interactions than is known about the development of children's comprehension of these interactions." (p. 377)

Table 6-1 presents the early intervention goals generated by these assumptions. They are from Bloom and Lahey's (1978) book *Language Development and Language Disorders.* This model places more emphasis on training semantic-syntactic structures than the other models, but there is also concern for facilitating content and use (a departure from earlier psycholinguistic models that concentrated exclusively on drilling syntactic structures or operations). At the same time, there is less emphasis on cognitive development than in the developmental model, and less concern for teaching the functional language features that the child needs to control the environment than in the behavioral model.

TABLE 6-1 Early intervention goals in a psycholinguistic program

I. Precursory goals
   A. for the development of language use:
      1. reciprocal gazing
      2. regulating the behaviors of others
      3. calling attention to objects and events
   B. for the development of content:
      1. searching for objects that disappear
      2. causing objects to disappear
      3. acting on different objects in similar ways
      4. acting on different objects in prescribed ways
      5. acting on two objects in relation to each other

TABLE 6-1   (continued)

C. for the development of form:
1. imitating movement and vocalization
2. producing linguistic signals that approximate the adult model

D. for the development of use that interacts with content/form:
1. producing utterances for the purpose of commenting, vocal play, regulating others, obtaining objects, calling attention to self or objects, and social interaction rituals
2. producing utterances about objects or events that are present or ongoing, and the child's own dynamic interactions with the environment
3. producing utterances following the utterances of others (but not necessarily contingent) and related to the prior utterances by the nonlinguistic context both share

E. for the development of content/use association:
1. producing single-word utterances to code existence, nonexistence, recurrence, rejection, denial, attribution, possession, action and locative action
2. producing two-word utterances (semantic-syntactic relations) to code the above meanings

II. **Later Goals**

A. for the development of use that interacts with content/form:
1. producing an increased number of utterances that serve the interpersonal functions (e.g., obtaining objects, regulating the behavior of others)
2. asking questions about location and identity
3. producing utterances about events that have just happened or are about to happen
4. producing utterances about persons and objects that are not perceptually present but are expected or have just previously been present
5. producing utterances about what other people are doing
6. producing an increased number of utterances that do not follow (are nonadjacent to) the utterances of others
7. producing an increased number of utterances that are related to both the form and content of the utterances of others

B. for the development of content/form associations
1. producing multiword utterances to code notice (direct someone's attention) and time
2. producing utterances which coordinate previously established content categories with action verb relations
3. producing utterances with recurrence and possession embedded within existence relations
4. producing the following grammatical morphemes—indefinite article "a" with the demonstrative pronoun, the present progressive verb inflection -*ing*, the prepositions "in" and "on" in locative state utterances, the modal verbs "wanna" and "gonna" to express

TABLE 6-1   (continued)

intended action or locative action, and the interrogative pronoun "where" to ask questions about location

5. producing utterances to code the new content categories—coordinate, causality, dative, and specification

6. producing old grammatical morphemes in new contexts—(e.g., possessive -s, third person -s)

7. producing an increased number of utterances and a greater variety of words

8. producing pronouns

Source: Bloom & Lahey, 1977.

A BEHAVIORAL APPROACH

The assumptions of Guess, Sailor and Baer's (1977) behavioral model are:

1. "If a child achieves some control, not only of the language teacher but also of much of the environment, through the language responses he has learned, then a motivation is established that could prompt the child to learn to attend to a language using environment, to learn from observation the skills of *asking* for language training from language users (e.g., "What's that?"); and to learn the skills of remembering these tactics for later productive use in gaining even more control of the environment. (p. 361)

> The Guess, Sailor, and Baer behavioral model emphasizes training of functional utterances.

2. "In essence, we depend extensively on the performance of severely handicapped children to tell us what they should be taught, the order in which it should be taught, and the most effective and efficient procedures to use in training . . . we have made no assumptions that the development of certain linguistic skills is necessarily dependent on the prior existence of other prerequisite behavior." (p. 364)

Table 6-2 represents goals (in sequence) of the Guess, Sailor, and Baer (1976) curriculum. The total program is available in four parts (Guess, Sailor & Baer, 1976 a, b, 1977 a, b, 1978).

Past behaviorist efforts (e.g., Lovaas, 1966) have been criticized on the grounds that (a) they teach children to produce meaningless sentences—that what they teach is less language than a response repertoire (Seibert & Oller, 1981), and (b) they fail to produce generalized initiated behavior because cognitive prerequisites are not required (Reichle & Yoder, 1979). Guess (1980) counters this argument, in part, with a review of studies where communicative structures were successfully taught to severely handicapped students in the absence of their presumed prerequisites.

TABLE 6-2   Intervention goals in a behavioral-remedial program

I. Persons and things content area

A. labeling common objects

B. identifying common objects receptively

C. requesting objects with "want _____"

D. asking "what's that?"

E. using "yes" and "no" as receptive indicators with object labels

F. chaining together previously learned responses

II. Action with persons and things content area

A. expressing and identifying common verb actions

B. using the second-person pronoun "you"

C. discriminating first and second person pronouns

D. asking questions to identify novel actions

E. increasing use of object labels

F. using "yes/no" concept to identify actions

G. increasing use of requests

H. producing longer and more varied utterances

III. Possessions content area

A. identifying the ownership of objects

B. using the pronouns "my" and "your"

C. identifying ownership receptively with "yes/no"

D. requesting objects with "I want my/your _____."

E. asking "Whose _____?" when object ownership is unknown

F. using possessive pronouns "my/your" with previously taught responses

IV. Color content area

A. labeling common colors

B. using color descriptor with object labels

C. identifying objects of various colors receptively

D. requesting actions involving various colors

E. identifying actions involving colors

F. using "yes/no" as indicators for correct responses

G. asking "what color?" when presented with unknown color labels

H. using color labels in conversation about coloring

V. Size content area

A. using "big" and "little" as size descriptors

B. identifying big and little objects

C. stating the location of objects placed in big or little boxes

D. using "yes/no" to identify receptively the location of items in big or little boxes

E. using size descriptors in requests and conversations

TABLE 6-2 (continued)

VI. Location/relation content area

    A. using "on/under" and "inside/outside" as reference labels

    B. identifying with "yes/no" the position and location of objects and persons

    C. requesting objects placed in the "on/under" position

    D. requesting a person to go inside/outside

    E. asking the questions "Where is my _____?" and "Where are you going?"

    F. using position/location concepts in conversation

Source: Guess, Sailor & Baer, 1977, 1976. This program has a total of 60 training steps—for the sake of brevity, this table combines some steps.

A DEVELOPMENTAL APPROACH

Bricker, Ruder, and Vincent (1976) state the following assumptions in support of their developmental model:

> 1. "Currently we believe the most satisfactory way to select the content and training sequence for language intervention is to draw on data provided by normal children. . . . The infant's early interaction with his environment . . . is the basis for later language development." (p. 303)
>
> 2. "Another basis for language development includes the imitative skills generally acquired during infancy." (p. 304)

The Bricker, Ruder, and Vincent model emphasizes training of cognitive prerequisites and imitative skills.

In a later description of the sequence of steps prerequisite to verbal behavior, Bricker and Dennison (1978) are more specific:

> 3. "In our opinion, basic cognitive structures or sensorimotor intelligence form the foundation for the development of a generative language system." (p. 158)
>
> 4. "For the severely impaired child, language dysfunctions do not begin at age 18 to 24 months when most children develop expressive language, but rather we believe that language problems arise because the child has failed to develop the prerequisite sensorimotor behavior." (p. 158)

Table 6-3 combines goals from two publications by Bricker and colleagues. The total program is presented in a monograph *A Language Intervention Program for Developmentally Young Children* (Bricker, Dennison, & Bricker, 1976). Note the emphasis upon cognitive **prerequisites** to the relative exclusion of social and affective development which has recently come to be viewed as equally important to language learning (e.g., Mahoney, Crawley, & Pullis, 1981; Uzgiris, 1981).

TABLE 6-3 Early intervention goals in a developmental program

---

I. **On-task behavior**
   A. sitting in chair
   B. looking at trainer
   C. working on a specific task

II. **Imitation**
   A. increasing vocalization
   B. imitating familiar and unfamiliar actions
   C. imitating self-initiated and model-initiated sounds
   D. producing closer approximations of English sounds

III. **Discriminative use of objects**
   A. establishing a variety of action patterns with different objects
   B. using objects appropriately

IV. **Word recognition**
   A. responding to simple words and phrases in relevant situations

V. **Single word training** (Bricker, Ruder, & Vincent, 1976)
   A. imitation of nouns, verbs
   B. comprehension of word-object and word-action associations
   C. production of nouns and verbs

VI. **Multiword constructions**
   A. imitation of 2, then 3 words
   B. comprehension of agent-action and action-object relations, then agent-action-object relations
   C. production of agent-action and action-object, then agent-action-object constructions

VII. **Modifications of agent-action-object structures**
   A. comprehension of modifying nouns (adjectives of size, color and number)
   B. production of adjective and noun phrases
   C. comprehension and production of prepositions
   D. comprehension and production of verb-adverb constructions
   E. comprehension and production of expanded agent-action-object strings
   F. comprehension and production of pronouns
   G. comprehension and production of *wh*-questions
   H. comprehension and production of negative forms

Source: Bricker, Ruder, & Vincent, 1976; Bricker and Dennison, 1978

COMPARISONS

Our reason for presenting programs developed in the early and mid-seventies, even though earlier programs were "purer" models (had less conceptual overlap), is that these particular programs and/or expanded versions are in general use. Each has many strengths. No one can state with any confidence that one or the other is the best approach. The major differences among the three models relate to (a) the issue of prerequisites, (b) the relative importance ascribed to development in other domains (e.g., cognitive, social), (c) the aspects of language that are emphasized, and (d) how much structure is imposed upon the training paradigm.

There are four major differences among the three intervention models.

Despite disavowal of the strict nativistic position, Bloom and Lahey assume some primacy for constitutional factors (a special inborn capacity to relate to speech and language events). Likewise, Bricker and colleagues emphasize prerequisites; however, their concern is more with early cognitive structures than with social or linguistic prerequisites. In contrast, Guess, Sailor, and Baer make "no assumptions that the development of certain linguistic skills is necessarily dependent on the prior existence of other prerequisite behavior" (p. 364).

To some extent, both the Bloom and Lahey and the Bricker models reflect the cognitive-semantic perspective described in Chapter One; both target content-form associations. However, Bloom and Lahey also target language use skills and the *association* of meaning (content), structure (form), and function (use). This concern for language use reflects the influence of the pragmatic-interactive perspective described in Chapter One, a concern which is also becoming more evident in developmental programs (e.g., Reichle & Yoder, 1979). Although Guess, Sailor, and Baer demonstrate no concern for cognitive or social prerequisites, they are emphatic about the importance of language use—training utterances that will aid the child in directing and controlling his environment.

Another difference among the three models relates to the comprehension-production issue. Bloom and Lahey target production only. Guess, Sailor, and Baer train production and comprehension *in that order*. Bricker and colleagues target imitation, comprehension, and *then* production.

Regarding teaching strategies and procedures, the primary difference among the three programs is degree of structure. All rely to some extent on behavioral procedures—modeling, reinforcement, shaping, fading, prompting and cuing, chaining, and discrimination training. However, the amount of structure imposed upon the training conditions and how systematically behavioral procedures are applied varies. On a continuum, the developmental model is somewhat less structured and the behavioral model is more structured. The psycholinguistic model falls somewhere in the middle.

AN INTEGRATIVE APPROACH

Most recent language intervention models incorporate pragmatic-interactive assumptions. In addition to psycholinguistic, behavioral, and/or developmental assumptions, these newer program models place heavy emphasis on intentions (what communicative function the utterance or

Most recent approaches incorporate pragmatic-interactive assumptions and goals.

nonverbal behavior serves) and social appropriateness. The concern is less with what the child can say and how he says it than with what he can accomplish with language. The effect of this trend is a tendency to define language very broadly as a mode of interaction; this essentially blurs the distinction between language and communication.

Representative of this trend are the following pragmatic-interactive assumptions (Rogers-Warren & Warren, in press):

1. Communicative language arises from a basis in other behaviors, especially the cognitive skills and social interaction repertoires of the child
2. Utterances have intentions or forces that define their contextually relevant meanings
3. There are rules which underlie the use of intention in conversational discourse
4. Meaning is determined by functions in context

At this time there is no intervention model or single set of goals that fully incorporate all of these tenets. However, the following reflect the movement toward pragmatic-interactive training goals:

1. *Ready, set, go: Talk to me* by Horstmeier and MacDonald (1978). This book is a component of *The Environmental Language Intervention Program,* also written by MacDonald.
2. *A Transactional Approach to Early Language Training,* a book by McLean and Snyder-McLean (1978).
3. *Communication Training Program* by Waryas and Stremel-Campbell (1982). This is a three-level training program which, in addition to psycholinguistic assumptions, incorporates some pragmatic-interactive tenets.
4. "A milieu approach to teaching language" by Hart and Rogers-Warren. In R.L. Schiefelbusch (Ed.), *Language Intervention Strategies,* 1978. This chapter describes an environmental approach to language training. This model suggests strategies for making language functional by arranging situations "in which the child works with language and by insuring that the child's language works to produce attention, things, and events" (p. 219).

This section has presented only a general comparison of approaches to intervention, not a detailed analysis. In actual practice, effective language and communication specialists and teachers draw from and combine aspects of different approaches. Among the factors influencing selection and combination of approaches are age and the severity and/or pervasiveness of the learner's impairments.

CHILD/STUDENT VARIABLES THAT AFFECT PROGRAMMING GOALS

The fact that an older severely handicapped student and a young child who is moderately or severely language delayed/deficient are functioning at the same developmental level does not mean they should have the same language training goals. A first and basic language intervention decision is whether to concentrate on (a) teaching specific behaviors that will maximize independent functioning, or (b) programming to facilitate more general communicative competence. Age and severity of handicapping condition will affect the type of objectives sought *and* the means by which these objectives are identified. The two sets of goals are not mutually exclusive, but they are based on different assumptions.

Generally speaking, the first set of goals—teaching the specific structures that will maximize independent functioning—is more suitable for older severely handicapped students, while the second is better suited to younger children. Selection of programming objectives, in all curricular areas, for older severely handicapped students should be judged against the "criterion of ultimate functioning." This concept, first introduced by Brown, Nietupski and Hamre-Nietupski in 1976, provides systematic guidelines for *what* to teach. (Other Brown et al. recommendations, described below, suggest *how* to teach severely handicapped students.) Brown et al. translated Wolfensberger's (1972) "normalization principle," which states that severely handicapped persons should be prepared for normal existence in the mainstream of society, to the injunction that all intervention efforts should be to prepare students "to function productively and independently in socially, vocationally, and domestically integrated community environments" (p. 8).

When applied to the sphere of language intervention, the "criterion of ultimate functioning" dictates a primary focus on teaching expressive behaviors that will maximize the student's potential for independent functioning in home, community and work settings. It has implications not only for selection of language training *goals* but also for selection of an output mode (e.g., speech, manual signing, communication board), and type of expressive system (e.g., pictures, phonemes, Blissymbols, etc.).

> When applied to language intervention with older severely handicapped students, the "criterion of ultimate functioning" dictates training of expressive behaviors that will maximize independent functioning in future environments.

Programming for infants and young children may have different priorities because there is the luxury of many years ahead for instruction. Particularly with young children who have less interference from sensory and motor impairments, intervention should focus on facilitating generative language and communicative competence. The broad goal of language intervention for this younger population is expression and understanding of an unlimited number of ideas and intentions in a range of contexts (generative language).

It should be emphasized that this difference between curricular priorities for older severely handicapped students and younger populations does not negate the usefulness of developmental information. Data concerning an older student's status compared to normal social, cognitive,

> The notion that program assumptions and goals will vary depending on age and severity of the child's handicap(s) is expanded later in the chapter.

and language development still have some value, and should be considered when you decide how to teach and weigh costs (in time and effort) and benefits.

THE ORCHESTRATION OF INSTRUCTION

The contexts of language teaching and learning have many functional elements. The responsibility for analyzing and evaluating these variables may fall on the language communication specialist, but, in the vast majority of school settings, the teacher is responsible for orchestrating them. Together, they should decide

1. *Who* will teach language
2. *Where* language instruction will take place
3. *When* language instruction will be scheduled
4. *What* materials and reinforcers to use

In the broadest sense, these elements *are* the intervention program; the success of training efforts will depend, to a great extent, on how these questions are answered.

WHO SHOULD TEACH LANGUAGE?

The optimal language learning environment includes a variety of language teachers and communicants.

In the natural learning environment many persons—parents, siblings, baby sitters, day care workers, neighbors, etc.—assume responsibility for language training. It may not be realistic to incorporate all the handicapped child's communicants into school instructional environments, but certainly all persons who *are* available (teachers, peers, aides, volunteers, and parents) should be involved.

The "isolated therapy model" is described in Chapter Eleven.

One basic problem with the so-called "isolated therapy model" (Sternat, Messina, Nietupski, Lyon & Brown, 1977), where children are removed from the classroom for therapy, is the implication that teachers and communication specialists have mutually exclusive responsibilities and separate instructional settings. This is not true. The language/communication specialist may function as a consultant for the design and implementation of language programming and assume responsibility for assessment, while sharing some direct service responsibilities. The orchestration and follow-through of activities to promote language learning and communication are usually teacher responsibilities (with continuous consultation from the language/communication specialist), but teachers must also share some assessment and program development responsibilities. They should plan together for (a) implementation of language training objectives, (b) organization and integration of language training activities into daily classroom routines, and (c) continuous monitoring of child progress.

WHERE SHOULD LANGUAGE BE TAUGHT?

The home is the primary language learning environment of the normal learner, but there is also considerable instruction in settings outside the home, such as the day care environment, playground, stores, neighbors' homes. All of these instructional settings contain varied stimuli that perform both discriminative and reinforcing functions for language.

Providing language instruction in *all* of the environments where a handicapped child presently functions or will function is rarely possible. However, with planning, at least some proportion of language programming can be implemented in the domestic, recreational, community, and vocational settings where older severely handicapped students will function. At school, language training environments should include halls, bathrooms, the lunchroom, the playground, and certainly the *entire* classroom. The discriminative and reinforcing stimuli of environments that are difficult to visit regularly may be inventoried (with the ecological inventory procedures described later in this chapter) and simulated in the classroom. Keep in mind, however, the generalization problems of severely handicapped students.

> Language instruction, to the extent possible, should be provided in all the environments where the child presently functions or will function.

WHEN SHOULD LANGUAGE BE TAUGHT?

No one has ever measured the exact amount of instructional time caregivers provide, but it is substantial. Normal learners receive language instruction almost continuously the entire day. Even when not directly involved with meeting their children's needs or in joint play routines, caregivers talk about what is happening and what they are doing at that moment.

Maximizing instructional time during the school day has only recently begun to receive some attention (e.g., McCormick & Goldman, 1979; McCormick, Cooper, & Goldman, 1979). One planning approach to assure opportunities for language and communication training and practice throughout the school day is a matrix format such as Figure 6-1 (also see Chapter Nine). Routine activities are listed on the left and the child's objectives are written across the top. This format can assist identifying and planning opportunities for the child to produce and practice targeted skills throughout the school day. If modified and/or enlarged to serve as a programming or data sheet, specific antecedents and desired responses or data can be written in the appropriate cells. The sample form includes only language and motor objectives; it could, of course, also include objectives in other domains.

> Use of a matrix planning form can help to assure opportunities to learn and practice language and communication skills throughout the school day.

WHAT ARE THE BEST MATERIALS AND REINFORCERS FOR TEACHING LANGUAGE?

As noted above, there are an enormous number of stimuli for the young child to manipulate and talk about in natural language learning environments. This means countless opportunities to practice language and communicative skills. Attention to and engagement with various objects

> Chapters Two and Five describe natural antecedents and reinforcers for language.

Planning Form

	Prepositions "in" and "on"	Plurals	"Wh" questions	Requests	Increase vocabulary	Standing/stand-up table	Sitting-with support			
Arrival 8:00 - 8:15	✓	✓	✓	✓	✓					
Toileting 8:15 - 8:30	✓		✓	✓						
Free Play 8:30 - 9:00	✓		✓	✓	✓					
Large Group 9:00 - 9:30	✓	✓	✓			✓	✓			
Snack 9:30 - 9:50	✓	✓	✓	✓	✓		✓			
Pre-Academic 9:50 - 11:30	✓	✓	✓	✓	✓		✓			
Music/Art 11:30 - 12:00	✓	✓	✓	✓	✓	✓				
Toileting 12:00 - 12:15	✓		✓	✓						
Lunch 12:15 - 12:40	✓	✓	✓		✓		✓			
Rest/Story 12:40 - 1:15			✓	✓						
Outside Play 1:15 - 1:30				✓	✓					
Bus Prep. 1:30 - 1:45	✓		✓	✓	✓					
Minimum trials per day	10	6	11	10	8	2	4			

Name: Bobby James

FIGURE 6-1 Planning Form

usually serves as a cue for caregivers to talk about those objects, and the child's attempts to communicate are generally responded to, regardless of whether the form (topography) of the communication is correct.

Unfortunately, this is not the case in many classrooms. Too often, language training centers around the concrete objects and discrete events depicted in pictures in commercially produced kits rather than the child's interests. There is little concern for whether the child is familiar with or interested in the training stimuli. The form of his responses receives more attention than meaning and intent.

This is very different from the natural learning environment where, if the child communicates what he intends, he is usually rewarded with attention—a verbal response and/or the desired object or event. If he says "doggie," for example (and he generally does so only in the presence of a dog if he is in the earliest stages of language acquisition), he is encouraged to pet the animal. When he says "more" and holds up his empty glass, he is given more of whatever he has just drunk. He is *not* given a piece of cookie or drink of juice for saying "doggie," and no one says, "good talking" or "say the whole thing" when he says "more." In natural communicative exchanges, the listener indicates in some way that he has received and understood the child's message, responds in kind (e.g., child says "Hi" and partner says "Hi"), or expands the child's utterance ("Hi, how are you?").

To arrange an optimal language teaching environment, select materials and reinforcers according to children's interests, cognitive capabilities, and functional needs. Let these same variables dictate the content of instruction and adult responses to the children's communicative efforts. Assure that even the most subtle attempts to communicate obtain confirming feedback and place primary emphasis on increasing the quantity and quality of communications to obtain desired objects or activities and regulate the actions of others. Most importantly, do not confuse the means with the ends. Syntactic knowledge and the use of syntactic devices such as word order and tense markers are means for communication; *communication itself is the end goal of training.*

> The child's interests, cognitive capabilities, and his functional needs should dictate the content of instruction, selection of training materials, and the way the child is responded to.

WHAT TO TEACH

Assessment for the purpose of selecting and individualizing instructional content was discussed in Chapters Four and Five. There we stressed that the goals and objectives on a child's IEP should be thought of as a set of hypotheses to be operationally defined, refined and/or expanded, and tested by the language/communication specialist and teacher once a placement has been made. In many cases, you will need to augment pre-IEP assessment information with additional observations collected under more varied and natural conditions. (If an IEP revision is called for, of course, a meeting for parental approval of the revisions is required.)

When analyzing pre-IEP assessment information, keep in mind the range of variables discussed in Chapters Four and Five (e.g., poor attention, lack of motivation, unfamiliar testing situation, behavioral problems) that may have affected the test results. Because much of the information collected during the initial assessment process was directed towards the function of classification/certification, it will probably be norm-referenced. (The child's behavior has been compared to that of normal learners and reported as an age-equivalent score.) Analysis of pre-IEP test protocols will provide some data on language strengths and deficits; however, it is unlikely to yield specific information about the child's communication strategies with different persons and in different settings. Additional observations to determine program content for young children and older severely handicapped students are outlined in the next section.

DETERMINING CONTENT FOR THE YOUNG CHILD

Teacher-made checklists and observation techniques are useful to verify pre-IEP information and pinpoint more precisely the young child's available communication strategies. Table 6-4 provides suggestions to guide these observations.

TABLE 6-4   Guidelines for pinpointing language and communication strategies

Observe:	Note:
1. Child's participation in routine activities (at relatively set times each day)	a. Extent of group participation b. Appropriateness of social interactions c. Attention and control strategies d. Following instructions
2. Child's involvement with different materials and objects (in structured and unstructured situations)	a. Material and object preferences b. Appropriateness of materials/object use c. Duration of materials/object manipulation
3. Child's interactions with adults and peers	a. Type of communication devices used to secure desired objects and events b. Whether child is primarily an initiator or a reactor c. Variations in frequency of vocalizations across adults d. Coordination/agreement between verbal and nonverbal communicative efforts e. Whether child takes turns in conversational exchanges f. Contexts which stimulate the most communication
4. Child's symbolic (representational) behavior in play contexts	a. Type of pretend play—whether based on child's own experiences or vicarious experiences b. Use of one object to represent another object c. Whether pretend activities are in logical sequence

Programming objectives, based on these observations and the other available information, may focus on the following communicative functions. These objectives should include both initiating and responding behaviors, and should be defined in terms of social contexts and conditions of appropriateness.

Here are suggested pragmatic-interactions goals

For the Preverbal Child (Dore, 1974; Bates, 1976):

1. *Requesting* an object, action or information
2. *Greeting* someone entering the immediate environment
3. *Giving* an object to another person
4. *Showing* off an action or object to another person
5. *Acknowledging* receipt of another person's message
6. *Responding/answering* another person's request

These functions, indicating communicative intent, can be achieved through gestures, eye gaze, and/or vocalizations.

For the Single-Word Level Child (Dore, 1974):

1. *Labeling* an object or event with a word or word approximation while looking at it
2. *Repeating* part or all of a prior adult utterance
3. *Answering* adult's questions
4. *Requesting* an object, action, or information with a word or vocalization
5. *Calling* adult's name loudly and waiting for a response
6. *Greeting* an adult or object upon its appearance
7. *Protesting* an adult's action with a word or cry
8. *Practicing* word prosodic patterns (in absence of the specific object or event)

A greater variety of discourse functions appear at the next level and the form of communications begins to vary according to the context and the persons present.

For the Multi-Word Level Child (Dore, 1977):

Training objectives at this third level should focus on the use of multi-word utterances to accomplish many of the same functions (Chapman, 1981).

1. *Requesting* information, action or acknowledgment
2. *Responding* to requests
3. *Describing* past and present events
4. *Stating* facts, rules, attitudes, feelings, and beliefs, and evaluating
5. *Acknowledging and evaluating* responses and nonrequests
6. *Regulating* contact and conversation
7. *Accomplishing* acts (e.g., warning, teasing, protesting)

There will be times when training of specific vocabulary is considered necessary. To the extent possible, this training should be incorporated into daily classroom routines and play activities rather than provided in a massed-trial format. Use these questions, suggested by Jens and Belmore (1976), to assist you in selecting specific words and phrases to train with young children.

1. What objects does the child come in contact with most frequently during routine activities?
2. What people does the child interact with most frequently?
3. What words and phrases does the child hear most often in school? At home?
4. What verbal responses will the child be expected to make most often in his environment?

Both young children and older students should be prepared to function in present and future environments with nonhandicapped peers. In the case of the preschool child, probably the most important future environment is the school; for the older student as discussed below, there should be substantial attention to the communication requirements of future work, community, recreational and domestic environments. In either case, the next step, after formulating a satisfactory list of goals and objectives, is to review, prioritize, and analyze these target behaviors. Highest priorities should be assigned to those goals and objectives that receive the most "yeses" when you ask these questions:

1. Is the skill chronologically age-appropriate? Is this a skill that is typically performed by same-age peers?
2. Will the skill be functional in future environments and will it increase the probability of transition to and maintenance in these environments?
3. Will the skill help the child to be viewed more favorably (and therefore treated better) by others?

DETERMINING CONTENT FOR OLDER SEVERELY HANDICAPPED STUDENTS

Curricula for the older student should be subdivided into skill sequences reflecting domains where the student is currently functioning or needs to function (Brown, Branston-McClean, Baumgart, Vincent, Falvey, & Schroeder, 1979). It is ideal if the IEP can be organized according to these skill domains (domestic, recreational/leisure, general community, vocational, and education) rather than the typical developmental skill areas (e.g., cognitive, social, language, etc.), but this may not be acceptable in some school systems.

The first step in specifying content for older severely handicapped students is to determine current and subsequent environments. Figure 6-2 is an example of this effort. Then identify sub-environments and the

FIGURE 6-2 Example of curricular domains for a severely handicapped student

Student: Mary Beth Branston   Age: 11

	Domestic	Recreational/leisure	General community functioning	Vocational	Other
Current environments	a. Natural home b. Home of a friend c. Respite care home	a. Neighborhood area b. School playground c. Home of friend d. Public parks/ beaches	a. Hospital waiting room b. Church c. Sidewalks/streets d. Shopping center	a. Bedroom b. Kitchen c. Laundry room d. Yard e. Basement workshop	a. Educational
Subsequent environments	a. Group home b. Natural home c. Home of friends	a. Bowling alley b. YWCA c. Public parks/ beaches d. Movies e. Home f. Shopping center	a. Public bus b. Sidewalks/streets c. Office of dentist	a. Motel room b. Home c. Simulated workshop d. Food preparation area in school	a. Educational

Source: L. Brown, M.B. Branston-McClean, D. Baumgart, L. Vincent, M. Falvey, and J. Schroeder. Using the characteristics of current and subsequent least restrictive environments in the development of curricular content for severely handicapped students. *AAESPH Review,* 1979, 4(4). Reprinted by permission.

The ecological inventory process yields a set of objectives directed toward independent functioning in present and future environments.

activities that occur in these settings (e.g., kitchen—eating, cooking, putting away groceries, setting the table, clearing the table, etc.). The final step of this ecological inventory strategy is to identify skills needed to participate in these activities. (Figure 6-3 illustrates analysis of skills for one of the activities in one sub-environment.) The final outcome of the ecological inventory process is a set of objectives directed toward the ultimate goal of independent functioning in relevant present and future environments. A summary of the steps in implementing an ecological inventory strategy to determine curricular content for severely handicapped students is presented in Table 6-5.

FIGURE 6-3   Example of activity analysis from an ecological inventory

Domain: *Recreational/leisure for a junior high age student*
   Environment: *Public park/beach*
      Subenvironment 1: *Refreshment stand*
         Activity: *Purchasing refreshments*
            Skills: 1. Locating the refreshment stand (by responding to location cues, printed words and/or symbols)
            2. Presenting the money needed for the purchase of a drink to the clerk
            3. Ordering the drink
            4. Putting change in a pocket
            5. Drinking the drink
            6. Putting empty cup in trash receptacle

Source: Adapted from L. Brown, M.B. Branston-McClean, D. Baumgart, L. Vincent, M. Falvey, and J. Schroeder. Using the characteristics of current and subsequent least restrictive environments in the development of curricular content for severely handicapped students. *AAESPH Review,* 1979, 4(4), p. 421. Reprinted by permission.

TABLE 6-5   Steps in the ecological inventory process

1. List the five domains for organization of curricular content.
2. List the most relevant and functional environments within each domain where the student is presently functioning.
3. List the most relevant and functional environments within each domain where future functioning is desired.
4. Analyze each environment into sub-environments where the most relevant and functional activities occur.
5. Delineate activities occurring in the sub-environments that the student should be prepared to participate in.
6. Determine the critical skill requirements of each activity.
7. Determine the critical dimensions of each skill and whether the topography of the response or the critical effect is more important.
8. Develop a skill checklist. (Behaviors should be operationally stated and sequenced according to the order in which they are performed.)
9. Determine precisely where the student is functioning relative to the listed skills.
10. Translate activity descriptions into goals.
11. Translate identified skill deficits into instructional objectives.

TABLE 6-6 Adaptations for severe sensory and/or motor impairments

1. **Providing personal assistance.** Instead of prohibiting participation in an activity because the student's sensory and/or motor difficulties preclude *full* participation, secure the necessary assistance from other persons for that portion of the skill sequence that is too difficult. Allow the student to participate as fully as possible and continually explore ways to increase his contributions.

2. **Providing different or adapted materials and/or assisting devices.** In many cases, simply adapting or changing materials will make it possible for the student to participate in an activity. The student who is not able to spread solid butter on a piece of bread without tearing up the bread may prove to be very successful at performing the skill with whipped margarine. The student who cannot pour from a half gallon milk carton may be able to manage very well with a quart size carton. Many students can perform dressing skills independently if some thought is given to the type of garments selected or if clothing is adapted (e.g., Velcro replacing snaps or buttons). An adaptive device such as a wheelchair or a pocket calculator can enable or enhance student participation in critical activities. Portable communication devices such as a picture booklet can make it possible for a nonverbal student to order food items at a restaurant or bakery.

3. **Rearranging the sequence of required skills and/or adapting the rules of the activity.** Most activities can be accomplished in a variety of ways. An excellent example of this type of adaptation is provided by Brown et al. (1979). A student who has difficulty deciding immediately what he wants to order in a fast-food restaurant could be taught to locate a seat first, sit down, locate the pictures of the desired food items in his communication booklet, and *then* proceed to the counter to order. Many behaviors that are potentially awkward and time-consuming when performed under one set of conditions (e.g., sorting and folding clothes at the laundromat) can be better accomplished in another, more familiar environment (clothes can be sorted before going to the laundromat and folded later at home). The rules of leisure time activities can be changed to permit the student to fully participate. For example, dice can be substituted for spinners or vice versa (depending upon the student's fine motor skills), so that the student can play a particular board game. A basketball hoop or a volleyball net can be lowered to allow the student to participate in these activities.

When the ecological inventory process is completed and the student's skill deficits have been translated into instructional objectives, you will find that a significant number of these objectives target communication skills. Each communication objective should specify what the student will be taught to communicate *about* and, more importantly, the critical effect that the communication should have. For example, if you look back to the activity analysis example presented in Figure 6-3, you will see that to get a desired drink (the critical effect) at the refreshment stand the student must make a request. Depending upon his sensory and/or motor impairment, the student may be taught to produce "I want (would like, need) a Coke," select and display the picture of a Coke in his communication booklet, or point to the picture of Coke (if one is on display at the refreshment stand).

Recognizing that many severely handicapped students with severe sensory and/or motor impairments are not able to perform the critical skills required by some activities as "normal people" do, Brown et al. (1979) suggest the adaptations presented in Table 6-6.

Additional factors to consider with the severely handicapped student (after specifying instructional objectives) include:

1. *How* will the student communicate? What type of output mode and symbol system is best suited to the student's communication needs in this particular activity? (Decision making related to augmentative communication is discussed in Chapter Ten.)
2. What are the less complex task components of the skill and how should they be arranged (ordered) for instruction? (Task analysis is described below.)
3. What is the student's status relative to important prerequisites for performing the component subskills of the task analysis?
4. Are there sensorimotor skill deficiencies (e.g., tracking, object permanence, functional object use, means-end skills) that will affect training? What training modifications (if any) will be required to accommodate these deficiencies?

TASK ANALYSIS

Task analysis is the process of isolating, sequencing and describing the component skills or steps toward mastery of an instructional objective. Task components, or subskills, are identified, arranged in a series, and then defined in terms of observable motor response to specific stimuli. Instructional techniques to teach each subskill are then identified and applied.

The same skill may be analyzed ("sliced") in a number of ways.

There is no one correct task analysis for a particular skill. Different analyses will "slice" the same skill differently because (a) of different conceptualizations of the task and the learning process, and (b) each student's behavioral strengths and deficits, and his unique needs and entry behaviors, are different. It is extremely rare to be able to use the same task analysis without modification for any two students.

Component subskills in a task analysis may be generated by (a) performing the task yourself and noting the skill requirements, (b) watching someone else perform it and recording their behavior, or (c) logical analysis. Williams (1975) recommends the logical analysis approach—simply asking the question "What must the student be able to do to master this skill?" Then, you visualize performance of the major task and subskills to arrive at a list of subskill components.

Once you have derived component subskills, you must identify critical prerequisite skills (entry behaviors). Skills are designated as prerequisite or entry skills if they are going to be taught separately, rather than as part of the program for which the task analysis has been done. For example, if a student is going to be taught to "request a desired drink" by pointing to a picture in his communication booklet, the ability to point is a prerequisite skill for the "request a desired drink" program. An alternative to identifying the motor behavior "pointing" as a prerequisite would be to include it as a component subskill and teach it as part of the instructional program. If a component subskill can be performed in a manner that does not require the prerequisite, then the prerequisite should be eliminated.

Because task analysis can be very time-consuming and tedious, you may want to try to locate an objective and subskill sequence that can be modified to meet your specifications. There are some 30 or so curriculum/training guides describing instructional programs for early childhood/special education and/or the severely handicapped that may be of some help. Many offer preformulated goals and field-tested skill sequences, but they vary widely in scope, specificity, empirical support and theoretical rationales.

HOW TO TEACH

Identifying or developing instructional experiences to facilitate acquisition of language and communication skills is the next step after determining *what* to teach. This section considers the following general issues related to *how* to teach:

1. Deciding whether to focus instruction upon comprehension or production first, or whether to work on the two concurrently
2. Selecting instructional strategies
3. Deciding among instructional arrangement alternatives
4. Curricular organization

THE COMPREHENSION-PRODUCTION ISSUE

Discussion of the comprehension-production relationship in Chapter Two emphasized that the premise that comprehension is always first in normal learning is no longer taken for granted. Although prior exposure is obviously necessary to know how to reproduce a word, phrase, or sentence, the learner need not necessarily understand the meaning of a word or the rules underlying a syntactic structure before producing it. For this reason, the normal development research cannot be of considerable help in guiding this curriculum issue.

The question is whether to train comprehension or production first. A third possibility, of course, is to train the two skills concurrently. We cannot rely on training of one to generalize to the other. Baer and Guess (1973) have reported a series of experiments suggesting that the two skill areas may be functionally independent. They contend that training in comprehension does not necessarily lead to correct production, nor can training in production be assumed to lead to comprehension.

These are the training alternatives:

Comprehension and production may be trained simultaneously, or one or the other may be trained first.

1. Elicit both types of responses concurrently, e.g., "Show me the _____." When the child has indicated the appropriate stimulus, then hold it up and ask "What is this?" or provide a model to be imitated ("Say _____"). In this case, the comprehension response is elicited first, followed by elicited production or imitation,

but it could as easily be sequenced with imitation and/or production and then the comprehension response (e.g., "Say _____" [model of the target form], "What is this?" and finally "Show me the _____").

2. Teach productive skills before comprehension skills as Guess Sailor, and Baer (1976a, 1976b, 1977a, 1977b, 1978) advocate. Verbal imitation is a necessary prerequisite in this approach.

3. Teach receptive skills (comprehension) before teaching production as Bricker, Dennison, and Bricker (1976) advocate. You remember that their program begins with strategies to establish attending, then teaches imitation, functional use, and word recognition (comprehension).

SELECTING INSTRUCTIONAL STRATEGIES

As discussed in an earlier section, almost all language training models, regardless of theoretical biases, use behavioral intervention strategies. Where the different models diverge is (a) the context for training—*where* modeling, reinforcement, shaping, fading, prompting, cuing, chaining, and discrimination training are provided, (b) the degree of consistency and (c) amount of structure. Past behavioral models tended to rely on rigid massed trial formats, while psycholinguistic and developmental models suggest less methodical applications. There is presently a trend away from dichotomizing developmental and behavioral procedures toward a search for overlapping and complementary strategies. Highly structured training procedures are gradually being supplanted by instructional strategies patterned after those of caregivers in naturally occurring caregiver-child interactions.

The important thing to remember about behavioral techniques is that they are just that—a technology, *not a curriculum.* The student's instructional curriculum goals and objectives should guide the selection of training strategies, not vice versa (Guess & Noonan, 1982).

Curriculum goals and objectives should guide selection of training strategies, *not* vice versa.

This section focuses on the behavioral strategies most often employed for language intervention. To better understand these elementary techniques and other, more sophisticated principles of instructional management (especially the appropriate use of reinforcement and punishment procedures), consult the following sources: Birnbrauer, 1977; Gardner, 1971; Kazdin, 1975; Alberto & Troutman, 1982. These instructional strategies are similar and, in some cases, identical to those used by caregivers. The main difference is that they are applied more loosely in the natural environment.

Modeling "Normal" learners may have a built-in propensity to reproduce what they see and hear. Think back to the many occasions when you have imitated the behavior of others in unfamiliar situations and you will realize the learning potential inherent in imitative skills. Verbal imitation is so important that when all attempts to teach it fail, communication in the speech mode may be ruled out. Verbal imitation is, in fact, one prognostic indicator for the success or failure of verbal language training.

The two terms "imitation" and "modeling" refer to distinctly different processes. Modeling is "showing how" behavior. When used as an instructional procedure, it means "providing a demonstration of the response (motor or verbal) expected of the learner." Usually the stimulus model is accompanied or preceded by a verbal direction (e.g., "Do this," "Say __"). When the word or sign is modeled, an instance of the concept being labeled (object, event, or appropriate picture) should also be presented.

> Modeling is "showing how" behavior, imitation is "matching" the stimulus behavior or model.

Imitation is the other side of the coin. It is a learning strategy: performance of a response that matches, or at least approximates, the stimulus behavior. Once learned, imitation skills can be used to establish an infinite range and variety of more complex skills. Imitation is also a learning process in and of itself. The child learns to take turns within a prescribed temporal dimension (Reichle & Yoder, 1979). The child learns to produce the appropriate topographical features of a behavior produced by another person, and, equally important, he learns to produce that copy at the right time (immediately after the model).

There are many approaches to establishing imitative responding so that modeling can be used as a teaching procedure. Some espouse developmental biases and others a behavioral-functional position. Developmental approaches to teaching imitation to nonspeaking children feature training that parallels stages in the normal development of imitative skills (e.g., Bricker, Dennison, & Bricker, 1976; Bricker & Dennison, 1978; Reichle & Yoder, 1979). Following the stages posited by Piaget (see Chapter Two, Table 2-4), training begins with mutual imitation if the child is nonimitative and proceeds through the various stages of development to spontaneous imitation of new models (the final stage). In the early training phases, motor and vocal models are selected from behaviors already in the child's repertoire. The main consideration is to begin imitation training at or near the child's entry functioning level.

> Developmental approaches advocate a training sequence that parallels the stages of normal development of imitative skills.

Reichle and Yoder (1979) also argue persuasively for viewing the establishment of mutual imitation as a first phase in the imitation training paradigm. The advantage is two-fold: in mutual imitation the child does not need to pay careful attention to and precisely match the topography of a new model, *and* he learns to be the initiator of turn-taking sequences. In other words, mutual imitation training teaches the child that he can initiate interactions and select the topography of turn-taking interactions.

Behavioral-functional approaches to teaching imitation to nonspeaking children place a high priority on assuring that modeled stimuli (motor or verbal) are (a) functional, and (b) provided in a meaningful context (e.g., Goetz, Schuler, & Sailor, 1979; Guess, Sailor, & Baer, 1978). Imitative responses that are natural and necessary to the child's daily activities (e.g., bringing a cup to the lips) and have the potential to result in positive, natural consequences (in the case of bringing a cup to the lips, the consequence is a taste of liquid) are identified and trained. These behaviors are what Guess, Sailor, and Baer (1978a) call *functional responses;* they are

> Behavioral approaches contend that modeled stimuli should be functional and provided in a meaningful context.

natural to the child's interaction with the environment and they produce an immediate consequence which is potentially reinforcing and specific.

Functional responses are behaviors natural to the child's environment that produce immediate and reinforcing consequences.

Selecting functional responses for imitation training has a definite advantage because it saves instructional time. In the past, there was a tendency to train imitation of such nonfunctional behaviors as nose touching, hand clapping, and arm raising. Training often required hundreds, or even thousands, of trials and the child had nothing to show for it except, presumably, a generalized response class (imitation). The child was not able to affect his environment with these nonfunctional responses. Committing the same amount of time to training functional responses such as activating a windup toy, twisting a door knob, turning on a record player, or unzipping a coat is appealing because these responses help the student gain some independence and control of the environment.

One recommendation of Reichle and Yoder (1979) crosses the line separating developmental and functional approaches—using manual signs as initial imitative training stimuli. Then, if the child is eventually determined to be unsuited for verbal language training, the basis for a manual signing program has already been established. If selection of stimulus signs is based on functional criteria, and if the child receives the object or event symbolized as a consequence for imitating the sign, this training would certainly qualify as a functional imitation training approach (illustrating the overlap between developmental and behavioral approaches).

Imitation training for echolalic children involves teaching discrimination of stimuli which *should* be imitated from stimuli which *should not* be reproduced.

Imitation training for echolalic children is somewhat different than for nonimitative children. Behavioral techniques (prompting, fading, reinforcing correct imitations, and ignoring echolalic ones) are applied to teach the child to discriminate speech that should be imitated from speech that should not be reproduced.

"Volume prompting" is one imitation training technique for echolalic children. The discriminative stimulus (e.g., "What is this?") is presented very softly (almost inaudibly), followed by a verbal model for the desired response (e.g., "a ball," said in a loud voice). The volume of the question is gradually increased while the model for the imitative response is decreased in volume.

Another technique for training imitation with echolalic children is reported by Freeman, Ritvo, and Miller (1975). The verbal model is presented before the question or instruction. For example, the teacher says, "Eating—what is the boy doing?" and provides reinforcement immediately when the child imitates "eating," before he has a chance to repeat the question.

Palyo, Cooke, Schuler, and Apolloni (1979) have developed an interesting variation of this technique. They trained three handicapped preschoolers exhibiting echolalia to respond to a series of questions by presenting taped models of the correct response. Prior to training, the three children consistently echoed each of the 25 questions, 12 of which were later used in the generalization probes. Each response targeted for training (responses were taught one at a time) was prerecorded on a cassette tape with 25 repetitions and a 1- to 2-second pause between repetitions. During training, after gaining the child's attention, the instructor presented the targeted stimulus question (e.g., "What's your name?"). If the child echoed the question, gave an incorrect response, or was silent for 10 seconds, the instructor said "No," removed the reinforcer from view, and turned away momentarily. Simultaneously, the tape recorder was switched on to play the correct response. When the child echoed the correct response, the recorder was switched off, and the child was provided with an edible and praise. If, following any of the 25 prerecorded repetitions, the child did not echo the taped response, the tape was rewound and training continued. Three to seven sessions (10 trials per session) were required before correct responses were emitted to the first stimulus question. However, each subsequent application of the procedure to a new question required fewer sessions. By completion of training on the first stimulus question, there was a noticeable decrease in echolalic responding to the three untrained questions in the set. Generalization of training to several new functional responses and increased spontaneous use of functional phrases were reported, in addition to generalization across settings and stimuli. The trained responses tended to remain over time and the children responded appropriately to untrained but similar questions at a 12-month followup.

Reinforcement Reinforcement is any event that immediately follows a response and has the effect of increasing the probability that the response will be repeated. When immediately following a response with some event strengthens the response (makes it occur more often in the future), only then can the consequent event be termed "reinforcement." The pervasive notion that provision of "goodies" (e.g., M&Ms, candy, trinkets, praise) after appropriate behavior is always reinforcement is simplistic and inaccurate. Reinforcement (positive or negative) can only be defined by its effect on the behavior that it follows.

> Any event that immediately follows a response and has the effect of increasing that response is a reinforcer.

When a response increases qualitatively or quantitatively because it is immediately followed by some particular event, a contingency arrangement is established. As discussed in Chapter Five, this association between response and subsequent event is termed a "functional relationship"; it has enormous implications for learning.

There are two types of reinforcement procedures—positive and negative. *Positive reinforcement* refers to the increased probability of a response resulting from the application of a positive event. *Negative reinforcement* has the same effect (a strengthened response), but it involves a different procedure. Instead of adding or providing a positive event, an aversive event (called a "negative reinforcer") is removed immediately following the target behavior. A good example of negative reinforcement can be found in cars that require fastening a seat belt to terminate an aversive alarm sound. Negative reinforcement occurs *if* cessation of the aversive sound (immediately following seat belt fastening) results in strengthening of the seat belt fastening response.

> Positive reinforcement is adding an event that strengthens a response; negative reinforcement is removing an event to strengthen a response.

There are two general classes of positive reinforcers—primary and secondary. *Primary reinforcers* are unlearned (unconditioned) (e.g., water if you are thirsty, sleep if you are tired). *Secondary reinforcers* are learned (conditioned); they have acquired their reinforcement value by being paired with already existing reinforcers (primary or secondary). An example is social praise, which is often established as a secondary reinforcer by pairing it with edibles (primary reinforcers). A third inclusive class of reinforcers are called "generalized reinforcers." *Generalized reinforcers* are secondary reinforcers that are particularly powerful because of their association with many established reinforcers. Examples of generalized reinforcers are money, tokens, attention, and approval.

The use of natural and response-specific reinforcers is relatively new and very pertinent to language training. Saunders and Sailor (1979) found that using a different ("specific") reinforcer for each response being trained resulted in more rapid acquisition of receptive labeling skills by three severely retarded children. The alternative is to use the same consequence for several responses. The degree to which stimulus and reinforcer are the same may also affect rate of learning. The child learning to say "cookie" when a cookie is displayed as the discriminative stimulus will acquire the label more rapidly if correct responses result in being allowed to eat pieces of cookies (provided, of course, that the child desires the cookie) than if correct responses result in some other event. This is the reason that labels for preferred foods are prominent in the normal learner's early vocabulary.

Reinforce the child's attempts to communicate *and* the meaningfulness and appropriateness of the communications.

Keep in mind that what is reinforced in the normal learning situation is the child's attempt to communicate and the relationship between form, content, and use (i.e., the meaningfulness and appropriateness of the child's communication). When a consequent event (effect) indicates to the child that he has communicated his intention, he is likely to communicate this particular intention in the same or similar way in the future. In other words, the communicative attempt has been reinforced and, therefore, strengthened.

The attention of a listener would seem to be the ultimate motivation for language; however, objects and events that the child considers desirable and important enough to be talked about and asked for are also powerful reinforcers. A positive implication of the recent focus on naturally occurring reinforcers is recognition of the need to identify the range and variety of potentially desirable consequences in the natural environment. This task, of course, is easier with some children than with others. Paradoxically (as discussed in Chapter Five), it is the children who are most in need of functional communication training (e.g., autistic children) who demonstrate the narrowest range of desires and needs.

Whenever possible, use naturally occurring events rather than contrived and artificial stimuli to reinforce desirable behaviors.

Whenever the use of contrived rewards and artificial reinforcement conditions can be avoided altogether in favor of naturally occurring events, this is the most desirable and effective approach. However, as discussed in Chapter Five, in the initial stages of instruction, particularly with the more severely handicapped child who has a narrow range of needs and desires, artificial reinforcers may be the only viable and effective resources. As training progresses, contrived consequences can be gradually replaced by, or faded toward, natural effects.

Children's developmental levels contribute to some of the variance in preferred events (individual preferences and deprivation state presumably account for the balance of this variance). Children appear to have different reinforcement preferences at different stages. As Cohen and Gross (1979) have pointed out, "The appeal of individual activities is developmental in nature ... certain sensory categories have a special appeal to the child, depending on the particular developmental level at which he is functioning" (p. 213).

Shaping   Shaping is the process of reinforcing gradually closer approximations of the desired terminal response. The skill is first broken down into component steps, and the steps are sequenced so that each is a closer approximation of the desired terminal response. Each step or approximation is reinforced until learned. At that point, the next behavior, an even closer approximation of the desired target, is reinforced, and reinforcement for the earlier step is withheld. Eventually, the child produces the desired form of the target response. For example, when shaping requesting behavior, the adult would initially provide the child with the desired (requested) object when he produces the most sophisticated requesting behavior in his repertoire, which might be staring, pointing, or grunting. Then a slightly more refined request form would be required and reinforced (by providing the requested object or event) until that behavior is produced at a high frequency. This process continues until the terminal requesting response (e.g., "want X") is produced at criterion level.

> Shaping is reinforcing closer and closer approximations to the target skill.

Prompting and cuing   There is considerable overlap and confusion in the definitions of prompts and cues. Because they both function to assist or "prime" a desired response, we have chosen to use the terms interchangeably and concentrate on the effect of these instructional supports rather than be concerned with semantic differentiation. Whether referred to as a prompt, cue, or direction, instructional assistance is not effective unless it occasions the desired response, and can be eventually removed or faded (Koegel, Egel, & Dunlap, 1980).

Falvey, Brown, Lyon, Baumgart and Schroeder (1980) describe various "priming" (they use the term "cuing") strategies. In each case, if the demonstration is provided after the child has responded incorrectly, it is considered a correction procedure.

1. *Modeled cues,* providing the student with a demonstration of the actions he is expected to perform
2. *Direct verbal cues,* providing the student with verbal directions or commands that require relatively specific actions
3. *Gestural cues,* providing the student with physical, nonverbal motions (e.g., shaking one's head, pointing) indicating that certain actions should be performed

> Fading is the gradual removal of assistance and supports until the desired behavior has been learned.

4. *Pictorial cues,* providing the student with representational, two-dimensional pictures, numbers, or other symbols to indicate that certain actions should be performed

The distinction between instructional cues (and correction procedures) and natural cues (and correction procedures) is more important, from a functional standpoint, than differentiation of the cuing strategies themselves. Falvey et al. extend Brown's ecological inventory strategy (presented earlier in this chapter) to include both procedures for identifying and the listing cues and correction procedures available in the student's natural environment. The reason for identifying naturally occurring cues and correction procedures is to insure generalization; these cues and correction procedures are the stimuli that must eventually control the student's behavior.

There are a number of ways to "prime" a response.

Naturally occurring cues and correction procedures in the student's environments and the skills required to participate in relevant activities in these environments can be observed and recorded with the ecological inventory procedures. The goal of instruction, then, is to teach the student to perform the relevant skills required when performing critical activities in response to naturally occurring cues and correction procedures.

Fading   Fading is the gradual removal of instructional supports and assistance so that the desired behavior is performed independently, or with only naturally occurring supports. Fading may involve shifting from complete to partial prompts and cues, or reduction of the amount of assistance. The important factor is continued maintenance of the learned behavior at acceptable criteria, without the instructional prompts and cues. Fading should never be haphazard. It should be planned in advance and implemented systematically to shift the control of newly acquired behaviors from instructional prompts and cues to those that occur naturally in the child's environments.

In time delay the prompt or cue is delayed so that the learner will anticipate and produce the desired response without assistance.

One useful method of fading prompts and cues in language training is time delay (Touchette, 1971). The provision of a prompt or cue is delayed by gradually increasing time increments to give the student an opportunity to anticipate and produce the response without assistance. For example, in teaching responding to the question "What do you want?" at snacktime, the child is asked the question, the juice is displayed as a cue, and a model "Say juice" is provided. When the child has learned to respond at criterion level, the teacher may reduce the cue to "ju" after asking the question and displaying the juice. Time delay procedures would dictate delaying the provision of "ju" for longer and longer intervals (perhaps one second longer after each correct trial), to allow the child to produce the response without assistance.

Applying fading procedures is more complicated when dealing with autistic children. As discussed in Chapter Five, many autistic children have a tendency to respond to only a very limited portion of the stimuli in a stimulus complex (called stimulus overselectivity)—a learning strategy problem that has particular implications for fading cues and prompts.

While most children are able to use the cues and prompts to assist learning to discriminate, autistic children often have difficulty shifting attention from the cues and/or prompts to the training stimuli. They tend to learn the "assistors" instead of the desired discrimination so that when prompts or cues are removed, they fail to perform the response or perform incorrectly.

Research dealing with the overselectivity problem has generally focused on two types of solutions (Koegel, Egel, & Dunlap, 1980): (a) procedures to avoid the overselectivity problem, and (b) procedures that attempt to remediate the problem. Schreibman's (1975) method of avoiding the overselectivity problem is to use prompts that are inherent within the training stimulus (called within-stimulus prompts). What this involves is simply exaggerating the relevant characteristic(s) of the training stimulus. If, for example, you are teaching the discrimination between a bus and a car, instead of adding an external prompt such as color (making the bus red and the car green), the curve of the top of the two vehicles would be exaggerated (possibly by a heavy black line that would then be gradually faded). Presumably, if color is added as a prompt, the child would learn to discriminate red and green but would not learn to discriminate the bus and the car.

Other investigations (e.g., Schover & Newsom, 1976) have considered techniques for working on the overselectivity problem directly. One method is to overtrain an already learned discrimination. Schreibman, Koegel, and Craig (1977) caution that overtraining alone may not be sufficient. They suggest interspersing unreinforced trials with prompts or cues among reinforced trials without the prompts or cues. To eliminate overselectivity, this procedure must be implemented for a prolonged period of time. After many trials some autistic children learn to respond to the complete stimulus complex (with both prompts and training stimuli).

Chaining Chaining, which in some ways resembles shaping, can be used to teach new behaviors or link together a series of responses already in the child's repertoire to form a more complex behavior. Chaining can be used very effectively to expand the length of utterances. The desired terminal behavior (e.g., a three-element sentence) should first be broken down into component parts. The parts are then sequenced as they will be taught, in either a forward or backward direction. In forward chaining, the first unit is taught first; in backward chaining, the last unit is taught first. As each successive step is mastered and performed along with the previous step, reinforcement is shifted to the next step of the chain.

McLean (McCormick) and McLean (1974) applied a backward chaining procedure to train three nonverbal autistic children to produce three-element sentences with small plywood shapes as words. The children were first reinforced for identifying the correct object-class word symbol and placing it after the symbol's agent-action already on a tray. After three object class symbols were taught to criterion level, identification and placement of the action-class word symbol and the object-class word symbol were reinforced (e.g., the child produced the two-element chain "give ball" when given a ball). In the third training condition the child identified (and placed on the tray in sequence) the entire three-element construction (agent-action-object) to describe different transactions. In all, the child learned through a chaining procedure to produce six three-element sentences to describe six discrete transactions.

Discrimination training   Premack (1970) suggests that to learn language a child must be able to (a) discriminate among various sets of symbols (words), (b) discriminate among various classes of objects and events, (c) discriminate among various sequential stimulus arrangements, and (d) associate different sequential arrangements with different meanings.

Discrimination, the opposite of generalization, can be defined as differential responding in accordance with the distinctive features and properties of stimuli. Desired responses are reinforced if produced in the presence of a particular stimulus (called a discriminative stimulus or S^D) or group of stimuli. Reinforcement is withheld if the response is produced in the presence of a second stimulus or group of stimuli. The ultimate goal of discrimination training is differential responding controlled by the relevant features of environmental stimuli or events.

INSTRUCTIONAL ARRANGEMENTS

Because young and/or severely handicapped students have special learning needs, they were thought to need one-to-one instructional arrangements.

Basically, there are three instructional arrangement alternatives: (a) one-to-one, (b) clustered individualized, where students are taught individually within the group, and (c) group instruction. In the past, many considered the one teacher-one student format ideal for instruction and therapy with any handicapped child, in almost all skill domains. Particularly with the very young and/or severely handicapped, the one-to-one format was advocated as the most appropriate arrangement because of heterogeneous skill deficits, attention deficits, and a range of disruptive behaviors. These assumptions are undoubtedly responsible for the popularity of the "isolated therapy model" (Sternat, Nietupski, Messina, Lyon & Brown, 1977) which is discussed in Chapter Eleven. In this model therapy services are one-to-one and provided in a segregated environment (usually a therapy room).

Recently, investigators have questioned the assumption that one-to-one instruction is the best instructional arrangement for handicapped students. They question it on two grounds—effectiveness and efficiency. Flavell, Flavell, and McGimsey (1978) found that learning rates for severely handicapped students on a word recognition task were as rapid under group instruction as in one-to-one training conditions. In addition, group training was three times more efficient in terms of teacher time. Alberto, Jobes, Sizemore, and Doran (1980) found no significant difference in acquisition of prepositions and color discriminations between individual and group formats, despite the fact that a smaller number of opportunities for direct responding were available in the group format. Storm and Willis (1978) obtained similar results with gross and fine motor tasks and Kohl, Wilcox, and Karlan (1978) found group instruction in motor imitation of manual signs provided acquisition of a greater number of signs. Work done by Dever (1978) and Miller and Yoder (1974) suggests that in tasks requiring a verbal response, responding in unison may enhance rate of acquisition. Frankel and Graham (1976) and Goldstein and Alberto (1979) found that group instruction of the severely handicapped in many cases can result in faster learning than one-to-one instruction. These findings have important implications for efficient use of classroom instructional time.

Problems related to generalization are another argument against exclusive reliance on one-to-one instructional arrangements in special education classrooms. Research with autistic children has found that responses such as attending, imitation, and communication that were learned in one-to-one training were rarely performed in a large group and only occasionally performed in 2:1 sessions (Koegel & Rincover, 1977).

Effective transition from early intervention programs to regular kindergarten classrooms, a major concern for preschool special education teachers, may be hampered by the use of one-to-one instructional arrangements. Regular kindergarten classrooms provide significantly less one-to-one instruction than special education classes (1% compared to 10%), and more small group activities (20% compared to 10% in early childhood/special education classes) (Vincent, Salisbury, Walter, Brown, Gruenewald, & Powers, 1980). Young children may not be able to generalize behaviors learned under very circumscribed one-to-one conditions in the special classrooms to more natural, ambiguous group instruction conditions in regular kindergarten or first grade settings.

Brown, Holvoet, Guess and Mulligan (1980) suggest three factors to help decide whether to implement one-to-one or group training:

> *Recent findings indicate that group instruction may be more effective than one-to-one arrangements.*

1. *Compatibility of students' needs*   A wide diversity of needs and instructional objectives is not sufficient reason to veto group instruction (because training can still be individualized), but it *is* a factor to consider

2. *Whether or not the skills to be taught are usually performed in a group or alone*   Some skills (e.g., most self-care skills) are performed alone as opposed to other skills (e.g., language and social skills) which depend on the presence of other persons

3. *The student's need for group interaction, observation, and communication skills*

An alternative to either one-to-one instruction or group arrangements is "clustered individualized." Students are individually instructed in a group context with no attempt to systematically structure peer interactions or observational learning. They may or may not be working on similar objectives. Stimuli are presented to one student at a time by the teacher, and individual response requirements are defined by the student's individualized program.

CURRICULAR ORGANIZATION

Traditionally, curricula have been arranged vertically by developmental areas—language training, social skills development, cognitive/preacademic instruction, motor training, and self-help training (Guess & Noonan, 1982). While this type of organization accommodates the scheduling needs of teachers and related service personnel, it may not be the most efficient or effective allocation of instructional time. In addition to perpetuating discipline boundaries, vertically arranged curricula have the potential to actually impede, rather than facilitate, acquisition and generalization.

When language and communication skill training is removed from the flow of daily living routines and instructional activities, it is like practicing chords without hearing the whole melody.

Separation of the curriculum and the school day into the traditional skill domains is unnatural and counterproductive. It is a bit like the repetitious practicing of chords on a musical instrument, rather than the whole song; you never hear the melody. The assumption has been that students will synthesize and generalize across skill domains and time periods. This assumption has rarely been supported with handicapped learners.

Brown and colleagues, working primarily with older students, define curricular domains in terms of "life spaces" where the student will need to function and train in these contexts. This method of curricula organization, and the one developed by Guess and colleagues (see Chapter Nine) for younger children, have several advantages:

1. Each target skill is directly relevant to increased independent functioning
2. Generalization is facilitated because target skills have been selected from, and are taught where they will be used—the natural environment

GENERALIZATION AND MAINTENANCE

The germane query about generalization is: How much, what, and where do we need to teach in order to guarantee the carryover and maintenance of trained skills in the natural environment? Because functional communication requires both response and stimulus generalization, both must be incorporated into curricular design. The ultimate goal is for students to produce newly learned responses (e.g., words, signs, gestures) in a range of contexts (with different persons, in different settings, with different stimuli, and removed in time from training). This type of carryover (stimulus generalization) is most readily achieved if the new persons, settings, and stimuli are very similar to those in the training context, and when the latency between training and the need for demonstration is very short. It becomes increasingly more elusive as demonstration contexts and time become more removed from the training context and time. In other words, the greater the differences between training and demonstration contexts, the greater the generalization challenge. Decreasing the disparity between these two contexts reduces the generalization demands on the child.

Stimulus generalization is production of learned responses in a range of contexts; response generalization is repertoire expansion.

Response generalization is equally important. Students should use newly acquired skills to expand their repertoire. If response generalization does not occur, the child taught to say "juice" would use the word only to request orange juice (as used in training) and not apple juice or other juices.

Response generalization is assessed by observing whether the child applies language knowledge and rules acquired during training in spontaneous communication. As you would imagine, response generalization research requires considerable resources and time. For this reason, there is a paucity of data concerning the response generalization of handicapped children.

TRAINING FOR GENERALIZATION AND MAINTENANCE

From an intervention perspective, it is best to begin with the premise that generalization will not occur naturally. It requires thoughtful planning. Warren, Rogers-Warren, Baer, and Guess (1980) suggest six procedures to promote generalizations. The first three are applied *during* training; the remaining three are to promote generalization in nontraining environments *after* training.

1. *Train sufficient exemplars*   Present sufficient concept or rule exemplars to demonstrate the scope of the stimulus class and continue training until generalized performance is demonstrated in the training context. Precisely how many exemplars will need to be trained will depend on the child, stimulus conditions, and the target responses.

2. *Train loosely*   During training, vary stimuli, instructors, and settings and be somewhat flexible about acceptable response forms. The premise here is that minimum control over the range of stimuli presented and responses accepted will promote transfer to a wide class of stimuli.

3. *Use intermittent schedules of reinforcement*   Reinforcement contingencies in the natural environment are unpredictable. Simulating these unpredictable conditions in training (after initial acquisition sessions) will make the response more resistent to extinction.

4. *Create opportunities for language*   Assure that the child has things to talk about and people to talk to in the natural environment. Arrange events to signal and encourage the use of language. The child with a limited repertoire obviously cannot talk about many objects and events. Unless the particular object and events he can talk about happen to be present in nontraining environments, he cannot be expected to talk. Also, keep in mind that there is no substitute for listeners. Environmental arrangements that make peer and adult listeners more readily available will have a positive effect on the rate of child verbalization.

5. *Make language functional for the child* Arrange interesting objects and events to be contingent upon verbal behavior. The child's attention focus should be a cue to request ("mand" in behavioral terms) the child to verbalize (e.g., "Tell me what you want"). If the child does not know the appropriate form or structure, provide a verbal model and insist upon imitation before providing the desired object or activity. There should be many opportunities during the school day (and at home) for the child to experience the "power" of language as a mediator of goods and services.

6. *Reward the use of language* Reinforce the use of trained responses and/or increase the overall rate of reinforcement for all language use. Provide attention, praise, desired objects, and services contingent upon talking to signal to the child that the non-training setting, like the training context, is a place where language is required and valued.

EVALUATING GENERALIZATION AND MAINTENANCE

Quantifying natural environment generalization may be time-consuming, but it is worth the effort. One or two 15-minute language samples a week should be taped or recorded in writing (at a time when the child is likely to talk), at home and/or in the classroom. List the goal(s) of the child's training program (e.g., object labeling, requesting, questioning, agent-action relations) on a checklist. Then listen to the tape or check through the written record and note whether there is generalization of trained responses.

If there are no natural opportunities or supports for trained responses, they are unlikely to generalize.

Keep in mind that, because of the situational specificity of some utterances, the context of the observation period may not provide an appropriate opportunity for the utterance to be demonstrated. When you suspect that this may be the reason why there appears to be a lack of generalization, change observation times and/or observe more frequently.

SUMMARY

1. Psycholinguistic, behavioral, and developmental models differ in the extent to which they ascribe importance to prior development and their programming focus.

2. The more recent pragmatic-interaction perspective de-emphasizes what the child can produce, focusing instead on what he can accomplish with language.

3. A basic decision in developing and/or selecting a language training program is how much emphasis to place on teaching specific communication behaviors versus targeting generative language and a broad class of communicative functions.

4. Curriculum content for older severely handicapped students should be based on the requirements for adaptation to, and independent functioning in, future environments.

5. Curriculum content for infants and young handicapped children should target generative language and the development of general communicative competence.

6. The success of language intervention efforts depends upon informed decisions (by the language/communication specialist and the teacher) about the *who, where, when,* and *what* of instruction.

7. Pre-IEP assessment information may not be sufficient to generate instructional content; additional natural environment observations are required.

8. Use activity adaptations, when necessary, to assist partial participation of students with severe sensory and/or motor impairments.

9. There are three ways to perform a task analysis—perform the skill yourself and list the skill requirements, watch someone else perform it and record his behavior, or use a logical analysis process.

10. Most language training programs, regardless of their theoretical orientation, apply the basic behavioral procedures—modeling, reinforcement, shaping, fading, prompting and cuing, chaining, and discrimination training.

11. There is some question about the effectiveness and efficiency of the traditional one-to-one training arrangement; it may hamper efforts to transfer students to regular education settings.

12. Separation of the curriculum and school day into traditional developmental skill domains may be unnatural and counterproductive.

13. Generalization and maintenance cannot be left to chance; they require thoughtful planning and the application of special procedures.

REFERENCES

ALBERTO, P.A., & TROUTMAN, A.C. *Applied behavior analysis for teachers.* Columbus: Charles E. Merrill, 1982.

ALBERTS, P., JOBES, N., SIZEMORE, A., and DORAN, D. A comparison of individual and group instruction across response tasks. *Journal of the Association for the Severely Handicapped,* 1980, 5(3), 285–293.

BAER, D.M., & GUESS, D. Teaching productive noun suffixes to severely retarded children. *American Journal of Mental Deficiency,* 1973, 77, 498–505.

BATES, E. *Language and context.* New York: Academic Press, 1976.

BIRNBRAUER, J.S. Mental retardation. In H. Leitenberg (Ed.), *Handbook of behavior modification.* New York: Appleton-Century-Crofts, 1977.

BLOOM, L., & LAHEY, M. *Language development and language disorders.* New York: John Wiley & Sons, 1978.

BRICKER, D.D., & DENNISON, L. Training prerequisites to verbal behavior. In M.E. Snell (Ed.), *Systematic instruction of the moderately and severely handicapped.* Columbus: Charles E. Merrill, 1978.

BRICKER, D.D., DENNISON, L., & BRICKER, W.A. *A language intervention program for developmentally young children.* Miami, Fla.: University of Miami, Mailman Center for Child Development, Monograph No. 1, 1976.

BRICKER, D.D., RUDER, K.F., & VINCENT, L. An intervention strategy for language deficient children. In N.G. Haring and R.L. Schiefelbusch (Eds.), *Teaching special children.* New York: McGraw-Hill, 1976.

BROWN, F., HOLVOET, J., GUESS, D., & MULLIGAN, M. The Individualized Curriculum Sequencing Model (III): Small group instruction. *Journal of the Association for the Severely Handicapped,* 1980, *5*(4), 352–367.

BROWN, L., BRANSTON-McCLEAN, M.B., BAUMGART, D., VINCENT, L., FALVEY, M., & SCHROEDER, J. Using the characteristics of current and subsequent least restrictive environments in the development of curricular content for severely handicapped students. *AAESPH Review,* 1979, *4*(4), 407–424.

BROWN, L., NIETUPSKI, J., & HAMRE-NIETUPSKI, S. The criterion of ultimate functioning and public school services for severely handicapped students. In M.A. Thomas (Ed.), *Hey don't forget about me: Education's investment in the severely, profoundly, and multiply handicapped.* Reston, Va.: Council for Exceptional Children, 1976.

CHAPMAN, R.S. Exploring children's communicative intent. In J.F. Miller (Ed.), *Assessing language production in children.* Baltimore: University Park Press, 1981.

CHOMSKY, N. *Aspects of the theory of syntax.* Cambridge, Mass.: MIT Press, 1965.

COHEN, M.A., & GROSS, P.J. *The developmental resource: Behavioral sequences for assessment and program planning* (Vol. 1 and 2). New York: Grune & Stratton, 1979.

DEVER, R.B. Language assessment through specification of goals and objectives. *Exceptional Children,* 1978,·*45*(2), 123–129.

DORE, J. A pragmatic description of early language development. *Journal of Psycholinguistic Research,* 1974, *3,* 343–350.

DORE, J. Children's illocutionary acts. In R. Feedle (Ed.), *Discourse relations: Comprehension and production.* Hillsdale, N.J.: Lawrence Erlbaum Associates, 1977.

FALVEY, M., BROWN, L., LYON, S., BAUMGART, D., & SCHROEDER, J. Strategies for using cues and correction procedures. In W. Sailor, B. Wilcox, & L. Brown (Eds.), *Methods of instruction for severely handicapped students.* Baltimore: Brookes Publishing Co., 1980.

FLAVELL, J.E., FLAVELL, J.E., & McGIMSEY, J.F. Relative effectiveness and efficiency of groups vs. individual training of severely retarded persons. *American Journal of Mental Deficiency,* 1978, *83,* 104–109.

FRANKEL, F., & GRAHAM, V. Systematic observation of classroom behavior of retarded and autistic preschool children. *American Journal of Mental Deficiency,* 1976, *81,* 73–84.

FREEMAN, B.J., RITVO, E., & MILLER, R. An operant procedure to teach an echolalic, autistic child to answer questions appropriately. *Journal of Autism and Childhood Schizophrenia,* 1975, *5,* 169–176.

GARDNER, W.I. *Behavior modification in mental retardation.* Chicago: Aldine/Atherton, 1971.

GOETZ, L., SCHULER, A., & SAILOR, W. Teaching functional speech to the severely handicapped. *Journal of Autism and Developmental Disorders,* *9*(4), 325–344.

GOLDSTEIN, D., & ALBERTO, P. *Matching appropriate instructional strategies to number of students and task.* Paper presented at the Sixth Annual Conference of the American Association for the Education of the Severely/ Profoundly Handicapped, Chicago, 1979.

GUESS, D. Methods in communication instruction. In W. Sailor, B. Wiley, & L. Brown (Eds.), *Methods of instruction for severely handicapped students.* Baltimore: Brookes Publishing Co., 1980.

GUESS, D., & NOONAN, M.J. Curricula and instructional procedures for severely handicapped children. *Focus on Exceptional Children,* Vol. 14, *5,* Jan. 1982, Love Publishing Co.

GUESS, D., SAILOR, W., & BAER, D.M. *Functional speech and language training for the severely handicapped (Part 1: Persons and Things).* Lawrence, Kans.: H & H Enterprises, 1976. (a)

GUESS, D., SAILOR, W., & BAER, D.M. *Functional speech and language training for the severely handicapped (Part 2: Actions with Persons and Things).* Lawrence, Kans.: H & H Enterprises, 1976. (b)

GUESS, D., SAILOR, W., & BAER, D.M. Language development programs for severely handicapped children. In N. Haring & L. Brown (Eds.), *Teaching the severely handicapped* (Vol. 1). New York: Grune & Stratton, 1976. (c)

GUESS, D., SAILOR, W., & BAER, D.M. *Functional speech and language training for the severely handicapped (Part 3: Possession and Color).* Lawrence, Kans.: H & H Enterprises, 1977. (a)

GUESS, D., SAILOR, W., & BAER, D. A behavioral-remedial approach to language training for the severely handicapped. In E. Sontag, J. Smith, & N. Certo (Eds.), *Educational programming for the severely and profoundly handicapped.* Reston, Va.: Council for Exceptional Children, 1977. (b)

GUESS, D., SAILOR, W., & BAER, D.M. *Functional speech and language training for the severely handicapped (Part 4: Size, Relation and Location).* Lawrence, Kans.: H & H Enterprises, 1978. (a)

GUESS, D., SAILOR, W., & BAER, D. Children with limited language. In R.L. Schiefelbusch (Ed.), *Language intervention strategies.* Baltimore: University Park Press, 1978. (b)

HART, B., & ROGERS-WARREN, A. Milieu approach to teaching language. In R.L. Schiefelbusch (Ed.), *Language intervention strategies.* Baltimore: University Park Press, 1978.

HORSTMEIER, D.S., & MacDONALD, J. *Ready, set, go: Talk to me.* Columbus: Charles E. Merrill, 1978.

JENS, K.G., & BELMORE, K. Language programming for the severely handicapped. *Focus on Exceptional Children,* Vol. 8, *3,* May, 1976. Love Publishing Co.

KAZDIN, A.E. *Behavior modification in applied settings.* Homewood, Ill.: Dorsey Press, 1975.

KOEGEL, R.L., EGEL, A.L., & DUNLAP, G. Learning characteristics of autistic children. In W.S. Sailor, B. Wilcox, & L.J. Brown (Eds.), *Methods of instruction with severely handicapped students.* Baltimore: Brookes Publishers, 1980.

KOEGEL, R.L., & RINCOVER, A. Research on the difference between generalization and maintenance in extra-therapy responding. *Journal of Applied Behavior Analysis,* 1977, *10,* 1–12.

KOHL, F., WILCOX, B., & KARLAN, G. Effects of training conditions on the generalization of manual signs with moderately handicapped students. *Education and Training of the Mentally Retarded,* 1978, *13,* 327–334.

LAZAR, I., & DARLINGTON, R. *Lasting effects after preschool.* Washington, D.C.: U.S. Department of Health, Education, and Welfare, Office of Human Development Services, Administration for Children, Youth and Families, DHEW Publication No. (OHO5) 79–30178, 1978.

LOVAAS, O.I. A program for the establishment of speech in psychotic children. In J.K. Wing (Ed.), *Childhood Autism.* Oxford: Pergamon Press, 1966.

MAHONEY, G., CRAWLEY, S., & PULLIS, M. Language intervention: Models and issues. In B.K. Keogh (Ed.), *Advances in special education: An annual compilation of research* (Vol. 2). Greenwich, Conn.: J.A.I. Press, 1981.

McCORMICK, L., COOPER, M., & GOLDMAN, R. Training teachers to maximize instructional time provided to severely and profoundly handicapped children. *AAESPH Review,* 1979, *4,* 301–310.

McCORMICK, L., & GOLDMAN, R. The transdisciplinary model: Implications for service delivery and personnel preparation for the severely and profoundly handicapped. *AAESPH Review,* 1979, *4*(2), 152–161.

McLEAN, J.E., & SNYDER-McLEAN, L.K. *Transactional approach to early language training.* Columbus: Charles E. Merrill, 1978.

McLEAN (McCORMICK), L., & McLEAN, J. A language training program for nonverbal autistic children. *Journal of Speech and Hearing Research,* 1974, *35,* 186–193.

MILLER, J.F., & YODER, D. An ontogenetic language teaching strategy for retarded children. In R.L. Schiefelbusch & L.L. Lloyd (Eds.), *Language perspectives—acquisition, retardation and intervention.* Baltimore: University Park Press, 1974.

PALYO, W., COOKE, T., SCHULER, A., & APOLLONI, T. Modifying echolalic speech in preschool children: Training and generalization. *American Journal of Mental Deficiency,* 1979, *83*(5), 480–489.

PREMACK, D. A functional analysis of language. *Journal of Experimental Analysis of Behavior.* 1970, *14,* 107–125.

REICHLE, J.E., & YODER, D.E. Assessment and early stimulation of communication in the severely and profoundly mentally retarded. In R.L. York & E. Edgar (Eds.), *Teaching the severely handicapped* (Vol. 4). Columbus: Special Press, 1979.

ROGERS-WARREN, A.K., & WARREN, S.F. Pragmatics and generalization. In R.L. Schiefelbusch and J. Pickar (Eds.), *Communicative Competence.* Baltimore: University Park Press, in press.

SAUNDERS, R.R., & SAILOR, W. A comparison of three strategies of reinforcement on two-choice learning problems with severely retarded children. *AAESPH Review,* 1979, *4,* 323–334.

SCHOVER, L.R., & NEWSOM, C.D. Overselectivity, developmental level and overtraining in autistic and normal children. *Journal of Abnormal Child Psychology,* 1976, *4,* 289–297.

SCHREIBMAN, L. Effects of within-stimulus and extra-stimulus prompting on discrimination learning in autistic children. *Journal of Applied Behavior Analysis,* 1975, *8,* 91–112.

SCHREIBMAN, L., KOEGEL, R.L., & CRAIG, M.S. Reducing stimulus overselectivity in autistic children. *Journal of Abnormal Child Psychology,* 1977, *5,* 425–436.

SEIBERT, J.M., & OLLER, D.K. Linguistic pragmatics and language intervention strategies. *Journal of Autism and Developmental Disorders,* 1981, 2(1), 75–88.

STERNAT, J., MESSINA, R., NIETUPSKI, J., LYON, S., & BROWN, L. Occupational and physical therapy services for severely handicapped students: Toward a naturalized public school service delivery model. In E. Sontag (Ed.), *Educational programming for the severely and profoundly handicapped.* Reston, Va.: Division on Mental Retardation, The Council for Exceptional Children, 1977.

STORM, R.H., & WILLIS, J.H. Small-group training as an alternative to individual programs for profoundly retarded persons. *American Journal of Mental Deficiency,* 1978, *83,* 283–288.

TOUCHETTE, P.E. Transfer of stimulus control: Measuring the moment of transfer. *Journal of the Experimental Analysis of Behavior,* 1971, *15,* 347–354.

UZGIRIS, I.C. Experience in the social context. In R.L. Schiefelbusch and D.D. Bricker (Eds.), *Early language: Acquisition and intervention.* Baltimore: University Park Press, 1981.

VINCENT, L., SALISBURY, C., WALTER, G., BROWN, P., GRUENEWALD, L., & POWERS, M. Program evaluation and curriculum development in early childhood/special education: Criteria of the next environment. In W. Sailor, B. Wilcox, & L. Brown (Eds.), *Methods of instruction for severely handicapped students.* Baltimore: Brookes Publishing Co., 1980.

WARREN, S.F., ROGERS-WARREN, A., BAER, D.M., & GUESS, D. Assessment and facilitation of language generalization. In W. Sailor, B. Wilcox, & L. Brown (Eds.), *Methods of instruction for severely handicapped students.* Baltimore: Brookes Publishing Co., 1980.

WARYAS, C.L., & STREMEL-CAMPBELL, K. *Communication training program: Levels 1, 2, and 3.* Hingham, Mass.: Teaching Resources, 1982.

WILLIAMS, W. Procedures of task analysis as related to developing instructional programs for the severely handicapped. In L. Brown, T. Crowner, W. Williams, & R. York (Eds.), *Madison's alternative for zero exclusion: A book of readings* (Vol. 5). Madison, Wisc.: Madison Public Schools, 1975.

WOLFENSBERGER, W. *The principle of normalization in human services.* Toronto, Canada: National Institute of Mental Retardation, 1972.

CHAPTER SEVEN

INFANTS AT-RISK

Diane Bricker and Richard L. Schiefelbusch

I nfants may be considered at-risk because of some factor present during the prenatal period, such as the age of the mother or inborn errors of metabolism. The at-risk label may also be applied after birth when the physical state of the infant and/or the prospects for adequate caregiving are in doubt. This chapter focuses on detection and intervention issues that relate primarily to the second group of at-risk factors. This emphasis is not meant to discount the importance of reducing prenatal risk factors. However, responsibility for activities related to those conditions is generally assumed by medical personnel, not teachers and/or communication specialists.

This chapter is specifically concerned with identifying and intervening with babies at-risk for developing communication problems. The primary focus is strategies for arranging the environment to enhance developmental progress.

PRE-INTERVENTION CONCERNS

The infant research literature provides a wealth of information about early "communicative" interactions.

To establish the appropriate rationale for communicative intervention with at-risk infants, it is useful to review several infant research findings touched on in earlier chapters. First, the young infant possesses a wealth of organized behaviors. An infant has the ability to discriminate among stimuli and to show preferences (Rheingold, 1967; Fagan, 1978), to initiate and respond to human interaction (Ainsworth, 1973), and to actively organize, integrate, and adapt to experience (Bruner, 1974, 1975). The infant's characteristics and behaviors elicit and influence the quality of caregiving she receives (Massie, 1980). Second, problems arising from prenatal and perinatal difficulties may be attenuated or intensified by the conditions of the environment (Braine, Heimer, Wortis, & Friedman, 1966). Third, increased understanding of mutual adaptations made by infants and families can make professional intervention more effective and increase the predictive validity of at-risk designations (Sameroff & Chandler, 1975). Four, communicative behaviors evolve during the period of early infancy from reciprocal exchanges between caregivers and infants.

Analyses of "communicative" interaction between mothers and infants show turn-taking to be both a force and a result of early socialization. The alternating interchange allows the mother to model or provide corrective feedback at a time when the child's attention is focused and lays the groundwork for later communicative interactions (Sugarman-Bell, 1978; Bricker & Carlson, 1981).

These findings have the following direct implications for early communication intervention with at-risk infants.

> Turn-taking routines are both the context and the desired outcome of early socialization.

1. *Effective intervention should be based upon the interactive functions found in reciprocal caregiving activities.* The research literature suggests that the turn-taking conversational format is an important early interaction pattern, and that developmentally delayed infants may have difficulty acquiring this basic interaction pattern (Jones, 1980). Vietze, Abernathy, Ashe and Faulstick (1978) describe differences between the interactions of typical infants and their mothers and atypical infants and their mothers. Atypical infants are often delayed and deficient in acquiring the elemental components of turn taking. If social interactions between caregivers and infants provide the critical context for language learning, difficulties in establishing reciprocal interactive patterns may produce or increase delays in language acquisition.

2. *Intervention procedures should be designed to stimulate the amount and the kind of natural contingencies that control normal infant-environment transactions.* Intervention activities should seek to enhance transactions between the infant and her environment. Mutual stimulation should be arranged for the caregiver and infant in recurring daily contexts (usually caregiving or play), where each partner can stimulate the responses of the other. Stimulation should be frequent and sustained, with the adult responding sensitively and directly to the infant's initiations. The adult should model and prompt responses to sustain and accelerate the infant's social-communication activities. The initial goal of intervention should not be to teach the infant specific words or other speech events, but to enhance the infant's reciprocal social-communication acts that are fundamental to the development of referential language. Without the necessary foundation skills for language, the infant may not be able to acquire subsequent formal linguistic structure or may take significantly longer to acquire such behavior.

> As emphasized in Chapters Five and Six, the initial goal of intervention is communicative function, not language form.

3. *Social-communicative exchanges between adult and infant can form the basis for training speech and language.* The basis for social-communicative exchanges is the partners' responsive-

ness to each other. Strategies for molding these exchanges may differ greatly if the child is handicapped. For impaired infants, programs of visual, tactile, kinesthetic, and auditory stimulation should be undertaken as soon as the caregiver is able to comfortably interact with the infant. Both the child's expressive and receptive capabilities should be enhanced by these transactional experiences. Early and continuous stimulation may do much to remediate developmental delays and maximize the infant's possibilities of acquiring a functional communicative system.

EXPRESSIVE CAPABILITIES

Some infants with neuro-muscular dysfunctions seem unable to develop the respiratory control necessary for intelligible speech. The effector processes that control the speech-producing mechanism consist of (a) the respiratory mechanism, which provides a source of power in the form of an airstream directed into the (b) larynx, where phonation occurs and pitch and loudness changes are effected, and (c) the supralaryngeal vocal tract where the sounds of speech—vowels and consonants—are formed. The normal speaker modifies the vegetative respiratory pattern for speech production, changing from a pattern in which inspiration and expiration are about equal in duration to a pattern where inspiration is quicker and expiration is longer and more controlled. The speech breathing pattern requires more neuromuscular integration than is required for breathing at rest. Further modifications of rest breathing patterns are required to produce the phrases and stress patterns for connected speech.

Speech production requires a complicated valving system in which the vocal folds are approximated with precisely the right amount of muscle tone for phonation to occur. Cerebral palsied infants may adduct the folds too tightly, preventing phonation. Poorly adducted folds produce a breathy quality and some infants have such poor control of the laryngeal valves that air escapes too rapidly, making it impossible to produce syllables. Malfunction of the supralaryngeal apparatus is sometimes so severe that even swallowing and chewing do not develop normally. An infant with grossly defective chewing, sucking, and swallowing is seldom able to produce intelligible speech (Shane, 1981).

Chapter Five also discusses the importance of considering output capabilities.

Careful observation and analysis of vocal behavior can reveal early signs of delayed or defective neuromuscular development (McDonald, 1980). The following are signs that the infant is at-risk for development of normal speech production:

About 1 to 2 Weeks: Failure to cry or peculiar vocal quality may indicate abnormal tone in laryngeal musculature

About 4 to 5 Weeks: Failure to produce differentiated sounds may signal difficulty in obtaining and maintaining articulatory control through action of the jaw and tongue muscles

About 2 Months: Failure to vocalize when stimulated may signal possible difficulty in developing the necessary muscular control

About 4 Months: Failure to produce consonant-vowel combinations or uttering one consonant-vowel syllable per exhalation

About 5 Months: Failure to utter simple vocalizations voluntarily and to use vocal signals to gain attention

About 6 Months: Failure to demonstrate speech-supporting breathing pattern. The vegetative respiratory patterns should be sufficiently modified to power production of continuous speech

About 7 to 8 Months: Failure to show adequate control of pitch variation and loudness on single vowels

About 9 Months: Failure to initiate vocalizations

About 12 Months: Failure to produce chains of syllables with various consonant-vowel combinations and have an expressive vocabulary of 2–3 words

In addition, the occurrence of persistent primitive reflex patterns, such as tonic reflexes which interfere with respiration, phonation, and articulation, are often associated with the failure to develop intelligible speech. Uncoordinated movements during sucking, chewing, and swallowing that remain over time are indications of pathology. Specifically, the infant may be suspected of poor speech development who sucks inefficiently past 1–2 weeks; who chokes on fluids past 1–2 weeks; who has jaw clonus past 6 weeks; who chokes on semi-solids past 28 weeks; who swallows excessive air past 40 weeks; who leaves the mouth open and drools past 40 weeks; or who fails to chew adequately past 18 months.

Infants who consistently show abnormalities or deficiencies of the nature described above demand thoughtful evaluation in selecting an intervention approach. There are two possibilities (McDonald, 1980): assume that although speech production is impaired, constrained, delayed, or uncertain, the infant will be able to learn to produce intelligible speech, or consider the infant/child a candidate for an augmentative communication system.

Chapter Ten also discusses variables which indicate that the child is at-risk for development of speech.

RECEPTIVE CAPABILITIES

Research on the auditory behavior of infants has established that most newborns (including premature infants and infants with known central nervous system abnormalities) can discriminate sound on at least seven parameters that are important for the decoding of speech signals (Eisenberg, 1976). Most research on these parameters has employed constant nonspeech auditory stimuli (e.g., pure tone). The configuration of the auditory signal may be of primary importance because available evidence indicates that infants may react differently to constant signals (e.g., pure tones and noise bands) than to patterned complex signals (e.g., tonal patterns and speech).

There is a growing awareness that consistent and discriminated auditory input during the first year of life is important for language and cognitive development (Horowitz & Leake, 1979). This is also an especially important period for auditory development. However, it coincides with an increased incidence of middle ear infections (Geibink & Quie, 1978), which may have deleterious effects on later language development and school performance and result in poorer performances on intelligence tests. While there is little detailed information about behavioral and developmental consequences of middle ear infections (Horowitz & Leake, 1979), our understanding of the effects of middle ear disease on an infant's language development is increasing with development of more refined early identification methods (Himelberg, Popelka & Shannon, 1979).

Most clinical procedures use variants of an operant discrimination paradigm for assessing threshold and suprathreshold auditory abilities in infants 6–12 months of age (Wilson, 1978). These procedures remedy some of the shortcomings of Behavioral Observation Audiometry (BOA), traditionally used for this age group. Two of these procedures, Visually Reinforced Audiometry (VRA) and Visually Reinforced Infant Speech Discrimination (VRISD), are based on findings indicating that when given an opportunity, infants will attempt to interact with and control their auditory environment (Butterfield & Cairns, 1976).

Research with the VRA procedure has several implications for clinical use in assessing auditory thresholds (Wilson, 1978). Thresholds obtained from normal infants are similar to those of adults tested using the same procedure. Also, the range of thresholds from the tested population was small, supporting their validity as clinical norms. Finally, the procedure is time-efficient and applicable with infants 6–12 months of age.

The VRISD procedure addresses developmental change in speech discrimination. At present, there is considerable research suggesting that infants as young as 2 months can discriminate various linguistic features in speech stimuli; however, the research procedures used to acquire these data are difficult to implement in a clinic and difficult to use with older infants. Conversely, the VRISD procedure opens up exciting possibilities for assessing speech discrimination abilities in disordered infants 6–12 months of age.

Work using masking techniques to assess an infant's ability to detect speech signals in noise (e.g., ongoing white noise) is now under way (Trehub, Bull, & Schneider, 1981). This task more closely approximates what the infant has to do in a typical environment—separate speech signals from other environmental sounds. Preliminary results suggest that with moderate background noise, 6-month-old infants require a signal 100 times more intense than an adult to detect the signal's presence. The intensity difference was not as great, however, when speech stimuli were used.

Unfortunately, much of the research literature on infant auditory functioning tends to ignore the importance of early reciprocal social-communicative exchanges. Such exchanges appear essential for the infant to learn to assign meaning to auditory signals that are created by the physical world, as well as those produced by the social world. For example, when the infant sees and hears a rattle that the caregiver is shaking, the

Review the discussion of auditory acuity in Chapter Five for other assessment information.

It is important to consider early auditory functioning in the context of caregiver-infant interactions.

caregiver may offer a label, demonstrate the toy's physical properties, or use it to attract the infant's attention. When the baby smiles and coos, the caregiver may respond by verbally noting the infant's contented state, labeling the social activity, or attending to the infant. The latter response is essential to assist the infant in learning that her vocal signals can attract adult attention. Caregivers also help infants focus on the topics of their verbal utterance; this eventually helps the infant "crack" the linguistic code of her particular language environment.

Development of both receptive and expressive communicative skills is highly dependent on the mutual exchanges and feedback provided by the social and physical environment. Research with at-risk and handicapped infants points to the adverse effects when such interactions are ineffective (Goldberg, 1979; Mahoney & Seely, 1976). The following section suggests an intervention approach designed to offset these problems.

GENERAL GUIDELINES FOR INFANT INTERVENTION

This section presents a discussion of (a) general guidelines for communicative intervention and (b) specific strategies for professionals working with caregivers to enhance communicative competence in the at-risk or handicapped infant. We begin with the general guidelines because they provide the context for developing and implementing a specific training plan.

Guideline 1 Early intervention is indicated if (a) the infant is thought to be in an environment that will not elicit and support the type of interactive behaviors described in Chapter Two, or (b) the infant's handicapping condition is sufficient to cause concern about the acquisition of early extra- and para-linguistic responses such as voice feature contrasts (i.e., angry-friendly, familiar-unfamiliar) and different intonation contours.

Guideline 2 An intervention program for infants should also be a training program for the adult caregiver. Intervention should focus on the primary caregivers because (a) the caregiver, usually the mother, is the individual with whom the infant generally spends the most time, (b) the primary caregiver, through the bonding and attachment processes, is usually the infant's most salient social reinforcer, and (c) diminishing resources in the area of social and educational programs make it less likely that sufficient professional workers will be available for direct intervention activities with at-risk and handicapped infants.

Guideline 3 During early intervention, stimulation should be provided in the form of mutual, reciprocal play. Play provides the primary context for developing of early attentional and reciprocal activities. The infant gains experience in both receptive and expressive functions by participating in simple play sequences. Interactions may include smiling, vocalizing, touching, reaching, gesturing, or object manipulation. The play should delight, interest, and attract the attention of the infant. The play activities should be selected to fit the appropriate wake state of the infant and should be woven throughout the day as opportunities arise (e.g., during diaper-changing time, or after feeding when the infant is relaxed and alert). The affective nature of the caregiver-infant relationship allows the infant to experience affection along with the perceptions of the ritualized play (Thoman, 1981). As important, the caregiver should perceive these interactions as positive and rewarding.

Guideline 4   Early communicative training should accommodate the infant who cannot use speech. Caregivers may need to use non-speech modes because some at-risk or handicapped infants may develop problems that reduce or eliminate their ability to use speech for communication. The action play of infant and adult can move naturally into a response board communication system. Such a system may be extremely functional in the child's daily life and may only require limited movement from a motorically impaired child. In like manner, the action systems of play could move easily into signing for children with severely impaired hearing but adequate motor integration.

We emphasize that the action play of infant and caregiver should provide a smooth transition into symbolic exchanges, as the child is able to make the necessary representational associations. The importance of a functional symbol system may be that it provides a means for this transition. Either a speech system or an alternative symbol system can be used for communication.

The assumption is that all children need a system of communication during the early years of life. It is late to begin teaching a transactional language after time and misspent efforts have revealed the child to be nonverbal. It is much better to effect a transition to language usage during the potentially creative play period of infancy. At this time, the functions of communication achieved during creative play, and the functions of language gained in the action-object-agent associations of the infancy period can be naturally and functionally combined by infants with or without speech. Such early stimulation may make a great difference in subsequent language acquisition.

These general guidelines set the stage for considering specific strategies to facilitate the acquisition of early communicative behavior in infants whose biological background and/or environment present conditions adverse to "natural" development. The following section suggests some specific training activities.

SPECIFIC STRATEGIES FOR INFANT INTERVENTION

Training activities have been divided into five interrelated phases: (a) strategies for enhancing the infant's general readiness for communicative exchanges, (b) strategies for enhancing reciprocity between the caregiver and infant, (c) strategies for enhancing the infant's social-communicative signaling, (d) strategies for enhancing the infant's comprehension skills, and (e) strategies for enhancing the infant's production skills. These strategies are appropriate for infants between the developmental range of approximately 4–30 months.

The format for the training phases includes: (a) definition of the target response or response class, (b) age when the behavior might be expected to emerge, (c) strategies for obtaining baseline or preintervention information on the frequency and, when possible, the quality of the response of interest, and (d) a few selected activities that can be considered by the caregiver/teacher for enhancing the target response.

PHASE ONE: GENERAL READINESS

A first consideration is whether the infant is ready for communicative exchanges. "The infant's degree of readiness to communicate is important because it provides the framework for nonverbal and/or verbal communication" (Stern, 1981). Before attempting to enhance communication, be sure the infant is aware of social stimuli signaling initiation of a communicative exchange, and look for evidence that she is ready to engage in a communicative exchange.

DEFINITION

Signals of readiness for communication vary across infants, but can include such responses as gazing at the adult, head orientation, body orientation, and distance reduction (Stern, 1981). For example, the infant may be quiet, turn the head toward the adult and gaze at the face, or, upon hearing a voice, stop an activity and poise the body in space, or lean forward toward the adult while vocalizing and gazing. All of these behaviors singularly or in combinations provide overt evidence that the infant is "ready" for a communicative exchange.

What is "communicative readiness?"

When to expect readiness behavior Although much individuality exists, infants generally gaze consistently at adult speakers around 4 months. They are able to orient their head to a speaker at about 5 months, and from 5 months on can begin to orient parts of their body in desired directions. Infants who fail to show these behaviors by the 9th-10th month are candidates for readiness stimulation.

At what age are readiness behaviors usually evident?

Assessment You can determine whether the infant provides signals of communicative readiness through systematic observation of daily activities (e.g., feeding, dressing, bathing, playing). Speak in a clearly audible voice while in front of and behind the infant and observe her responses. Also observe responses when other adults talk to her. Does the baby generally quiet and gaze at the face of the speaker, or does she generally ap-

How can baseline information on readiness behaviors be collected?

pear not to notice the communication directed towards her? Remember that there are times when the infant will fail to respond to communicative bids from the adult; it may be a sign the infant is not ready for an exchange. Ignoring or averting behavior is often observed also in normally developing infants. You should only be concerned when infants rarely give readiness signals when in an appropriate state (e.g., awake, alert), or when they are significantly delayed in acquiring such signals.

ENHANCEMENT ACTIVITIES

What are some activities to enhance readiness? Before beginning any activity to enhance attentiveness or readiness, it is important to assess the infant's state. In general, if the baby is crying, drowsy, or sleeping, do not attempt to encourage communication: consider these behaviors signs that she is not ready for such exchanges. In addition, if the infant makes clear moves away from the adult through gaze aversion or body orientation (e.g., turns away), do not force an interaction. For extremely difficult infants, the caregiver may have to learn how to "gentle" the infant into a relaxed state.

Gazing or visual attention After determining that the infant is in a receptive state, the caregiver should be positioned in front of the infant, with her face at the infant's eye level and within the infant's reach. Have the caregiver smile and talk to the infant. Generally it is most effective to use short phrases, raise the pitch of the voice, and/or alter the pitch contour. Infants appear to be particularly sensitive to changes in pitch contour (Fernald, in press). If the infant fails to maintain her gaze, gently direct the face back toward the caregiver. If the infant initially gives even the most fleeting glance, have the caregiver provide some positive feedback. The nature of such feedback will be infant-specific. For some babies, tactile stimulation may be a reinforcer, while for others auditory or visual spectacles may be more effective. Gradually reduce the physical prompts for gazing at the caregiver, and eventually the infant should begin gazing at the adult, which should in turn elicit appropriate responses from the caregiver.

Head-body orientation A key to effective intervention is the selection of objects/sounds that have saliency for the infant (i.e., persons, objects, or events that attract the infant's attention). Appropriate selection may require considerable experimentation with a variety of stimuli. Variations in pitch and intensity may attract some babies, while others will respond better to more sustained sounds.

After the initial training objective—to get attention and localization to nonspeech sounds or visual events—has been achieved, the next objective is to get the infant to orient to a human speaker. Have the caregiver present the chosen object, event, or person slightly out of the range of the infant's gaze so that a small change in head orientation is necessary to focus on the eliciting stimulus. When the infant changes her orientation, the caregiver should provide some immediate pleasurable feedback. Such feedback may be continued activation of the stimulus item the infant has oriented towards (e.g., the caregiver continues talking to the infant, a sound-making toy is activated again, or a visually colorful toy is offered to the child). If the infant does not orient towards the stimulus source, physically prompt the response by gently turning the infant's head. Gradually decrease prompts and change placements of the stimulus source to require more head turning by the infant.

Once the infant learns to turn toward her caregiver's voice, then introduce activities that will require the infant to change the body orientation to locate the sound source. Procedures similar to those employed for shaping head turning can be used.

Reduction of distance   Leaning toward the caregiver is a signal that the infant is ready to engage in a communicative exchange. If she does not begin moving toward the caregiver during the training activities selected for gazing or orientation, have the caregiver initiate specific activities to encourage this response. When the infant is gazing at the caregiver, the adult can move her head back slightly to see if the infant will then lean forward to compensate for the adult's shift away. If not, the infant can be prompted to do so. The adult could offer a toy just beyond the infant's reach and, when the infant strains to acquire the toy, move toward the infant while talking and reducing the distance between the infant and caregiver. The caregiver could place her face close to the infant's and then slowly move away, hoping the infant will move with the adult or imitate the action during the next interaction. Again the infant's responsiveness will determine selection of activities.

PHASE TWO: RECIPROCAL ACTIONS

Piaget calls the period between 8 and 12 months sensorimotor stage IV. When caregiver and infant play together, they attend to objects simultaneously. The caregiver looks at and talks about what the infant looks at, and the child follows the caregiver's line of regard to attend to the same thing (Bruner, 1975). This is a period of increased receptive and expressive processing by the infant.

Since infants at this stage can imitate head shaking, lip pursing, hand clapping, and facial gestures, they *seem* to understand what the parent is saying as an accompaniment to these imitation games. However, in reality, the infant is only responding to the imitation, the context, and the affect. The receptivity of the infant is a diffuse, but highly responsive, system that leads to the more specific speech functions soon to follow. The infant participates actively during this stage and is led by the caregiver's actions, which are, in turn, tied to the infant's responding. In the context of communication games and joint attention to objects, the child experiences a variety of social behaviors in addition to simple, well-formed, repetitious, expressive speech (Chapman, 1981).

Infants and adults display organized interactions which appear as structured cycles of affective and attentional responses. These cycles, which reflect periods of adult-infant activity and engagement as well as inactivity and disengagement, strike a balance between the mode and intensity of the behavior of both partners. They typically consist of the following sequence of responses:

1. *Initiation:* Infant vocalizes while looking at adult to attract attention
2. *Mutual Orientation:* Infant vocalizes and adult focuses on her face
3. *Recognition:* Infant smiles when seeing adult, establishing a joint reference
4. *Reciprocal Play-Dialogue:* Adult vocalizes and infant vocalizes
5. *Disengagement:* Adult vocalizes and infant looks away (Brazelton, Koslowski & Main, 1974)

There are clearly identifiable cycles or response sequences in caregiver-infant exchanges.

The disengagement, or looking away, phase probably reflects the infant's need to control the amount of stimulation she can process during a period of intense social interaction. These cycles or response sequences cannot be characterized as having a fixed pattern or behavioral content, but rather exhibit substitutability (Uzgiris, 1981). That is, infants and adults can enter the cycle at any point with widely varying behavioral content and still obtain the desired outcome.

To successfully engage in a synchronous interaction, certain prerequisites are required of the dyad's participants. Children's caregivers contribute their unique sensitivities and environmental experiences to the interaction when reading and responding to the infant's signals. Equally important, the infant must clearly and predictably signal her state and needs, as well as remain receptive and responsive to the caregiver's feedback. Without the establishment of a match between initiator and respondent, the dyadic relationship may not evolve into a healthy context for the infant's social-communicative development.

DEFINITIONS

What are "reciprocal actions?"

Reciprocal actions refer to the synchrony of action between the infant and the caregiver. This interactional process may be conceptualized as a jointly or mutually regulated system in which each member of the dyad modifies and adapts her behavior to dovetail with the other. For communication to occur, the child and adult must assume the roles of initiator and responder, each influencing the other's behavior in a reciprocal manner. The balance of reciprocity changes over time, with the infant's participation increasing with age. The adult reduces dominance in the interaction as the infant becomes capable of initiating activities.

At what age do infants engage in reciprocal actions?

When to expect reciprocal behavior Most infants begin engaging in reciprocal actions with caregivers during the latter part of the first year. An infant who is more than 12 months of age and shows little mutuality of play when given ample opportunity should be thoroughly evaluated to determine if intervention is needed.

Assessment   Baseline data can be collected in a variety of ways. Encourage the caregiver to stimulate reciprocal play by marking an object (shaking, pointing, or gazing at it). If the infant follows the adult's eye gaze and looks toward the marked object, training is not necessary. If this does not occur, plan to implement enhancement activities.

How can baseline information on reciprocal actions be collected?

ENHANCEMENT ACTIVITIES

The establishment of joint attention or a mutual topic by speaker and listener is essential to communication; communication depends on some mutuality of focus. Once the infant is able to locate a sound source, the next step is to help her focus on an object, event, or person that is the topic of the adult's "conversation." Joint attention teaches the infant (a) that the adult's words are related to "here and now" events, and (b) the relationship between words and the concepts they represent.

What are some activities to enhance reciprocal actions?

Activities involving objects are particularly useful for establishing joint attention. Again, the selected event and training strategies need to be individualized, but we outline here a general procedure. While seated beside the infant, select a desired object and place it in front of the infant. The caregiver should look at the object and comment on it. If the infant looks toward the object, make sure some pleasurable activity occurs (e.g., give the object to the infant or activate it). Comments should be relevant to the most salient aspects of the object and should be redundant. If the infant does not look in the direction of the object for a sustained period, then point to the object and shake it if necessary. If the infant still does not focus on the object, gently prompt the response by turning the infant's head. If this procedure is unsuccessful, then follow the infant's gaze; notice what attracts the infant's attention, then point to that object and label it. For example, before giving an infant a glass of juice, hold it up and comment, "This is juice." Wait for the infant to focus attention on the cup before offering it.

Once the caregiver can get the infant to focus on particular targets, the next step is to establish reciprocal responding. To reach this target, the following procedure is recommended. When the infant responds, the interventionist/caregiver should wait briefly and then imitate the infant's response.[1] Upon completion of the imitative response, the caregiver should provide a positive social response and then wait for the baby to respond again. When the next response occurs, the caregiver should again imitate the response, accompanied by some positive affective behavior. For example, if the infant says, "Ah" when waving an object, the caregiver should immediately copy the infant's behavior by using the same vocalization while waving a similar object. If the baby reproduces the action, the care-

---

[1]Initially choose responses that are visible to the infant. Imitation of visible behavior (e.g., *hands together*) is easier for most infants than imitation of invisible behavior (e.g., *hands on head*).

giver should imitate the sequence and then demonstrate some obvious pleasure, such as smiling or laughing while looking at the baby. Such a paradigm should be effective for a number of reasons. First, imitation of the infant forces the caregiver to attend closely to the infant's behavior to imitate her previous response. Second, the infant's behavior precedes the caregiver's and forces her to follow the infant's lead. Third, it can be presumed that the infant is engaging in self-reinforcing behavior and fourth is a contingency control factor. The infant discovers that her behavior elicits some systematic, predictable effect from the environment. Allowing the infant to control the speed of initiating responses should permit establishment of an optimal flow for producing and assimilating responses.

Once the caregiver has established a chain of reciprocal responses, attempts should be made to expand the infant's repertoire. For example, if the baby and caregiver have initiated and maintained a vocal imitation pattern, the caregiver may introduce a minor variation in the imitated response, from "ba-ba" to "be-be," and watch to see if the baby responds differently. When retrieving objects that are being dropped, the caregiver could introduce slightly different ways of returning the desired object so that the infant will have to accommodate the reach and grasp response a little each time. It is easy to develop other simple extensions of the imitation method.

Following training on reciprocal interaction chains, social ritual games can be introduced. Such games as "up we go," "pat-a-cake," "peekaboo" (you need to select other more appropriate games for older children) provide opportunities for the infant to learn to participate in activities in which partners have mutually reciprocal roles. The types of games should be individually determined based on the infant's motor capabilities and on the game's reinforcement value. The form is unimportant, but the infant should be assisted in gradually assuming independence in participating in more of the activity. The caregiver should introduce systematic variation to enhance the infant's imitative repertoire.

As the baby and caregiver reciprocally interact with each other in the environment, their social-communicative interactive exchanges should be associated and mutually contingent. Social stimulation successfully elicits social-communicative feedback from the infant, just as the infant's expanding communicative repertoire effectively elicits adult attention and communicative responses. The contingent feedback provided by the adult to the infant's signals appears to be instrumental in fostering the development of communication, just as it increases the infant's ability to control the environment.

PHASE THREE: SOCIAL-COMMUNICATIVE SIGNALS

Prior to comprehension and production of referential words, most infants enter a developmental phase in which they use nonconventional and conventional vocalizations and/or gestures for a variety of communicative functions. Because these vocalizations and gestures are not always conventional symbols (e.g., words), they have been termed social-communicative or prelinguistic communicative signals. The appearance of these prelinguistic signals generally precedes the onset of initial referential language.

DEFINITION

Social-communicative signals are any nonsymbolic vocal or gestural response used to communicate. For example, such responses can include pointing to indicate a desired object, vocalizing to gain an adult's attention, or standing beside the door to show the wish to go outside. During the first year, infants often begin to vocalize to attract the adult's attention. Observing a prelinguistic infant generally reveals a repertoire of a variety of gestures and vocalizations used to communicate.

What are "social-communicative signals?"

When to expect social-communicative signals   Most infants begin to use vocalizations and/or gestures for communicative purposes before their first birthday. Infants who do not demonstrate such responses frequently by 15 to 17 months should be a source of concern.

At what age are "social-communicative signals" usually evident?

Assessment   The most useful assessment data can be obtained through observing the infant in her environment. Record the frequency and the form of any systematic vocalization or gesture produced by the infant and specify the conditions present when the vocalization/gesture was produced.

How can baseline information on social-communicative signals be collected?

ENHANCEMENT ACTIVITIES

Training strategies should be appropriate for the infant and caregiver. Although it may be preferable to have a simultaneous vocalization and gesture, initially either is acceptable separately. Baseline data will suggest what responses are likely training targets. For example, if the infant tends to look towards a desired object and wave, this can be an appropriate target. Any looking, vocalization, or motoric gesture that can be shaped into a social-communicative signal should be encouraged. Even seriously motorically impaired infants may have simple communicative signals such as eye points. Discovering these may require sensitive observation of the infant in a variety of environmental settings and events. For the nonmotorically impaired infant, pointing is often an appropriate target. This response tends to occur naturally and is easy to prompt.

What are some activities to enhance learning of social-communicative signals?

     The most important aspect of training is to establish a contingent relationship between the vocal/gestural action used by the infant (e.g., pointing) and some response from the environment (e.g., receiving the object pointed at). If a pointing response is selected, it may be useful to place favorite or desired objects around the room. Keep these objects visible, but out of the infant's reach. When the baby indicates a desired object, be sure and retrieve it immediately. As the signal begins to occur regularly, shape it into a more conventional form.

The importance of establishing functional relationships between child responses and environmental effects is also discussed in Chapters Five and Six.

Infant vocal/gestural actions may initially be idiosyncratic, setting-specific, and rather general in nature. That is, the infant may use the same vocalization to obtain her caregiver's attention and to have the adult retrieve a desired object. She must be assisted to develop conventional social-communicative signals, and to discriminate the use of signals across settings or changing conditions (e.g., the signal used to gain attention is different than that used for refusal).

Communication training at home, like that provided in the classroom, should be embedded in daily routines.

Arranging the environment so the infant must use a variety of social-communicative signals is necessary for the infant to learn the discriminated use of different signals. The caregiver should be encouraged to demand more explicit communicative gestures and vocalizations over time. For example, initially the baby may point and say, "da" when requesting an object. Once this pattern is established, the caregiver should change the criteria so the infant must say "want (or wa) da" or imitate the name of the requested object—"ball" rather than "da." If refusal is indicated by head shakes, the infant should be prompted to use the vocalization, "no" or "na." The infant who is using a standard vocal production, such as "na" to indicate label-seeking ("What's that?") or denial functions, should be encouraged to differentiate the two communicative functions. "Na" or "no" can be paired with a head shake to indicate denial or rejection while an alternative sound combination, with a visual point, might be encouraged for seeking object names.

PHASE FOUR: EARLY COMPREHENSION

If the infant is to learn to associate sounds in her environment with persons, objects, and events, she must hear the names or labels for such items or events while interacting with them or when they attract her attention. Language will not be meaningful for the infant or young child unless it is relevant and directly related to ongoing experiences. Therefore, it is essential to talk about what the infant sees and does in simple, consistent language.

Initially, the infant becomes aware that certain events and objects always occur simultaneously or immediately concurrent to one another. For example, juice is associated with "Do you want a drink?"; sweaters are associated with going outside. Infants indicate that they are making such associations by their anticipatory behavior (e.g., excitement when a sweater is taken from the drawer).

DEFINITION

What is comprehension?

Comprehension refers to an infant's ability to relate or associate a referent with its symbol. The infant comes to "know" that the word or sign "ball" refers to the round, red object that bounces.

At what age is comprehension of words and phrases evident?

When to expect comprehension   Infants under a year of age may give some evidence of comprehending words or phrases in a familiar context.

In the second year, they become more adept at understanding the meaning of words apart from a specific or familiar context. Infants who fail to show any comprehension skills by 16 to 18 months are possible candidates for intervention.

Assessment   Prior to training, observe the infant's environmental interactions and select a group of training words that meet these criteria:

How can baseline information on comprehension be collected?

1. Select words that represent objects, persons, or events with which the infant has frequent contact. Frequent opportunities to hear the word in relation to its referent should facilitate learning
2. Select words that refer to objects, persons, or events that are important to the infant: for example, favorite toys or foods
3. Select words that have functional value for the infant. Learning names of common environmental items and events should assist the infant to adapt to the environment and should have some intrinsically rewarding features
4. Select words that are relatively easy-to-produce sound combinations. Although the objective of this training phase is comprehension, training of word production should follow or occur simultaneously. Selecting easy-to-produce words may enhance production training.

Using the above criteria, select a group of items (e.g., words) and then determine whether the infant gives indications of associating these words with their appropriate referents. If not, training should be initiated.

ENHANCEMENT ACTIVITIES

Training involves teaching appropriate responses to selected words or commands. For example, when training the infant to respond to the word "up," prompt her to raise her arms when you say, "Do you want up?" Then immediately pick her up to establish a genuine communicative exchange. Remember that the primary objective of this phase is not production, but comprehension or word recognition. Do not expect the infant to repeat the words or sounds, but encourage any form of expression that occurs.

What are some activities to enhance comprehension?

Once the infant is responding appropriately to a few selected words or phrases presented in context, the caregiver can begin to expand the youngster's repertoire in two ways. First, begin to fade the contextual cues so the infant is required to respond to the word alone. Second, continue to add new words and phrases to the infant's training repertoire.

Training can either be conducted in a more formal manner or continued using a naturalistic approach. It is often appropriate to do both. During formal training the infant can be seated on the floor with the selected training objects. The caregiver asks the child to select the objects one at a time, varying requests to include such phrases as "touch," "point to," "show me," "get," "take," "give me," or "find." The caregiver may begin teaching a new word-object association by placing only one item in front of the child and asking her to touch that object. Imitation and physical prompts should be used if necessary. After the child has touched the first training object on command, a second object is introduced so the child must make a choice between two objects. The child should be encouraged to play with the objects in a functionally appropriate way after selecting the correct object, and the caregiver should continue to label the items frequently as the child plays with them. Once the child has learned to attach a verbal label to an object, the caregiver can begin to expand the class of objects encompassed by that label. For example, if the object used to train "cup" has been a white coffee cup, other cups of varying size, shape, and color should be introduced and labeled to broaden the child's concept of cup.

Training action words (verbs) or events differs somewhat. For example, if targeting the verbs, "eat" and "ride," place a cookie, apple, boat, and wagon on the table and give the child a toy dog and doll. Suggest the child "Make the doggie eat," or "Make the doll ride." Use motor imitation and physical prompts until the child indicates the ability to discriminate between the action words. Maximize learning opportunities by having alternative training stimuli available (e.g., other dogs and boats) in the form of objects and pictures. If these stimuli are available, opportunities should arise when the caregiver can ask a child to "get the apple," "point to the boat," or "bring the wagon."

PHASE FIVE: EARLY PRODUCTION

The ability to control the environment in both a social and informational sense depends largely on communicative competence. In our culture the most desirable form of communication is oral language; it should be the programming target unless serious sensory or motor problems preclude development of speech. In such cases, nonvocal language modes such as signing or communication boards must be substituted.

DEFINITION

What is production?

Production refers to the use of a symbol (e.g., word) or signal for the purpose of communication with the social environment. The training activities described are for oral production; however, an interventionist can make adjustments in the activities to accommodate other production or expressive modes.

At what age does the infant begin to produce words and word approximations?

When to expect production   Even the neonate vocalizes. The nature of the vocal behavior changes over time, until at about 8 to 10 months most infants babble. Shortly after, word approximations appear, and then between 12 and 16 months most infants begin producing single words. Infants who show a 4 to 5 month delay in production are candidates for a comprehensive evaluation.

Assessment   Observe frequency of the child's vocalizations, sounds, or word production, what conditions affect frequency and, when possible, quality of her productions. Assessment can be informal, structured, or both.

How can baseline information on production be collected?

ENHANCEMENT ACTIVITIES

Begin language production training by attending to all of the infant's appropriate vocalizations. Either imitate her vocalizations, answer in some way, or provide requested objects and events. Schedule play periods with as many opportunities as possible to evoke vocal responses. Make these situations fun and exciting; making noises and sounds should be an enjoyable experience. Appropriate times for these training periods can be identified within the infant's normal routine (e.g., mealtime or bath time).

What are some activities to enhance production?

Physical stimulation such as tickling is a good way to increase vocalizations. Have the caregiver make pleasurable sounds while engaging in these activities and stimulate the infant to make "happy" vocalizations, such as laughing and babbling in return. These vocalizations can then be rewarded with more tickling, touching, or roughhousing as well as imitation to stimulate repetitions.

Over time the infant will begin to produce closer approximations to English sounds, for example "ma" and "da." She will also begin using intonation patterns that match adult intonation patterns. The objective is to have the baby produce sounds that make up the phonologic components of English.

Begin sound training with sounds the infant can already produce and gradually introduce new sounds, one at a time. Sometimes a mirror helps the infant focus on her oral motor movements. One efficient training strategy for this phase is an imitative approach, though some infants may resist this approach; and if so, use other strategies. Over a period of a few days when the infant is alert and vocalizing, have the caregiver stand or sit where the infant can see and touch her face. Wait until the baby has been silent for a few seconds and then present one of the training items. Be sure to keep track of the infant's success in imitating the selected training sounds or syllables and continue training until reasonable approximations of the target sound are produced. If the infant is motivated and has been working on some specific sounds without reaching criterion for several days, consider changing the sounds selected for training and/or the training procedures.

Once the infant is producing a variety of consonants and vowels (e.g., babbling), the caregiver can begin working on word production. Again training can proceed using either a formal or informal procedure, or both. Encourage the caregiver to use every opportunity throughout the day to ask the infant the names of the objects, events, or people targeted for training. Most of the activities that have been suggested in the earlier phases are also appropriate for this phase, with appropriate content modifications.

Before training production of action words (verbs), determine the child's skill level by demonstrating an activity (e.g., the dog eating dog food) and then ask the child, "What's the dog doing?" The child should respond with some form of the correct verb such as "eating," "eat," or "eats." Action words that assist the child to control her environment should be priority training targets. Words such as "go" (meaning *go out* or *go down*), "up" (meaning *pick me up* or *pick it up*), "want" (meaning *get me the thing I am pointing at*), "give" (meaning *put it in my hand*), and the like should be included in this training phase if the child is not frequently using these words.

Once the child is able to produce single content and action words, the interventionist should encourage the caregiver to begin training the child to sequence words into simple phrases such as, "want drink," "go outside," "baby sleep," etc.

Assessment procedures are the same as those used in previous phases, except the length of target responses is recorded. Target verbs should be presented in combination with target objects to determine where to begin training. Demonstrate an activity (push truck) and then ask the child, "What am I doing?" or "What's happening?" The child's response should be some form of the correct verb combined with the correct object (e.g., "pushes truck," "pushing truck," or "push truck").

The caregiver can also ask, "What is happening?" when the child is demonstrating an action with the stimulus objects. Appropriate responses can be prompted using imitation. The caregiver should begin by using one object and one verb, then one object and two verbs and so on; then introduce another object with one verb, two verbs, etc. The two objects should be alternated with the four verbs. The third and fourth objects should be added in the same manner until children can identify any of the four objects with any of four verbs.

Planning for generalization of multi-word responses to other environments is essential. One advantage of the two-word action-object phrases is that they constitute simple requests that can be "naturally" reinforced. For example, if the child says, "want drink," she can be given a glass of milk. The phrase, "go out" can be reinforced by taking the child outside. "Give ball," should result in the child receiving the ball. "No car" conveys the child's rejection of an object or event. Learning such phrases provides control over the environment, if the caregiver responds appropriately. The ability to communicate desires and needs more precisely should have natural and powerful consequences that lead the child to the acquisition of more formal linguistic responses. These responses will eventually allow her to cope successfully with increasing societal demands.

SUMMARY

1. Once an infant is identified as at-risk, intervention takes the form of assisting the caregiver to develop compensating arrangements for the identified environmental or organismic deficiencies.

2. Atypical infants are often delayed and deficient in acquiring the elemental components of turn taking.

3. The context of intervention for at-risk infants should be caregiver-child shared experiences, where each partner stimulates the responses of the other.

4. An infant may be considered at-risk for speech if she sucks inefficiently or chokes on fluids past 1–2 weeks, has jaw clonus past 6 weeks, chokes on semi-solids past 28 weeks, swallows excessive air, breathes with mouth open, or drools past 40 weeks, or fails to chew adequately past 18 months.

5. Because they help the infant to learn to assign meaning to auditory signals, reciprocal social-communicative exchanges play a critical role in development of auditory discrimination skills.

6. Early intervention is indicated if there is evidence of an environment which provides minimal or adverse learning conditions *or* if the infant is organismically vulnerable.

7. Early intervention should focus on the primary caregivers and the context of intervention should be play.

8. The assumption that all children need some means of communication as early as possible suggests introduction of augmentative communication modes as early as possible.

9. Early communication training activities, for infants functioning between 4 and 30 months of age, include readiness activities, reciprocal action activities, strategies for enhancing social-communicative signaling, comprehension activities, and production activities.

REFERENCES

AINSWORTH, M.D. The development of infant-mother attachment. In B. Caldwell & H. Riciutti (Eds.), *Review of Child Development Research,* Vol. III. Chicago: University of Chicago Press, 1973.

BATES, E. *Language and context: The acquisition of pragmatics.* New York: Academic Press, 1976.

BAUMEISTER, A.A. AND BROOKS, P.H. Cognitive deficits in mental retardation. In J.E. Kauffman and D.P. Hallahan (Eds.), *Handbook of special education.* Englewood Cliffs, New Jersey: Prentice Hall, 1980.

BELL, S.M. AND AINSWORTH, M.D. Infant crying and maternal responsiveness. *Child Development,* 1972, *43,* 1171–1190.

BRAINE, M., HEIMER, C., WORTIS, H., AND FRIEDMAN, A. Factors associated with impairment of the early development of prematures. *Monographs of the Society for Research in Child Development,* 1966, *31*(4), 92.

BRAZELTON, T.B. Joint regulation of neonate-parent behavior. In E.Z. Tronick (Ed.), *Social interchange in infancy: Affect, cognition, and communication.* Baltimore: University Park Press, 1982.

BRAZELTON, T.B., KOSLOWSKI, B., MAIN, B. AND M. The origins of reciprocity: The early mother-infant interaction. In M. Lewis and L. Rosenblum (Eds.), *The effect of the infant on the caregiver.* New York: John Wiley and Sons, 1974.

BRICKER, D. AND CARLSON, L. Issues in early language intervention. In R.L. Schiefelbusch and D. Bricker (Eds.), *Early language: Acquisition and intervention.* Baltimore: University Park Press, 1981.

BRUNER, J. From communication to language—A psychological perspective. *Cognition,* 1974, *3*(3), 255–287.

BRUNER, J. The ontogenesis of speech acts. *Journal of Child Language,* 1975, *2*, 1–119.

BUTTERFIELD, E. AND CAIRNS, G. The infant's auditory environment. In T.D. Tjossem (Ed.), *Intervention strategies for high risk infants and young children.* Baltimore: University Park Press, 1976.

CHAPMAN, R. Mother-child interaction in the second year of life: Its role in language development. In R.L. Schiefelbusch and D. Bricker (Eds.), *Early language: Acquisition and intervention.* Baltimore: University Park Press, 1981.

EISENBERG, R.B. *Auditory competence in early life.* Baltimore: University Park Press, 1976.

FAGAN, J. Infant recognition memory and early cognitive ability: Empirical theoretical and remedial considerations. In F. Minifie and L. Lloyd (Eds.), *Communicative and cognitive abilities—Early behavioral assessment.* Baltimore: University Park Press, 1978.

FERNALD, A. The perceptual and affective salient of mothers' speech to infants. In L. Feagans, C. Garvey & R. Golinkoff (Eds.) *The origins and growth of communication.* New Brunswick, N.J.: Alkex Publishing, in press.

GEIBINK, G.S. AND QUIE, P.G. Otitis media: The spectrum of middle ear inflammation. *Annual Review of Medicine,* 1978, *29,* 285–306.

GOLDBERG, S. Premature birth: Consequences for the parent-infant relationship. *American Scientist,* 1979, *67,* 214–220.

HIMELBERG, M.A., POPELKA, G.R., AND SHANNON, E. Tympanometry in normal neonates. *Journal of Speech and Hearing Research,* 1979, *22*: 179–191.

HOROWITZ, F.D. AND LEAKE, H. The effects of otitis media on cognitive development. Unpublished manuscript, 1979.

JONES, O. Prelinguistic communication skills in Down's syndrome and normal infants. In T. Field (Ed.), *High-risk infants and children.* New York: Academic Press, 1980.

MAHONEY, G.J. AND SEELY, P.B. The role of the social agent in language acquisition: Implications for language intervention. In N.R. Ellis (Ed.), *International review of research in mental retardation.* New York: Academic Press, 1976.

MASSIE, H.N. Pathological interactions in infancy. In T.M. Field, S. Goldberg, D. Stern & A.M. Sostik (Eds.), *High risk infants and children: Adult and peer interactions.* New York: Academic Press, 1980.

McDONALD, E.T. Early identification and treatment of children at risk for speech development. In R.L. Schiefelbusch (Ed.), *Nonspeech language and communication: Analysis and intervention.* Baltimore: University Park Press, 1980.

RHEINGOLD, H.L. A comparative psychology of development. In H.W. Stevenson, E.H. Hess & H.L. Rheingold (Eds.), *Early behavior: Comparative and developmental approaches.* New York: Wiley and Sons, 1967.

SAMEROFF, A. AND CHANDLER, M. Reproductive risk and the continuum of the caretaking causality. In F.D. Horowitz (Ed.), *Review of Child Development Research,* Vol. IV. Chicago: University of Chicago Press, 1975.

SHANE, H. Decision making in early augmentative communication system use. In R.L. Schiefelbusch & D. Bricker (Eds.), *Early language: Acquisition and intervention.* Baltimore: University Park Press, 1981.

STERN, D.N. The development of biologically determined signals of readiness to communicate which are language "resistant." In R. Stark (Ed.), Language behavior in infancy and early childhood. New York: Elsevier/North-Holland, 1981.

SUGARMAN-BELL, S. Some organizational aspects of pre-verbal communication. In I. Markova (Ed.), *The social context of language.* London: Wiley and Sons, 1978.

THOMAN, E.B. Affective communication as the prelude and context for language learning. In R.L. Schiefelbusch and D. Bricker (Eds.), *Early language: Acquisition and intervention.* Baltimore: University Park Press, 1981.

TREHUB, S., BULL, D., AND SCHNEIDER, B.A. Infant speech and nonspeech perception: A review and evaluation. In R.L. Schiefelbusch and D. Bricker, (Eds.), *Early language: Acquisition and intervention.* Baltimore: University Park Press, 1981.

UZGIRIS, I. Experience in the social context. In R.L. Schiefelbusch and D. Bricker (Eds.), *Early language: Acquisition and intervention.* Baltimore: University Park Press, 1981.

VIETZ, P.M., ABERNATHY, S.W., ASHE, M.L., AND FAULSTICK, G. Contingency interaction between mothers and their developmentally delayed infants. In G.P. Sachett (Ed.), *Observing behavior,* Vol. I. Baltimore: University Park Press, 1978.

WILSON, W.R. Behavioral assessment of auditory function in infants. In F.D. Minifie and L.L. Lloyd (Eds.), *Communication and cognitive abilities: Early behavioral assessment.* Baltimore: University Park Press, 1978.

CHAPTER EIGHT

LANGUAGE INTERVENTION IN A PRESCHOOL/ CLASSROOM SETTING

Kenneth F. Ruder, Betty H. Bunce, and Charlotte C. Ruder

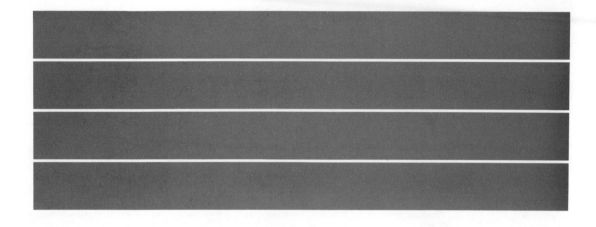

T his chapter describes a language training program for language deficient/delayed children, ages 3 to 6. The goal and rationale of the program is to help the children learn to use language in real-world environments. Rather than initially training the child in clinical isolation and hoping for generalization to different contexts and individuals, this program faces the problem of generalization training at the outset. Speech and language are trained directly in the school and home—the child's significant environments. Most of the child's communicative and social needs and interactions occur in these environments; why not begin speech and language training in these highly personalized and meaningful contexts?

Most of this chapter is about a single program developed at the University of Kansas, but the chapter also draws from other programs and general guidelines accumulated over 10 years of language training research. While the program is for preschool age children, variations of the principles can also be applied to older language-impaired children. The principles and methodologies can be extended to other environments.

This chapter describes the Preschool Language Training Project, Bureau of Child Research at the University of Kansas.

The Preschool Language Training approach grew out of research on the content, structure, and methodology of language training. There are four features to this service delivery model: (a) the language training is performed in the preschool classroom in the context of academic and preacademic activities; (b) the language training is both intensive and generalized (In our model program we see children five days a week for at least three hours daily and incorporate language training into all preschool activities); (c) the teacher assumes responsibility for classroom management as well as language training; and (d) parents are an integral part of the intervention. Normal language learners are included in the program as role models. A half-day program is provided for all twelve children (eight language-impaired and four nonhandicapped).

Intensive language instruction is provided in the context of academic and preacademic activities.

Admission to the preschool is generally by referral from school officials, physicians, psychologists and/or speech and language pathologists.

However, direct parent contacts, Head Start, and "Count your Kid In" programs have also provided a steady source of referrals. Children are placed in the program on a month's trial basis, following an intake interview with the parents and collection of preliminary evaluation data.

The following descriptions of some of the children served during the development of the preschool program demonstrate the nature and variety of their language handicaps.

1. **S.S.** At age 4, this child demonstrated average intelligence and a severe expressive language delay. He produced sounds but no intelligible words (except for the word "bye"). Comprehension of language was good; he was able to follow directions and understand most of what was said to him. As he learned to say and combine words, some anomia (word finding difficulties) was apparent. His pattern of articulation was inconsistent. These difficulties suggested a diagnosis of apraxia, a problem of motor patterning for speech production. Now, at 6 years 10 months, he is attending a regular first grade and doing average work in the class. He has only a mild articulation problem and normal productive language skills.

2. **J.F.** At age 5, this child's productive language was limited to 2–3-word sentences. Her receptive language and vocabulary were also delayed, and she made many articulation errors. She also demonstrated visual acuity and gross-motor problems. Her home environment provided little appropriate stimulation. She is now 6 years old and using 4- and 5-word sentences which are usually intelligible. Her receptive vocabulary is near age-level. She attends a regular first grade, but is doing below average work.

3. **M.H.** At age 2½, this child's expressive language development was delayed, but receptive language was adequate. He communicated with grunts and pointing. At 4 his receptive and expressive language and articulation are considered adequate, though he still has some difficulty attending, following directions, and scanning his environment for meaningful information. His behavior suggests that there are risk factors for learning.

4. **C.C.** At 4, this child speaks only in 2-word sentences with multiple articulation errors. He has difficulty sequencing sounds and words. He is a bright youngster, however, with good comprehension.

5. **A.O.** At 5 years of age, this child was delayed in both productive and receptive language, but articulation was good. Her medical diagnosis is cerebellar ataxia. She has poor gross and fine motor coordination. Emotional and behavioral problems were evident as productive language increased. Her pragmatic use of language was often inappropriate. At age 8 she is attending a regular second grade with resource room help.

The one characteristic common to all handicapped children in this program is language difficulties.

The handicaps and/or underlying causes of the language impairments of these children are very different. However, they had one thing in common at the time they were accepted into the program—all were *functionally* noncommunicative.

ASSESSMENT

The purpose of the intake evaluation is to formulate placement recommendations and determine in-depth assessment needs.

Evaluations are undertaken to determine the nature and extent of the child's language handicap at the time of referral. The first step is an intake evaluation, which includes an interview with the parents, and some preliminary speech and language testing. Data collected during the intake evaluation lead to placement recommendations and/or further in-depth evaluations.

After the intake evaluations, a program is designed and implemented. Ongoing evaluations then probe specific training results. Periodic language sampling checks the child's progress and provides information about the transfer of trained structures to spontaneous language. Tests and observation checklists used in the initial evaluations are readministered again at the end of the year (or semester) to evaluate the child's progress and the program's effectiveness.

EVALUATIONS: INTAKE AND IN-DEPTH

Intake data are one component of the in-depth evaluations, except in cases where preschool placement does not seem advisable. In these cases, the intake evaluation terminates with "no preschool recommendation." The complete intake evaluation procedure may take from a one afternoon evaluation to one month (trial placement in the preschool). The type of testing, including parent interviews, does not differ substantially in content or structure for intake and in-depth evaluation; only the scope and depth of the testing differentiate them. We discuss below the major areas and procedures involved in intake and in-depth evaluations.

Preliminary evaluation procedures include (a) a parent interview, (b) observations, (c) a language sample, and (d) formal and informal testing.

Parent interview   The primary purposes of the parent interview are to obtain information about the child, and give the parents an opportunity to ask questions about the child's development and our program. The parent's statement of the problem is extremely important. The parent is asked to give specific examples of the child's situational communication behavior and information about the child's developmental history. The parents gain knowledge about the staff and program, and staff members get to know the parents during this interview. It sets the stage for subsequent coordination with the parents to develop the child's program, the home program, and the parent training program.

Initial observation of play and communication   During the initial evaluations, the clinician makes some informal observations of the child's interactions with others during play. The child may be observed playing alone and with an adult or another child. Of particular interest is how the child expresses his needs and wants, what he appears to comprehend, and how he uses toys and other equipment (does he use symbolic play?). In this way, an observer can form an initial impression of the child's speech and language, as well as his cognitive and social development.

Informal observation of structured activities   Subsequent in-depth evaluation includes observations of the child in the preschool setting. We are particularly interested in how the child reacts to other children and to his teachers, and what skills and weaknesses he may have in preacademic and academic areas. Sometimes a child will do very poorly on formal tests, yet manage to communicate effectively with his peers or in "real," in contrast to picture situations. This information is crucial to devising the child's program. For example, we may need to use object stimuli rather than the picture stimuli, may have another child demonstrate, or may use gestures or signs as cues. To help structure the observations, we use a short checklist to note behavior during preschool activities. In addition, we note the child's ability to match, categorize, and sequence both auditorily and visually, and we test the child's writing skills, counting and number skills, and knowledge of the alphabet. These data are marked three more times during the year as a progress report of preacademic skills.

Informal observation of unstructured activities   Clinicians can gain a great deal of comprehensive information concerning the child's linguistic and cognitive abilities simply by observing unstructured activities, including free play. The observation period may range anywhere from the initial half-hour observation to an extended evaluation lasting four to six weeks.

In the free play observation, the clinician observes and records the child's behavior in three general areas: (a) interpersonal communication, (b) verbal and nonverbal communication skills, and (c) play skills. This observation session requires, in addition to the child and his parents, other children about the same age as the target child, an adult supervisor (evaluator), and a variety of toys.

In the area of interpersonal communication, the evaluator observes the child's methods of requesting, demanding, questioning, and responding to questions. These communication events are observed in at least three interpersonal paradigms to note the manner in which the child communicates with his parents, with other children, and with other adults.

A major aim of this informal observation is to determine the quality and quantity of the communications in each of the three interpersonal/social paradigms. The type and degree of verbal and nonverbal behaviors the child uses to communicate in these situations, and also the types of communication events which he will respond to, are of concern. The goal of this informal observation is to obtain a baseline record of the child's interactions with other individuals in his environment.

The third category of observations is assessment of play skills. How does the child play? What toys does he play with? Does he play with toys appropriately? Imaginatively? The manner in which the child uses toys provides important information about cognitive functioning. A child demonstrates understanding of the function of a toy by playing with it appropriately. The more cognitively advanced child plays in a conventional, socially acceptable manner, and may also create novel, imaginative uses for the toys. He may use toy blocks to build a tower or pretend that the block is a toy car. This imaginative play demonstrates a degree of mental representation that is basic to language use in communicative contexts. Pretending without objects is an even more complex manifestation of mental representation. The lack of "imaginative" displays in the play behaviors of communicatively handicapped children can be valuable diagnostic information.

When informal observation of free play activities does not provide opportunities to observe all the types of interactions and communication events targeted, activities may be arranged to elicit the desired interactions. One way to arrange observation of demanding behavior is to provide some children with cookies and then observe how the target child goes about obtaining one for himself.

Another strategy is to have parents, teachers, or peers model behaviors (e.g., folding paper or playing with a novel toy) for the target child to imitate, or communicate with the child entirely with gestures in a play context to assess how well the child responds to nonverbal communication. Still another technique is to ask the child to pretend that an object has a function other than that with which the child is familiar (i.e., give the child a block and instruct him to "play car").

These informal observations are not intended to replace formal cognitive and language assessments. Rather, their purpose is to supplement and provide validation for formal test results. They are also an important aspect of the ongoing intervention process. In practice, the informal observations provide both formative and summative program evaluation data.

Language sampling   A language sample is taken during the initial evaluation while the child is engaged in play. Utterances are recorded in writing and also tape recorded, if possible, to be analyzed at a later time. Usually one teacher interacts with the child while another records what the child says and, when possible, what the adult says. Generally, standard orthography is used, but international phonetic symbols may be necessary if the recorder is unsure what the child is saying or needs to note articulation problems. Being careful not to fill in articles, verb tense endings, etc. unless the child uses them, the recorder notes the context (i.e., playing with blocks) of utterances and, if possible, whatever communicative functions they serve (i.e., answer, question, statement, greeting).

The use of MLU for comparative research is discussed in Chapter Two.

Language sample analysis may consist of nothing more than counting the number and type of vocabulary items used, or it may be a complex grammatical analysis. In most cases, we begin by determining the Mean

Length of Utterance for the sample. The first step is to determine the utterance boundaries (where does one utterance end and another begin?), and count the total number of utterances in the sample. Then morphemes are identified and counted in accordance with Brown's (1973) rules. Generally, this procedure can be reduced to identifying as morphemes all intelligible words, as well as any prefixes or suffixes which the child utilizes in a functional manner. The total number of morphemes in the language sample is then divided by the number of utterances, yielding the Mean (average) Length of the child's Utterance (MLU) for that sample. For younger children, at least, MLU is considered to be a fairly valid index of language production capability; comparing MLUs taken early in training with those taken later provides a general indication of the child's language growth. We may also analyze the language sample to determine the absence or presence of specific linguistic structures.

Informal language testing   Informal tests help to complete our picture of the child's linguistic strengths and weaknesses. Waryas and Stremel-Campbell (1978) and Chapter Four of this volume describe this type of testing in detail. It consists of presenting stimulus items picturing the target structure and distractors (called foils). The distractor pictures are chosen to contrast the subject, object, and verb of the target structure. In addition, for reversible S-V-O (Subject-Verb-Object) structures the subject and object of the sentence must be equally likely to occur as either a subject or an object. For the structure "girl push boy," the foils could be "boy push girl" and "girl kick boy." To make the correct choice, the child must understand all of the structures. We test production using a similar format. If the child fails the reversible Subject-Verb-Object test, then he is tested again using nonreversible Subject-Verb-Object pictures. If this is still too difficult, Verb-Object testing is done. In this way, we formulate an accurate picture of the child's ability to comprehend and produce syntax.

Formal Language Tests   Formal assessment instruments are usually administered during the one month trial placement, but some may be included in the intake evaluation (e.g., the *Goldman-Fristoe Test of Articulation* [Goldman & Fristoe, 1972] the *Northwestern Syntax Screening Test* [Lee, 1969], the *Temple University Short Syntax Inventory* [Gerber & Goehl, in press], the *Assessment of Children's Language Comprehension* [Carrow, 1977]). In addition, the *Peabody Picture Vocabulary Test* (Dunn, 1965) is usually administered to provide information about the child's receptive vocabulary. We use these particular tests because they provide an overview of the child's problem and help us decide whether additional in-depth testing is needed and, if so, what kind. These tests do not take long to administer and most children readily respond to them as "games" because of their picture formats.

   After we analyze the intake evaluation and the child has adjusted to the preschool routine, we do further testing of articulation, language comprehension and language production. Information from these evaluations guides development of the child's individualized training program. The formal language tests we use most frequently are:

1. **McDonald Deep Test of Articulation** (McDonald, 1964), used to test a specific speech sound within a variety of contexts.
2. **Test for Auditory Comprehension of Language** (Carrow, 1977)
3. **The Test of Language Development** (Newcomer & Hammill, 1977)
4. **Sequenced Inventory of Communication Development** (Hedrick, Prather, & Tobin, 1975), used for children who are not capable of attending and responding to some of the tests involving picture stimuli
5. **Preschool Language Assessment Instrument** (Blank, Rose, & Berlin, 1978b), to check the child's ability to understand the "language of learning" (Find one like this, why is that different?, how are these the same?, etc.)
6. **Boehm Test of Basic Concepts** (Boehm, 1971)

After testing is completed, the child's scores are listed on the Test Summary Chart (see Figure 8-1 for example chart). In addition to profiling the child's initial performance on intake evaluations, we use the Test Summary Chart to profile regular progress evaluations. Each time a test is administered, we list the scores on the chart. The result is a cumulative record such as the one in Figure 8-2, which provides an overview of the child's progress and facilitates discussion of his development with parents and other professionals.

Other summary forms are used to record assessment data and developmental progress in gross-motor skills, fine-motor skills, speech and language, cognition, behavior, and preacademic skills. Figure 8-3 is a sample of a completed summary form for one child in the program.

When all language assessment data have been collected and analyzed, they are reported on a skill progress report. Structures the child is using (and in what situations he uses them), transpositions, omissions and other incorrect usages of language structure are identified and the child's program is planned accordingly. Preacademic progress is also recorded and charted regularly.

THERAPY PROBES

After we complete the initial and in-depth evaluations, we devise the child's program. We administer probes periodically and collect daily data to monitor progress and evaluate the training's effectiveness. The parents may also take data on the child's home performance. In the case of articulation, probes are taken at the sound, syllable, bisyllable, word, and phrase level. Here again, daily data is graphed and a home program may be used.

FIGURE 8-1 Test summary for intake assessment and annual progress evaluation

DATE:

Hearing Test

Mean Length of Utterance

Peabody Picture Vocabulary Test

Chronological Age   Language Vocabulary Age

Temple University Syntax Screening Inventory

Articles	Nouns	Pronoun	Verbs	Prep.	Conj.	Adj.
/20	/38	/8	/28	/4	/2	/4

Preschool Language Assessment Instrument (Profile of child's discourse skills)

Level I   Level II   Level III   Level IV

above 2.0—strong discourse skill   Level I & II—perceptual
1.5–2.0—moderately strong   Level III & IV—thinking skills involving "how" and "why"
1.0–1.4—moderately weak
below 1.0—weak

Articulation Testing

Omissions: Substitutions: Distortions:

Preacademic Skills

1. Alphabet   4. Counting to 10
2. Writing of Name   5. Labeling Numbers to 10
3. Sight Word Vocabulary   6. One-to-One Matching

FIGURE 8-2   Test summary: an example

Date:

Sept. 1983: Hearing screening test indicated normal hearing, bilaterally.

Peabody Picture Vocabulary Test

	Chronological age	Language Vocabulary Age
9-14-82	6-4	5-1
1-23-83	6-8	5-7
5-15-83	7-0	5-7

Temple University Syntax Screening Test

	Art.	Noun	Pron.	Verb	Prep.	Conj.	Adj.
9-19-82	0/30	23/38	3/8	3/27	1/4	0/2	4/4
1-24-83	3/30	36/38	4/8	6/27	4/4	0/2	4/4
5-15-83	6/30	37/38	8/8	16/27	4/4	1/2	4/4

Mean Length of Responses

Sept. 1982	1.8
May 1983	4.1

Preschool Language Assessment Instrument

	Level I	Level II	Level III	Level IV
1-24-83	1.8	2.5	1.9	1.1
5-14-83	2.2	2.3	2.3	1.4

Above 2.0	—strong discourse skill	Level I & II—perceptual
1.5–2.0	—moderately strong discourse skill	Level III & IV—thinking skills involving
1.0–1.4	—moderately weak	"how" and "why"
below 1.0	—weak	

Articulation Testing: Goldman-Fristoe Test of Articulation

9-14-82   Omissions: v, θ, ð, s, z, ʃ, tʃ, dʒ, l, r, j, and g.
Substitutions: d/k (I), d/g (IF), d/f (M), d/θ (IM), d/ʃ (M), d/s (I), d/z (I), t/s (M), t/z (M), n/d (M), n/j (I), n/dʒ (M), and s/ʃ (MF)
Distortions: some vowels distorted particularly OI = UI
Blends: none produced correctly

5-8-83   Omissions: /j/
Substitutions: n/d (M), l/j, w/l (I), d/l (M), b/v (M), s/tʃ (M), t/ð (M)
Distortions: OI = UI
Blends: 3/12 produced correctly

OTHER TESTING AND REFERRALS

Hearing and oral peripheral examinations may be done if there are concerns in these areas. Other evaluations include tests or observations of fine- and gross-motor movements, adaptive skills, and preacademic skills (discussed in curriculum section). Collecting daily data on large group preschool activities is precluded by personnel limitations, but probe data is collected at least three times a year. In addition, we might take daily data

FIGURE 8-3   Development chart for one child in the program across all skill areas

	Four Years Old 1979-80	Five Years Old 1980-8	Six Years Old 1981-82	Seven Years Old 1982-83
Gross-Motor	Walked slowly, did not run. Unable to use gym equipment. Did not ride trike.	Walked at normal rate. Does run. Can jump, but not hop. Beginning to do finger plays. Tries to climb on jungle gym. Can ride trike.	Walked at normal rate. Does run. Still can't hop. Has trouble catching a ball. Likes to play jungle gym.	Walks and runs normally. Enjoys playing "tag." Still has difficulty hopping or catching a ball.
Fine-Motor	Had difficulty in holding pencil or crayon. Muscles were very limp. Had difficulty placing puzzle pieces.	Can paste if helped. Pencil held better. Can color on paper but not within a defined area. Had difficulty using scissors. Can assemble (difficult) interlocking puzzles.	Hand dominance still not established. Would hold pencil and attempt to write. Can assemble 25–30 piece puzzles. Can stack 7–8 1-in. blocks. Did *intricate* creative building with blocks.	Hand dominance not firmly established. Usually used right. Still often held pencil with palm grip, unless reminded. Can trace slanted and vertical lines. Can make a "T" and "H" to represent name. Made intricate items out of blocks and legos.
Speech & Language	Mostly echolalic. Could produce most sounds used in English. Said only a few words in Vietnamese.	Mean Length Utterance 1.6. Usually used 2-word sentences. Often gave function not label. Spontaneous speech often inappropriate to situation.	Recep. Vocabulary Age 2–7 (C.A. 6–5). Usually used 3-word sentences, sometimes used 4 & 5 word combinations. Beginning to use questions spontaneously.	Mean Length Utterance 2.65. Recep. Vocabulary Age 3–5 (C.A. 7–5). Often produced 5–6 word utterances. Used "ing," plural "s," possessive "s," articles, some prepositions & adjectives, & contractible copula. Expressed range of functions: requests, questions, labels, protests, states. Absent was function of answering.

FIGURE 8-3 (continued)

	Four Years Old 1979-80	Five Years Old 1980-8	Six Years Old 1981-82	Seven Years Old 1982-83
Cognition	Had difficulty following simple directions. Did learn routine of classroom.	Had difficulty in following directions except during creative activities. Learned to match identical & similar obj. Liked to look at books.	Could match identical & similar pictures. Could match colors, but not labels. Could arrange 3 picture sequence if story very familiar. Liked books. Creative skills far in advance of other skills. Learned names of dinosaurs.	Knew some shapes and colors. Could count objects to three. Knew some of the alphabet. Learned 35 vocabulary words which were paired w/ a picture. Knew 3 other words minus the picture. Liked books. Liked to retell stories. Did creative art work.
Behavior	Inconsistent. Appeared not to hear or notice attempts to gain his attention auditorily, visually, or tactually. No crying behavior. Periods of blank staring. Attention worse in individual session. Would respond sometimes in a group.	Often lethargic, may be related to diet. When diet improved, became more spontaneous. Still withdrawn around strangers. Inconsistent attending behaviors of blank staring. Periods of good progress, then inattentiveness, with passive body posture. Unusual crying behavior.	Still inconsistent. Not as much blank staring, now will chew knuckles and shake body. Teachers able to stop this after 3 wks. Liked singing & stories. Most consistent, appropriate behavior when in a small group. Did not interact much with peers except to defend toys. Tattled on peers. Follows direction in creative activities the best.	New inappropriate behavior was running away from group. Stopped after 2 mos. Liked teacher attention and would initiate interaction. Had to be encouraged to interact with peers. Sometimes waits turn, often interrupts. Rocking behavior often occurs when waiting turn. Stopped when name called loudly. Language sometimes inappropriate to situation. Liked to initiate learning activity.

on one or two children if there is a specific need (i.e., child is not progressing, another agency wants information, etc.). If the child has a visual or motor disability or we suspect perceptual motor problems, we make appropriate referrals for in-depth testing.

PROGRAM EVALUATION

At the end of each year and sometimes each semester, tests originally administered during the intake evaluation (and possibly some of the in-depth tests) are readministered and another language sample is analyzed. This helps us evaluate the program and chart child progress. In addition, feedback from parents is elicited (both verbally and with an evaluation checklist).

To reiterate, the program includes four types of evaluations: (a) an initial evaluation and observation, (b) in-depth evaluations, including language sampling and observations, (c) probes of specific therapy results, and (d) evaluations of the effectiveness of our program.

GENERAL LANGUAGE PROGRAMMING PROCEDURES

After the intake and in-depth evaluations are completed, we discuss the results of all tests and observations with the parent(s) and any other professional who may be seeing the child. Parent feedback and questions concerning the accuracy of the data are encouraged. Then, we use this information, together with the parents' (and other professionals') input, to develop an individualized speech and language program. An Individualized Educational Plan (IEP) may be formally filled out if the child is attending both our program and a school district program.

Whenever possible, we use a group training format. This type of instructional arrangement has several advantages. For example, it is much easier to teach pronouns, "him," "her," "them," etc., if there are more people available than just "you" and "me." Training at different levels within the same group also has advantages; children learn from watching their peers respond and interest is maintained by the variety of responses.

Our comprehension training format utilizes a verbal rehearsal strategy. The teacher or communication specialist presents the stimulus, the child repeats it (verbal rehearsal), and then makes a comprehension response (following the direction, pointing to an object or picture, etc.). If the child makes an incorrect comprehension response, the correct response is modeled and the trial is repeated.

The general approach in production training is to provide the stimulus (e.g., a picture) and model the correct response. After several models have been provided, the stimulus item is presented without a model, and the child is requested to make the verbal response. For example, when training subject-verb-object production, the teacher or communication specialist might show a picture of a boy throwing a ball, ask the question,

The general approach is to provide a stimulus and model the correct response.

"What is happening in this picture?" and immediately model the correct verbal response. Later trials present the stimulus item and the question (no model).

If the child makes an incorrect response, it is corrected and the trial is repeated. Correct responses are reinforced and expanded. For example, the teacher or communication specialist would expand the response "boy walk" by adding the progressive marker -*ing* (the next structure to be taught) to the verb. Expansion reinforces the child's response and prepares him for the next structure to be trained, e.g., "That's right, boy walk-*ing*." For a detailed description of this method, see Stremel and Waryas (1974), Stremel-Campbell and Waryas (1978), and Ruder and Stremel (1975).

TRAINING CONTENT

Our program teaches (a) concepts, (b) vocabulary, (c) grammar, and (d) language use. Each requires a different instructional context and somewhat different procedures.

Chapter Two describes the process through which an infant comes to "know" an object.

Concepts   A major thrust of language training is teaching concepts, both at home and at school. Both the teacher and the parents concentrate on expanding and developing the child's conceptual experiences. We encourage children to handle and play with many objects, explore the environment, and think about objects and events in different ways. Teaching the functional use of objects is a priority. During play the child is taught to roll or throw balls, push cars, rock, feed, and change babies, build with blocks, and chatter on a play phone, etc. We provide him with such objects as a cup, spoon, pin, key, soap, crayons, comb, wooden hammer, sock, and mirror, and encourage him to demonstrate the appropriate use of each.

After the child demonstrates understanding of the functional use of the objects and plays appropriately with toys, the sequence in training concepts is: (a) matching similar objects, (b) matching objects to identical pictures, (c) matching objects to similar pictures, (d) sorting, (e) categorizing according to function, (f) regrouping according to physical attributes, (g) eliminating odd items in an array, and (h) sorting by association.

Initial sorting activities include sorting dolls, blocks, trucks, balls into piles, helping with the washing by sorting socks, pants, shirts, and sorting knives, forks, spoons, etc. Later the child is taught to categorize objects and pictures according to their functions, e.g., things we eat, wear, wash with, ride, play with, use as furniture or tools, things found outside or inside, things we wear in cold weather and hot weather. Training then focuses on teaching him to regroup objects according to shape, color, size, and texture, to eliminate the different objects from an array, and sort objects by association (that is, things that go together: pencil and paper, socks and shoes, a bird and a nest, a lamp and a light bullb, a glass and some milk, a pin and a diaper, a wheel and a bike).

Children must also learn patterning and sequencing. The sequencing of language elements (phoneme sequence, word order, etc.) is crucial to the understanding and production of language. Similarly, much of our environment is ordered (temporal order, hierarchical categorization, etc.) so that ability to sequence and perceive order in the environment is crucial to acquiring and developing concepts and the language that maps them. Some specific sequencing activities (taught in the center and at home) include (a) completing two patterns of objects, color blocks, beads, shapes, and pictures, (b) following visual sequences in finger plays and action games, (c) following auditory patterns, e.g., beating a drum, (d) activities which build auditory memory by following simple or complex commands, and (e) visually sequencing the pictures of a story or acting out or telling a story in sequence.

Vocabulary-training We consider the child's language needs, interests, and concepts in choosing vocabulary words to teach. He is more likely to learn words that he has frequent experiences with and opportunities to use. Because one of the natural consequences of language is to control the behavior of others, there is also a concern for selecting words that have high interest and natural reinforcement value for the child.

> Selection of initial training forms is also discussed in Chapter Six.

The names of small familiar objects which the child can handle and interact with are taught first. Next come verbs that he can perform or verbs and adjectives that will help him get something he wants. Early verbs might include, "eat," "drink," "sleep," "walk," "crawl," "open," "come," "want," "go," and "give." Adjectives and adverbs might include "more," "hot," "big," "no," and "allgone."

Selection of vocabulary words at the two-word level is based on the language functions expressed in normal language acquisition. These include recurrence, rejection, location, interrogation, possession, attribution, agent-object, agent-action, and action-object. We teach the child words that will help him express these functions.

> Chapter Two (Table 2–5) provides a list of semantic functions at Stage I.

Grammar The pivotal unit of language in our approach to language training is the *agent-action-object* relation, expressed by the *subject-verb-object* word order. The language training program has two parts. The first part of the program helps the child learn to express the basic semantic relations of agent-action-object. The second part helps him expand these relations.

During the first phase of training, the child is trained to express single-word utterances that represent agents, actions, or objects. Then he learns to express two-word utterances that combine these relations (agent-action and action-object). The last step is to teach him to express three-word utterances that combine into the agent-action-object relation.

> The goal is development of the basic grammatical relations (agent-action-object) and then expanding them.

The purpose of the second phase of training is to teach the child two ways to modify the basic agent-action-object sentence. One type of operation modifies the nouns or verbs in the subject-verb-object string by adding adjectives ("big ball," "happy girl"), adverbs ("run fast," "eat slow"), or prepositional phrases ("walk to school"). These additions do not change the propositional meaning of the sentence. The other type of operation on the subject-verb-object sentence changes the propositional meaning in some way. These operations train the child to make negative statements ("No, boy push car," or, later, "The boy didn't push car"), to ask questions ("I eat cookie?" or, later, "Can I eat a cookie?"), and to express tense relationships (i.e., "The girl is falling," "The girl fell," or "The girl will fall").

In normal language acquisition, a child uses language structures at different levels of complexity. This same phenomenon is reflected in our training sequence. We train several language structures at the same time, but, since each structure has its own sequence of development, the child may progress at a different rate in the different sequences. The specific language structure trained at a given time depends on the individual child's language needs; we do not follow a rigid sequence of training.

Training language use   The child experiences many opportunities for social interaction in the context of the preschool activities. Structured special activities such as free play, snack time, and show and tell are ideal contexts for teaching the appropriate use of language. At snack time, for example, we train use of polite forms (please, thank you), asking questions, and answering questions. Arts and crafts and play activities provide numerous opportunities to structure turn taking, question and answer activities, and requesting behavior. Show and tell affords the child opportunities for conversational turn taking, question and answer behavior, requesting information, and relating information. These activities provide opportunities to train the child how and when to use the communication and grammar skills that are the focus of the other, more structured, specific language training sequences.

HOW TO STRUCTURE TRAINING

We have discussed the content of our training program (concepts, vocabulary, grammar, and language): this section considers procedures. One way to look at language training is to focus on the three events that comprise each training task. Each task has: (a) an antecedent event—what you plan to do with and say to the child; (b) a response—what the child does or says; and (c) a subsequent event—your response to the child. This section will discuss some training procedures in for the three categories of events.

> Every training task has an antecedent, a response, and a subsequent event.

Antecedent events   The purpose of structuring and planning antecedent events is to maximize the child's opportunities to respond correctly. Antecedent events include (a) behavior control procedures, (b) where and when training occurs, (c) materials, (d) training sequences, and (e) training structure. The following are suggestions for arranging these events.

> Chapters Five and Six also discuss arrangements for antecedent, response, and consequent events.

1. **Establish behavioral control of the child**   The child must be able to sit in a chair (initially for at least five-minute periods), attend to

verbal stimuli and to the objects and actions used in training, and match objects that are the same.

2. **Maintain control of the stimulus materials**   Place the objects or pictures the child is to respond to on a response board that can be easily moved from one side of the table to the other. With the array of toys or pictures on the board in front of you, give the verbal directions, and then slide the board in front of the child for his response.

3. **Stop training before the child gets tired or bored**   Early sessions may last only five minutes or so, but they can be gradually lengthened as the child learns to attend longer. At first it is best to have two short sessions a day to which the child can give good attention. An older child may spend a half hour to 40 minutes a day in specific language training, but no more than 10 minutes is devoted to teaching any one language structure.

4. **Select materials that are of interest to the child**   If you choose vocabulary words which name small common objects that the child can manipulate and do things with, then your materials will probably be interesting to the child. Later in training, use pictures and/or objects to represent various nouns, verbs, adjectives, prepositions, and subject-verb-object structures. Be sure that the pictures are simple representations of the structure you are training.

Another aspect of structuring the antecedent events for language training involves training in comprehension and/or production of language. Comprehension of language is a receptive learning task; production is an expressive language task. Comprehension of language is knowing that the word "ball" means *that round thing that just rolled off the table*. Production is the ability to say "ball" when asked, "What is this?"

During comprehension training we teach the child to indicate understanding of the verbal stimulus by performing the action or pointing to the named object or picture. If comprehension of language is limited, training should be structured to maximize the probability that whatever behavior the child emits will be the desired response. Place an item in front of the child and give a command that coincides with the way the child usually interacts with the object. For example, if a child usually plays with a small ball by throwing it, hold a ball in front of him and say, "Throw ball." When he throws the ball, say "Good, you throw ball." Then, after several trials with only the ball, place the ball and a block on the table and say, "Throw block." If the child throws the ball instead, say, "No, throw block," and show him how to throw the block. Then train the child to differentiate between the directions "throw ball" and "throw block." Add more objects or actions to the task after the child masters the first discrimination. Other commands which capitalize on the child's typical way of responding in-

The purpose of comprehension training is to teach the child to link a verbal stimulus with the concept it represents.

clude "eat cookie, cereal, and raisins"; "drink water, milk and juice"; "push car, doll and chair."

Train vocabulary words by having the child select the labeled stimulus from an array of objects or pictures. If teaching the word "shoe" for example, place a sock, shoe, cup, and shirt in front of the child and say, "shoe." Consistent indication of the shoe when named is evidence that he understands the word.

Comprehension training of verbs consists of requesting the child to perform an action that is already in his repertoire. It is useful to incorporate an object in the command for verb training (e.g., "walk or run to the door," "push chair or box"). If the child's response is incorrect, the action should be demonstrated.

The major comprehension training strategies are rehearsal and prompting.

Another useful strategy, as noted in an earlier section, is to combine rehearsal of the stimulus with comprehension training. Display pictures or objects in front of the child as described in the comprehension task. Ask him to rehearse (repeat) your verbal stimulus ("shoe," "tiger," "push box," "boy push chair") before pointing to the object, picture, or performing the action.

Prompts can be used during comprehension training to help structure the task for the child. One method of prompting is to use manual signs. The sign is paired with the auditory stimulus to help the child remember the target word or language structure (e.g., an -*ing* ending, a preposition, or pronoun).

Procedures to structure production training are somewhat different than those for comprehension training. Production training may begin as verbal rehearsal during the comprehension training task. An array of objects or pictures is placed in front of the child, or he is directed to perform an action (as we described during the discussion of comprehension training). However, before the child is allowed to point to the picture or object or perform the action, he is required to rehearse your verbal stimulus. For example, when teaching the word "shoe" say to the child, "Shoe. Look for shoe." As he is scanning the array of objects, ask him to imitate the stimulus word "shoe." After he has rehearsed the word, push the tray of toys within his reach and say, "Find shoe."

The major production training strategies are rehearsal, imitation plus referent, questions plus prompts, questions alone, and story telling.

The child's rehearsal behavior need not be a perfect imitation of the verbal stimulus. Because he is learning a new structure in comprehension, do not expect him to be able to produce it correctly. The purpose of rehearsal training during the comprehension task is to provide many opportunities to practice production of the targeted structure. Verbal rehearsal also assists the child in the comprehension task because it helps him keep in mind the object or picture he is to find or the command he is to follow.

Another production training procedure is imitation training with a referent. Hold up the shoe and say, "What is this?" or "Say, *shoe*," or point to a picture and ask, "What is the boy doing? Say, *Boy push chair*." The child should imitate the three-element sentence. After several correct imitation trials, pause after the questions to give the child an opportunity to spontaneously produce the correct answer.

Another procedure used in production training is to combine the question form with prompts. There are many kinds of prompts. Gestures or hand signs may be used to cue words or word endings (verb tense or plural forms). If the sign for "shoe" was used during comprehension training of "shoe," signing the word "shoe" may help the child recall "shoe" when you ask "What is this?" Or, signing of the word "push" may help the child insert the word "push" in his response to the question "What is boy doing?" ("Boy push chair"). There are some simple visual and auditory prompts to help the child sequence a word or sentence. For example, three lines marked on a paper or three taps on the table may help the child remember how many words he has to say in the sentence, "Boy push chair."

Intraverbal prompts are also used in production training to help the child start a sentence. Say to the child, "What is the boy doing? Boy _____." The child responds, "Boy pushing chair." At an earlier training level (when training the production of verbs), begin the sentence and require the child to add the verb: "What is boy doing? Boy _____." The child should respond, "Sleep."

Another production training procedure consists of asking the child for spontaneous response: "Tell me about the picture", or "Tell me what's happening." If the child's response is incorrect or partially incorrect, use the procedures (imitation and prompts) from the lower levels of production training. This type of production training without cues gives the child practice using newly acquired words or language structures.

A final production procedure which can also be used to train generalization of newly acquired structures is story telling. Story telling gives the child an opportunity to practice production of a sequence of sentences. After ordering a series of pictures, he is required to tell the story. Or, after listening to or acting out a familiar story, he may be required to *retell* it.

The structure for concept training is similar to that for comprehension and production training. In all three types of training the child is required to learn many types of match-to-sample activities. During comprehension training, he must match pictures, objects, or his actions to an auditory stimulus. In production training he must match his verbal response to an auditory model (during imitation or rehearsal training), or a visual sample (when you ask him "Tell me about the picture?" or "What is this?"). Conceptual training requires him to match one visual stimulus to one or more other visual stimuli.

> Conceptual training focuses upon matching, categorizing, and sequencing.

Categorizing objects and pictures of objects and actions helps a child think about the relationship of one object to another or one action to another. It also helps him think about how an object is used or functions; this aids construction of concepts about objects and events.

Categorization tasks include (a) sorting pictures and objects according to their function (pictures of things we eat, wear, ride, use as furniture or tools, things we play with, use in grooming, use inside or outside the house, wear on hot or cold days, use on a farm or in town, and animals), (b) sorting objects according to association (matching objects that go together such as shoe and shoe lace, baby and a bottle, pencil and paper, bread and butter, hammer and a nail), (c) sorting along physical dimensions (by size, shape, color, texture, e.g., things that are smooth or rough, hot or cold, new and old, and long and short).

Sequencing activities teach the child to sequence objects, shapes, pictures, actions, and sounds, follow one-, two-, and three-part commands, and sequence events in stories. The child may be asked to complete a pattern of objects, shapes, or pictures. Action songs and finger plays can provide experience sequencing actions. For example, having him imitate a tapping pattern on a drum is one way to practice auditory sequencing. Another way to train auditory memory and sequencing is to have the child practice following one-, two-, and later three-part commands. Arranging up to five pictures that represent the events of a story, or acting out the events of a familiar story or nursery rhyme are other strategies to develop sequencing skills.

Response events   Response events are essentially what the child replies (actions or words) to antecedent events. The response of a child in comprehension training may be pointing to the named object or picture, or performing a directed action. In both cases the response might also include rehearsal of a target word or sentence. If the child is in production training, his response might be a word, phrase, or sentence.

Many times a child's verbal response (either imitative or spontaneous) will not be intelligible; however, articulation training is not begun until the child has developed a considerable amount of language. As a child progresses in training, his sound combinations for certain words are shaped by successive approximations. For example, early in training a child's acceptable word for *cookie* might be "oo." Later he is only reinforced when he says "koo." Still later only a closer approxmation to the word is acceptable, "kook," and finally, only the correct production of "cookie" is reinforced. The objective, at each level in training, is to gradually move the child's production closer to your model and provide the child with maximum success at each stage.

Concept training requires the child to respond in ways that demonstrate how he thinks about objects. How he plays with dolls, toy furniture, cars, trucks, and airplanes and how he uses a comb, toothbrush, cup, spoon, hammer, and phone provide information about his concepts of these objects. Placing identical or similar items or pictures into piles or containers, or grouping them in some way during matching or categorizing activities and putting a paper X or a cloth over the different item during oddity matching are other conceptual training responses. Responses during visual sequencing activities include laying out objects, pictures, or shapes to complete a pattern on display, or following the sequence of actions demonstrated by another.

Subsequent events   Subsequent events are the behaviors that follow a child's response: reinforcing events, expansions, explanations, and corrective feedback are examples of subsequent events. The natural, and usually most powerful, reinforcer for the child's verbal response is control of the attention and behavior of another person: having his requests for an action or object fulfilled and his questions answered. Another type of reinforcement is praise for attempts at talking during production tasks, listening during comprehension tasks, and performance in matching or categorizing activities. Give praise when a child performs well or is trying hard. If a child does not respond correctly or at the level he is capable of, simply say, "That's not quite right," or "I know you can say that better."

Initially, in language training it may be necessary to use food reinforcers (cereal, raisins, a favorite food) to establish desired behaviors. Later, tokens may be substituted for the food reinforcers. They can be traded for trinkets, toys, coins or desired events.

Expansion of the child's responses to the next level of linguistic complexity is also a subsequent event. For example, a verb-object statement may be expanded to a subject-verb-object statement: the statement "Boy pushing girl," can be expanded to "Yes, boy is pushing girl." As noted earlier, this type of grammatical expansion also highlights the next step in training for the child and may help him acquire the new structure without direct training.

Explanation is a subsequent event most often used with older children. An explanation may even describe the appropriate linguistic rule. For example, when training the third person plural objective pronoun, an explanation would be "When there is more than one person, we say *them* instead of *him* or *her*."

This section has provided some basic perspectives on structuring and implementing a preschool language intervention program. Many of the procedures we have described are most easily implemented in a one-to-one format, but this is not to say that they cannot be used in small group arrangements. Language should be taught within a number of social and educational contexts. The next section describes the integration of language training into the broader curriculum.

CURRICULUM DESIGN

RATIONALE

Many language-delayed children demonstrate skill deficiencies in areas other than language (e.g., fine- and gross-motor control, behavioral control, self-care skills, and perceptual and conceptual skills). Later success in school (and life) might depend not only on the attainment of speech and language skills, but also on these other abilities. A major reason for having the language-delayed child attend a special preschool is to teach him skills which will help him adjust to and function in subsequent school environments.

Behaviors which may help a child adjust better in a kindergarten class include (a) fine-motor control, (b) gross-motor control, (c) personal-social skills, (d) listening and attending skills, (e) language, communication and conceptual skills, and (f) specific preacademic skills including prereading and prearithmetic activities. These categories are arbitrary (and many preschool activities will teach more than one kind of skill), but this grouping facilitiates organization and discussion of these skills.

Fine motor skills   The main goal of fine-motor control is the development of eye-hand coordination so that the child will be able to perform such activities as working puzzles, manipulating objects, holding a pencil or crayon, using scissors, pasting, tracing lines with firm movements, making letters and numbers, drawing, and painting. There are two reasons why the language-delayed child needs these skills. He will succeed at routine classroom activities and he will be able to communicate his ideas and feelings through creative drawings, painting, and other endeavors. The child who is not able to communicate well through talking may be able to "talk" through his art work.

Gross-motor skills   If the child's gross-motor problems are major, some kind of prosthetic device may be necessary. If the problem is relatively minor and the child seems just clumsy, the preschool environment can encourage development of gross-motor coordination through activities using such equipment as tricycles, jungle gyms, climbing toys, balls, walking boards, and blocks. In addition to helping the child learn to use his large muscles, these activities provide a natural context for language training.

Personal-social skills   Specific aims under personal-social behaviors include (a) self-care skills (the ability to take care of toileting needs, clothing changes, etc.), and (b) interactive/social skills (the ability to get along with peers, teachers, and other significant persons). Training in these areas will help the child attain adaptive and independent functioning, in addition to providing opportunities for language learning. A child is motivated to communicate when he needs or wants something, or when he wants to control someone else's behavior.

Listening and attending skills   Attending skills are extremely important, not only for school, but also for appropriate functioning in a nonschool environment. Visual and auditory discrimination tasks, command-following and direction-following tasks, and music and finger play activities can be used to improve attending skills.

Language and conceptual skills   Language and conceptual targets include (a) specific syntactic structures such as verb-object, noun-verb-object, copula, and auxiliary usage, pronouns, prepositions, and adjectives, questions, plurals, and tense markers, (b) classifying according to a variety of categories such as use, size, shape, texture, color, number, and kind, (c) understanding *same* and *different,* (d) new vocabulary words, and (e) making associations between items (part-whole, opposites, and items that go together), and (f) sequencing items according to size, shape, or color, or sequencing stories. Music activities involving sequencing of actions, lyrics, or rhythm can be helpful in developing sequencing abilities. Other activities might include questions such as how, why, when, and where, which require the child to give reasons or explanations for occurrences.

Preacademic skills   Basic preacademic skills such as counting, number and alphabet recognition and recall, phonics, and left-to-right orientation will help the language-delayed child achieve early success in the kindergarten class. This is important not only for the child's self-image, but because it will demonstrate to others that difficulty in talking and using language does not necessarily mean intellectual impairment.

SCHEDULING

The above separation of the skills into six categories is not meant to suggest that they are separated this way in the curriculum. The following activity descriptions illustrate how the various parts are integrated in the daily routine. Keep in mind that the communication specialists are teachers as well as language trainers in the Preschool Language Training Project.

Free play   A typical day begins with free play time. The children enter the classroom, remove their outer garments, and select free play activities. A child may choose from a variety of items. He may choose to play alone or with others, to talk or be silent; the point is that he controls his own behavior during this period. Children initiate interactions and develop or practice a variety of skills, such as self-help behaviors, communication of needs and wants, and fine-motor control. Perceptual and conceptual skills are developed as the child sorts, stacks, aligns, counts, identifies, classifies, and in general manipulates the toys and other materials available to him. Materials involving specific preacademic activities such as tracing, matching, or writing letters and numbers are also available.

   Free play time is also very important for the teacher or communication specialist because it provides an opportunity to collect data on spontaneous production of trained items. If generalization is not occurring, specific activities and materials may be made available to stimulate production of specific utterances in a natural interchange. For example, if prepositions are being trained, a box with a lid or a block bridge or some other prop might stimulate the child's producing "in," "on," or "under." Also, analyses of language sample data taken during free play provide ongoing evaluations of the child's language use. Finally, free play time provides opportunities for the teacher to interact with the children on a more casual basis. It can be a special time for shared confidences or shared activities such as building something together, or it can be a time for the child to demonstrate new skills.

Show and Tell   After the toys and materials used in free play have been put away, the children form a circle for Show and Tell. Children show and discuss toys, clothes, and objects they have brought, or talk about recent experiences. The procedure is for one child to be chosen as the question-er and another to be the responder. Questions such as "What do you have?", "What do you do with it?", "Where did you get it?", "How does it work?", and "What is that?" are asked. At first some children are able to produce only one or two words, such as "have" or "what have" with question intonation, but as their language ability improves, the length and complexity of questions also increases. If necessary the teacher may prompt or provide a stimulus for the child, but most children soon learn to produce the questions spontaneously.

The child who is describing the object is required to reply appropriately to the questions. Other children are required to listen and sometimes take part in the discussion. For example, if a child has brought several small cars, these may be counted by the group, or colors may be labeled.

When one set of children has finished, a second set is chosen. This continues until all children who have Show and Tell items have had a turn, or until the end of the allotted time. At first children use the "learned" set of questions only at Show and Tell time, but as the year progresses, they begin to use these questions spontaneously during other activities. Parents also report increases in question behavior at home.

Music   After Show and Tell, there is a music and finger play time. The children sing a variety of songs, some of which involve actions, and do some finger plays. Examples of songs include "Six Little Ducks," "Old MacDonald," "The Wheels on the Bus," "Mr. Alligator," "Five Little Mon-keys," "Five Little Babies," "Open and Shut Them," and "Had a Little Turtle." The teacher or another child will lead the songs and finger plays.

We have found that some children will respond to songs and finger plays when they will not respond in any other activity. Also, it appears to help them in auditory discrimination and in sequencing of sounds and words. Often, a child's first intelligible two-word combinations occur during the singing or chanting of songs and finger plays. The action activities also help develop attending skills, gross- and fine-motor coordination, and vocabulary expansion, particularly verbs. Singing also helps vocal quality and use of pitch, rhythm, and dynamics. Children love to sing and enjoy these activities immensely.

Language and conceptual activities   After music time, the children are divided into smaller groups. Some receive specific speech and language therapy, and others receive perceptual and conceptual training which also involves more general language usage. Group assignments are based on data from formal and informal evaluations. All of the children receive some specific language therapy and participate in some activities to enhance their perceptual, conceptual, and thinking skills. In addition, some children receive articulation therapy.

Specific language training targets were discussed in a previous section (verb-object, noun-verb-object, prepositions, adjectives, etc.). Perceptual and conceptual activities include tasks involving auditory and visual discrimination, auditory and visual memory, classification and cate-gorizing, and some tasks involving reasoning and thinking skills which may or may not be closely aligned with immediate perceptions.

We do not expect all children to achieve the same level of compe-tence; we require different children to give different responses within the same activity. In addition, a variety of skills (tasks) might be incorporated into one activity. For example, a specific lesson might involve sequencing skills, classifying skills, and visual and auditory memory skills. The teacher might require one child to replicate a patterned sequence with colored cubes or objects, while another child might be required to name colors or describe objects according to color, size, shape, or kind. Another in the group might be asked to produce the pattern from memory. We might ask still another child to form a pattern from verbal instructions (place the yel-low cube in the middle of four blue cubes). Another might be required to tell how one pattern is different from another. The range and variety of re-sponses allows children to learn by watching others as well as by doing. The child who may be just beginning to learn to label colors will have suc-cess on his level, yet he also will be able to gain knowledge in other areas by watching. Later, he may be able to do the more difficult tasks because of the experience of a peer model.

Another type of activity targets story sequencing. One child may be required to retell the story from stimulus pictures, another may sequence some of the story pictures, and a third child may sequence all the pictures. Other children may act out the story, provide a new ending, or tell what might happen next. This permits the children to systematically progress from talking about the here and now, to talking about what happened, to making generalizations about what will happen.

In vocabulary expansion and classification tasks, the children may initially classify according to broad categories such as food, clothes, or an-imals. Later, they deal with more specific categories: fruits and vegetables, clothes worn in winter and clothes worn in summer, or zoo animals and farm animals.

These activities have a broader focus than just increasing the chil-dren's knowledge; they are designed to provide the children with positive feelings about their ability to manipulate objects, follow directions, and communicate. At first, only imitative responses may be required. The teacher starts where the child can be successful.

Sometimes the children end a session by marking or completing papers related to the activity. At this time the children may also do the writing-program activities, which begin with making vertical lines within a defined area and extend to horizontal lines, half-circles, circles, and finally letters.

Another method of teaching used during the language and concept sessions is modeled on the methods described by Marion Blank et al.

(1978a, 1979). They suggest arranging materials and activities so that the child can see the consequences of his response. The goal is to increase a child's thinking skills beyond an immediate perceptual level. For example, we roll a big red ball across the floor and ask the child why it rolls. One child's responses were particularly interesting. First he said it rolled "because it was red." The teacher then tried to roll a red block. The child paused, and then said it rolled "because it was big." The teacher then rolled a little ball. The child thought awhile, seemed to focus on the shape of the ball, and then said it rolled "because it was round." But instead of just saying "yes," the teacher picked up something else that was round, a roll of masking tape, and rolled it. (Other objects could also be rolled). The child and the rest of the group then agreed that the ball rolled because it was round.

This kind of activity helps children follow through on their reasoning and correct themselves. The challenge to the teacher is to have items available to demonstrate the effects of the answers and be able to reduce the complexity of the questions. Some children may not be able to handle a "why" question at first and will need to be guided to the answer by shifting to more concrete questions like "What shape is the ball?"

Outdoor play/snack time Outdoor play and a snack are scheduled after language and conceptual activities. The importance of outdoor play is not only the exercise and fresh air; it is another short period of free play when children can initiate interactions and teachers can observe spontaneous productions.

The focus during snack time is on personal-social language. Some children pass out the snacks and use polite language forms such as "What do you want?" or "Do you want juice?" The other children respond by saying "Cracker, please," "Yes," or "I want water, please."

Preacademic activities The next period of time is devoted to preacademic activities. Again, the children are not all expected to reach the same level of competence. Since preacademic activities are also included in conceptual language sessions, the focus at this time is on teaching the alphabet, phonics, numbers, and number concepts. Whenever possible, we incorporate number concepts into activities such as counting in songs or counting items. Also, writing numbers and letters may be done at the earlier writing sessions. Alphabet-learning activities include matching, recognizing, and recalling letters in a game format. We do similar activities with the numerals.

Phonics work includes matching letters and sounds and blending sounds into words. In addition, a sight reading vocabulary is developed, with each child selecting his own words to learn. For example, one child might choose "Superman," "Big Bird," or "dog." Eventually, the child's words are combined into a story that he can read for himself. There are two reasons why we teach an initial sight reading vocabulary: it helps the child understand what a word is and it gives him an opportunity to demonstrate a special language skill. He may not be able to say all the sounds in a word, but reading the word makes others aware of his abilities as well as his disabilities.

Arts and crafts The final session of the day is arts and crafts. These activities are quite varied; some emphasize art media while others are more related to particular concepts (e.g., circle pictures when we are discussing shapes). These activities may use paints, crayons, scissors and paste and different kinds of paper, cloth, modeling clay, and other materials. Some of the activities require following directions (paper folding), while others are relatively free of directions. During the latter ones, the child may express whatever he wants. Media used for these activities include finger paint, tempera paint, drawing materials, and clay.

Arts and craft activities are particularly important for language-delayed children because they provide a context for expression without the need for sounds. They also train eye-hand coordination and give experience with various kinds of art media. As ability to use the various media improves, so does self-confidence. Since these same skills are used in kindergarten, the ability to do the activities without help may contribute to better adjustment in these environments. And finally, the arts and crafts items produced can provide a topic of conversation for the child and his parents. It gives the child an answer for the question "What did you do in school today?"

Behavioral control Controlling behavior is rarely a problem. We give much social reinforcement for appropriate behavior, incuding praise, hugs, kisses, and pats. Occasionally, children earn edibles or trinkets during the specific language therapy time. For inappropriate behavior, the child is separated from the group and ongoing activity for a brief period. If inappropriate behavior continues to be a problem, we develop a specific program for that child.

Teacher/specialist training One unique aspect of the Preschool Language Training is that the communication specialists have also had training and experience teaching in normal classrooms (kindergarten and 3rd grade levels). They were teachers prior to training and certification as speech/language pathologists or audiologists. With this type of background, they know what will be expected of a child when he leaves preschool; they also know how to relate to school personnel.

THE PARENT PROGRAM

As emphasized throughout this chapter, a basic premise of the preschool language intervention program is that language is best trained in context. The context we have described is a preschool environment in which teachers are the focal point for both training and initiating communicative interactions. However, the instructional context is incomplete unless it includes the most significant individuals in the child's communicative environment—his parents. The parent program is an integral component of our overall intervention plan. Parents are involved from the beginning, planning their child's program (writing an IEP) and subsequently implementing the intervention procedures in daily interactions with the child.

PLANNING THE IEP

The teacher/specialist, in consultation with the parents, draws up an initial draft of the IEP, explains it to the parents in detail, and then provides them with a copy to study and revise. Once the parents and the teachers arrive at an acceptable intervention plan, the parents play a central role in program implementation. They are kept informed of their child's problems and progress through regularly scheduled meetings and counseling sessions, and they take an active role in training and charting the child's progress.

PARENT TRAINING PROCEDURES

Parents need to be reassured that they are not the cause of their child's language problem, and that there are many things they can do to enhance their child's language development. The initial focus of our parent training is general activities to make the home conducive to language learning. Parents are taught the training techniques listed in Figure 8-4.

Parents are given procedures relating to these techniques to read prior to a parent night discussion session. Then they view a videotape demonstrating each technique and discuss its application.

Parents learn to score adult-child interactions on the *Talking Effectively Rating Sheet.*

The *Talking Effectively Rating Sheet* (see Figure 8–4) is also discussed. All of the parents score segments of the videotape which depict a teacher-child interaction and then discuss their ratings. After this initial training, parents are scheduled to observe a teacher interacting with their child. They observe the teacher and child engaged in a typical home activity (dressing or toileting, preparing food, making sandwiches, preparing breakfast, looking at a story book, fixing a toy, or playing with a toy). The session is also videotaped so the parent and teacher can score the interactions together on the Talking Effectively Rating Sheet.

Then a parent demonstration is scheduled. Parents prepare an activity similar to the one used by the teacher. This session is also videotaped. The parent(s) and teacher view the tape, score the interactions and discuss their ratings. Depending upon the parents' understanding and use of the techniques, additional sessions may be scheduled. We make periodic rechecks of parents' skills as the child's language skills increase to insure that the parents continue to use appropriate expansions and proper directions.

The parents are also encouraged to use the rating sheet in the home to check themselves on talking effectively. Parent progress in the training component is assessed periodically, both in terms of carrying out assign-

FIGURE 8-4   Talking effectively rating (1 to 4 words)

A check indicates need for improvement.
          DID   **NOT**

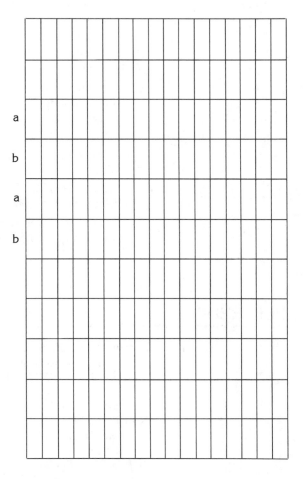

1. Get child's attention before talking.

2. Talk about the here and now.

3. a) Label objects (nouns) repeatedly, b) then
       talk about objects in different ways (verbs +
       adjectives, etc.).

4. a) Coordinate your sentences with actions,
       labeling the action (verb), b) then add other
       elements (agent, object, location, etc.).

5. Pause to give child an opportunity to imitate
       words.

6. Respond to child's utterances meaningfully.

7. Expand child's utterances to next level of
       linguistic difficulty.

8. Ask child meaningful questions.

9. Require child's speech to be at appropriate
       levels of production.

ments and in terms of the child's progress. The nine-point program is
further supplemented by additional specific activities assigned by the
teacher/specialist for the parents to implement at home. Such activities
may involve direct training of language structures being worked on in the
preschool, or simply charting and recoding data in the home. In any case,
the teacher/specialist first instructs the parents about the task in the preschool (clinic) setting before assigning it as part of the home program.
Evaluation of the parents' participation by both the parents and the
teacher/clinician is pivotal in determining the future shape and direction of
the child's total intervention program.

SUMMARY

1. This chapter describes the Preschool Language Training Project at the University of Kansas.
2. The purpose of intake evaluation is to collect data for placement recommendations and/or to decide directions for further in-depth evaluations.
3. Language training targets concept development, vocabulary, grammar, and language use in a variety of daily activities.
4. In addition to language and conceptual skills, the program attempts to develop fine- and gross-motor skills, personal-social skills, listening and attending skills, and preacademic skills.
5. Scheduled activities, all of which integrate language training tasks, include free play, show and tell, music, language and conceptual activities, outdoor play/snack time, and arts and crafts.
6. Parents are involved in a range of planning, program implementation, and generalization activities.

REFERENCES

BLANK, M., ROSE, S., & BERLIN, L. *The language of learning-The preschool years*. New York: Grune & Stratton, 1978. (a)

BLANK, M., ROSE, S., & BERLIN, L. *Preschool language assessment instrument-The language of learning in practice*. New York: Grune & Stratton, 1978. (b)

BLANK, M., ROSE, S., & BERLIN, L. Testing communication skills in children with language and learning disabilities. Short course, American Speech and Hearing Association Convention, Atlanta, Ga., 1979.

BOEHM, A.E. *Boehm test of basic concepts*. New York: Psychological Corp., 1971.

BROWN, R. *A first language*. Cambridge, Mass.: Harvard University Press, 1973.

CARROW, E. *Test for auditory comprehension of language*. Austin, Tex.: Learning Concepts, 1973 and 1977.

DUNN, L. *Peabody picture vocabulary test*. Circle Pines, Minn.: American Guidance Service, Inc., 1965.

GERBER, A., & GOEHL, R. *Temple university syntax screening test*. Baltimore: University Park Press, in press.

GOLDMAN, R., & FRISTOE, M. *Goldman-Fristoe test of articulation*. Circle Pines, Minn.: American Guidance Service, Inc., 1969, 1972.

HEDRICK, E.P., PRATHER, E.M., & TOBIN, A. *Sequenced inventory of communications development*. Seattle, Wash.: University of Washington Press, 1975.

LEE, L. *Northwestern syntax screening test*. Evanston, Ill.: Northwestern University Press, 1969, 1971.

McDONALD, E. *A deep test of articulation-picture form.* Pittsburgh, Pa.: Stanwix House, Inc., 1964.

MILLER, J., & YODER, D. *Miller-Yoder test of grammatical comprehension.* University of Wisconsin-Madison: Experimental Edition, 1977.

NEWCOMER, P.L., & HAMMILL, D.D. *Test of language development.* Austin, Tex.: Empiric Press, 1977.

RUDER, K. Planning and programming for language intervention. In R.L. Schiefelbusch (Ed.), *The bases of language intervention.* Baltimore: University Park Press, 1978.

RUDER, K., SMITH, M., & HERMANN, P. Effects of verbal imitation and comprehension on verbal production of lexical items. In L.V. McReynolds, (Ed.), *Developing systematic procedures for training children's language.* American Speech and Hearing Association Monograph #18, 1974, 15–29.

RUDER, K., & STREMEL, K. *Perspectives on language training* (16mm film). Lawrence, Kans.: Bureau of Child Research, University of Kansas, 1975.

STREMEL, K., & WARYAS, C. A behavioral psycholinguistic approach to language training. In L. McReynolds (Ed.), *Developing systematic procedures for training children's language.* ASHA Monograph #18, 1974.

STREMEL-CAMPBELL, K., & WARYAS, C. Grammatical training for the language delayed child: A new perspective. In R.L. Schiefelbusch (Ed.), *Language intervention strategies.* Baltimore: University Park Press, 1978.

CHAPTER NINE

USING AN INDIVIDUALIZED CURRICULUM SEQUENCING MODEL

Marilyn Mulligan and Douglas Guess

The Individualized Curriculum Sequencing (ICS) model described in this chapter is the result of over four years of research and program development in classrooms for severely handicapped students. The basic premises were first presented in 1978 in a series of articles by Guess and colleagues (Guess, Horner, Utley, Maxon, Tucker, & Warren, 1978). Since then the model has been further developed and refined in a number of articles (Brown, Holvoet, Guess, & Mulligan, 1980; Holvoet, Guess, Mulligan, & Brown, 1980; Mulligan, Guess, Holvoet, & Brown, 1980) and a recent book (Sailor & Guess, 1983).

The ICS model has several unique characteristics: (a) the teaching of skills in functional sets, called clusters, and (b) arrangement of skill clusters in a natural fashion across traditional content domains (e.g., social, language, self help). The key words in this model are *functional* and *natural*. Classroom activities are planned to increase the child's functional interactions in the natural environment. Generalization training is an integral part of the training process. The ICS program recommends changing trainers, instructional cues, materials, body positions, settings, and other antecedent events across training sessions.

A strength of this approach is its incorporation of, and ability to accommodate to, divergent theoretical approaches. Based on the premise that no one set of techniques has been proven to be superior, the ICS draws from all available information—from Piagetian, behavioral, remedial, and neurodevelopmental systems. A consequence of this broad theoretical base is a model which lends itself particularly well to the transdisciplinary team model as described by Lyon and Lyon (1980).

The transdisciplinary team approach is described in Chapter Eleven.

HOW IT WORKS

The ICS model emphasizes the importance of teaching more than an assortment of splinter skills; a basic goal is to teach children how skills relate to one another, and where and when they should be performed. It is not difficult to see how this approach differs from more traditional methods which provide isolated, repeated trials (called a massed trial training) on tasks which may be irrelevant to the student's immediate needs and/or the requirements of her surroundings (Guess, Horner, Utley, Holvoet, Maxon, Tucker, & Warren, 1978). For example, in other approaches it is common to find students being provided with 10 or more repetitions of "shirt off," or requested to imitate a particular sound 10 times in a single training session. The ICS would schedule trials on these skills (if they are determined to be functional and necessary for the child) throughout the day, in combination with other related skills, in different locations, and with different trainers. This is the distributed trial strategy described below.

A basic goal of the ICS model is to teach children how skills relate to one another, and where and when they should be performed.

TRAINING CONDITIONS

The ICS approach is based on research in experimental psychology and recent findings related to the learning characteristics of severely handicapped children. Data generated in the field of experimental psychology suggest that skills taught with a spaced or distributed trial sequence are learned better than skills learned in a massed trial format (Deese, 1958). After initial learning, performance becomes a negatively accelerating function (the learning curve climbs less dramatically over time) of both the length of the rest period (Kimble, 1949; Kientzle, 1946) and of the number of trials (Adams, 1952; Duncan, 1951). The general conclusion is that the overall effect of massed trials is a depression in performance at the high point of the learning curve.

Additional factors that seem to affect cognitive performance under different conditions of practice are (a) criterion levels of responding, (b) the difficulty of the task, and (c) the similarity of items being learned. Underwood, Kapelak, and Malmi (1976) report superior performance under spaced trial conditions when subjects had high or difficult criteria levels for responding (as opposed to low criteria levels). Elmes, Sanders, and Dovel (1973) demonstrated that when the cues for trials in a massed trial format were conspicuously different from ongoing activities, then performance was similar to that in a spaced trial format where cues were not distinguishable from ongoing activities. In other words, the more unfamiliar or demanding the task, the more a spaced or distributed trial strategy assists performance.

The more unfamiliar or difficult a task, the more spaced or distributed trial strategies improve performance.

Studies dealing with acquisition and retention of motor skills have also demonstrated superiority for a distributed trial sequence over massed trials. Typically these studies trained college students on nonfunctional tasks and measured performance in terms of number of trials to criterion or number correct per session. Chasey's (1976) work with retarded boys is possibly more relevant. Not only did his students learn the target fine-motor task with fewer trials to criterion under distributed trial conditions, they also demonstrated significantly better retention (than other students taught with massed trials).

The difference between massed, distributed, and spaced trial formats centers on what occupies the time between two trials from the same program (see Figure 9-1). Trials are *massed* if repeated so closely that no other behavior can occur between trials. Both spaced and distributed trial sequencing have separated trials: there are periods of time between two trials from the same program. Trials are *spaced* if a rest period, or pause, occurs between two repeated trials from the program (Underwood, Kapelak, & Malmi, 1976). Trials are *distributed* if a trial from another program or programs occurs between two repeated trials from the same program.

PROGRAM DEVELOPMENT

The ICS model recommends teaching *skill clusters,* as opposed to individual skills. A skill cluster (discussed in more detail later) is a group of target behaviors which comprise a functional and natural skill sequence. For example, a particular child's objectives (from her IEP) might include (a) holding head erect and arms stable (gross-motor objective); (b) vocalizing to gain attention (language/communication objective); (c) scanning items on a communication board (cognitive objective); (d) pointing/ indicating items on a communication board to indicate needs (language objective); and (e) reaching and grasping (fine-motor objective). These skills, grouped naturally together as a unit, would be trained across a variety of settings, persons, and materials: they would be trained at lunch (to gain food), at grooming times (to ask for a wash cloth), and at leisure activity time (to request use of the tape recorder).

Instructional as well as natural cues may be used to teach the skill clusters. If, for example, a student is being taught to ask for help (e.g., materials are out of reach or a toy is dropped), and does not respond to the natural cues, there are several possible alternatives. Say "What do you need?" or "Point to the _____," and then either model the desired reponse or physically prompt the correct response (Brown & Alderson, 1978; Lent & McLean, 1976). A second possibility is to use a time delay procedure (Halle, Baer, & Spradlin, 1981; Snell & Gast, 1981).

Time delay procedures are described in Chapter Six.

The interests, activities, and daily routines of a nonhandicapped same-age peer are one reference for selection of materials and training locations for a severely handicapped student. This will assure age-appropriate materials and activities. Another source of ideas for identifica-

Trial distribution	Three types of schedules
XXXXXXXXXX YYYYYYYYYY (time)	**Massed** trial sequence for programs X and Y.
X X X X X X X X X X (time)	**Spaced** trial sequence for program X.
XYXYXYXYXYXYXYXYXYXYXYXY (time)	**Distributed** trial sequence for programs X and Y.

FIGURE 9-1 Different trials arrangements over time for massed, spaced, and distributed trial training

tion of training materials, activities, and locations is an inventory of the student's present, and possibly future, environments as suggested by Brown and colleagues (e.g., Brown, Branston-McClean, Baumgart, Vincent, Falvey, & Schroeder, 1979). (The ecological inventory approach to generating curricular content is described at length in Chapter Six.)

Figure 9-2 outlines ICS program development activities after initial assessments have been completed. The first nine steps have to do with ICS planning, design, and implementation of skill sequences: the program evaluation/review process begins with Step 10. The following sections will discuss Steps 1 through 4 (planning and program development) and Step 13 (program revisions).

Assessment and development of objectives   Some assessment instruments focus on specific age ranges or areas of development; others focus on particular characteristics and cover the entire school age population. The strategy of assessment may be (a) to identify the student's deficits relative to normal development milestones, or (b) to identify strengths and deficits in relation to some set of prespecified criteria. (See Bayley, 1969; Frankenburg & Dodds, 1969; Guess, Rues, Warren, & Lyon, 1980; Haring, 1976; and Somerton & Turner, 1974 for reviews of the applications of different types of assessment tools with severely handicapped and deaf/blind students.) Selection of assessment devices to generate program objectives depends on the age and handicapping condition of the student and the expertise of the professional.

The ICS model does not stipulate which assessment tools to use as long as all functioning domains and developmental areas are evaluated, thoroughly and comprehensively. One of the most effective procedures for generating functional and age-appropriate objectives is to conduct environmental inventories. As noted above, these inventories assist identification of the skills (as well as materials, activities, and training activities) necessary for independent functioning in present (and possibly future) settings. Settings to be assessed include domestic, school/vocational, community, and leisure environments (Brown, Branston-McClean, Baumgart, Vincent, Falvey, & Schroeder, 1979).

The ICS does not specify particular assessment procedures.

The results of both student and environmental assessments are combined to formulate instructional objectives. For example, if fine-motor assessments indicate the need to work on directed reach and grasp, and an environmental inventory suggests the need for training to grasp doorknobs and eating utensils, and reach and obtain items from shelves, then one of the student's objectives might be to "reach and grasp items at ¾ arm's distance." Appropriate training materials would include doorknobs, eating utensils, clothing, and vocational sorting items. If student assessments indicate the need to teach a greeting response and environmental inventories suggest that the student should communicate (to announce her presence) when entering the kitchen, vocational setting, and classroom, then an objective should address greeting (with a single hand wave and/or vocalization) in these locations.

Combine student and environmental assessment results to formulate instructional objectives.

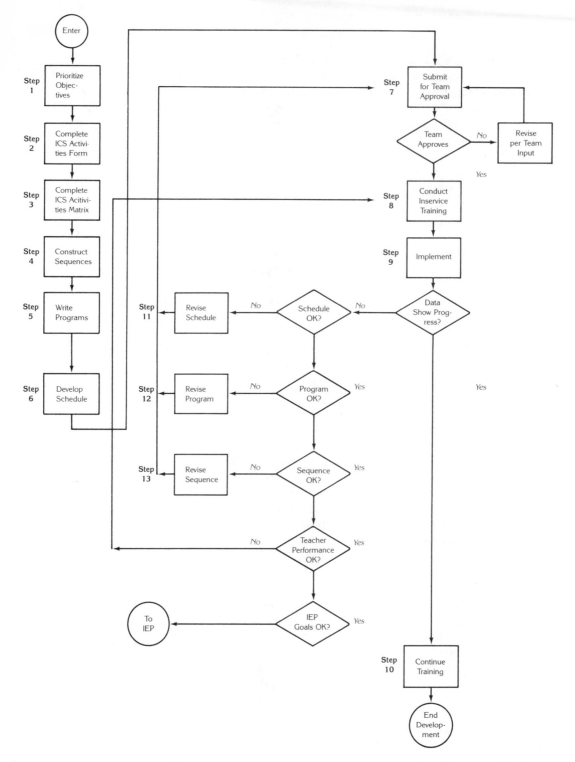

FIGURE 9-2 Procedure for developing, implementing, and evaluating the ICS model

After objectives have been formulated and agreed upon, enter the flowchart (Figure 9-2) at Step 1 and rank order the instructional objectives based on knowledge of the student's functional needs, her family's concerns, and environmental requirements. Skills that will be used the most frequently within and across training settings, persons, and materials should be assigned higher priorities.

Instructional objectives may be prioritized on the IEP form.

Selecting daily activities   The next step is to complete an ICS Activities Worksheet (such as the sample presented in Figure 9-3) for the classroom. Reproductions of this form with "classroom" deleted can be used to plan for nonschool activities. In the first column list activities in the various categories.

Classroom routines are just what the name implies—daily events. Functional daily activities are for the purpose of increasing independent functioning. Age-appropriate activities include activities designed to teach age-appropriate social, leisure, and work skills. The sample form presented in Figure 9-3 is completed for a preschool child. An ICS Activities Worksheet for an adolescent or young adult would look very different. For example, age-appropriate leisure time activities for an older student might include using a tape recorder or radio, work activities would target vocational skills, and social skills training might include playing board games or group singing.

The amount of time each day committed to each activity should be noted in the second column. Persons available in the classroom to act as trainers (e.g., aide, foster grandparent) are noted in the third column, and, the desired adult-student ratio (instructional arrangement) for the activity is indicated in the last column. This information, together with the student's prioritized objectives, is then used to develop an individualized curriculum.

Sequencing objectives across activities   Step 3, completion of the ICS Activities Matrix (Figure 9-4) is a means of combining activity information with prioritized objectives to develop a daily schedule. List the student's priority objectives across the top and daily classroom activities on the left. An ICS Activities Matrix indicating skills that can be logically taught during the school day should be prepared for each student. In essence, this form represents an individualized curriculum outline. (The ICS matrix presented in Figure 9-4 is for a half-day schedule.)

The ICS matrix in Figure 9-4 is essentially an individualized curriculum: its use is also discussed in Chapter Six.

Daily activities and the approximate amount of time each requires depends, to a large extent, on the age and functioning level of the student and the particular setting. There are, however, some considerations applicable for all students. The sequence of daily activities (first vertical column) should reflect the school routine of a nonhandicapped student of the same age. For example, young children usually have individual work periods, group periods, indoor and outdoor play situations, snack and lunch routines; a similar schedule should be devised for the special education classroom.

ICS Activities Worksheet

Activities	Estimated time	Trainers available	Student-trainer ratio
Classroom routines			
Physical health check-in	15 min.	Health aide, teacher aide,	1:1
Hanging up coat in locker	10 min.	foster grandmother and teacher	1:1
Snack time	20 min.	Same	Group
Good-morning group	20 min.	Same	Group
Functional daily activities			
Going to the bathroom	15 min. (Twice daily)	Aide, foster grandmother, and teacher	1:1
Eating lunch	30 min. (Total)	Aide, teacher	Group
Waiting for the bus	10 min.	Aide	Group
Moving from one place to another	20 min.	Aide, foster grandmother	1:1
Cleaning up the work area	10 min.	Aide	Group
Age-appropriate activities			
Assembling puzzles (leisure)	30 min.	Aide, foster grandmother, and teacher	Group
Sitting at desk (school)	30 min.	Aide	Group
Singing nursery rhymes (social)	20 min.	Foster grandmother	Group
Other activities			
Weekly assembly	45 min.	Aide, teacher	Group
Adaptive P.E.	45 min.	Adaptive P.E. teacher and aide	Group

FIGURE 9-3 The ICS activities worksheet for a preschool severely handicapped student

ICS Activities Matrix
IEP Objectives in Order of Priority

Schedule of daily activity & approximate time req.	Vocal imitation "ah," "bah"	Reach and grasp	Indicate desired item on communication board	Roll for mobility	Toilet regulation	Drink from cup	Type of activity
Entry/health check (15 min)	X			X			Routine
Bathroom (15 min)		X	X		X		Functional, low
Activity of daily living (30 min)	X	X	X				Age-appropriate, low
Snack/leisure (30 min)	X	X	X	X		X	Age-appropriate, high
Academics (30 min)	X	X	X				Age-appropriate, low
Bathroom (15 min)		X	X		X		Functional, low
Lunch (30 min)	X	X	X	X		X	Functional, high
Total training opportunities	5	6	6	3	2	2	

FIGURE 9-4 ICS matrix showing IEP objectives (in order of priority) and when training can be provided in the classroom routine

There are three considerations when planning daily activities: (a) alternate low and high interest/difficulty activities; (b) natural sequencing of skill training/practice trials within activities; and (c) the logical order of events. The ordering of daily activities should apply the *Premack Principle* (Premack, 1965), which suggests alternating low and high probability events. Periods of work on more difficult activities could be alternated contingently or noncontingently with periods of more enjoyable activities. For example, if the activity is functioning in a group (sitting independently, and taking turns pointing to pictures in a book), and this activity is difficult for most of the children involved, then schedule it before an easier and more enjoyable activity such as a leisure or snack time activity. Sequencing skills in a natural order during the group activity—e.g., head up, look at the book, point to the picture—will also reward appropriate responding.

Finally, daily activities should be scheduled in logical order reflecting what might occur in the natural environment. For example, bathroom activities should be scheduled after arrival, and before lunch, going home, or into the community. Work activities should be scheduled before play or leisure, and snacks should be provided 1½ hours before or after lunch.

Figure 9-5 shows three sample schedules.

Figure 9-5 provides three sample schedules for preschool or early elementary-aged children: schedule A is for older, less physically handicapped children; schedules B and C might be used for more physically or sensory handicapped older students or preschool children. The schedules incorporate the requirements of normalizing, rewarding, and logical sequencing.

Now, look at Figure 9-4 again. The column to the far right of the ICS Activities Matrix, under the heading "Type of activity," is included to remind the teacher to be sure that all activities are functional, age-appropriate, and sequenced appropriately. The teacher indicates whether an activity is routine, functional, or age-appropriate, and whether it is a high or low probability event. The majority of activities should be functional and/or age-appropriate and the high and low probability activities should be alternated.

The ICS Activities Matrix shows which objectives are appropriately taught during which activities. Objectives and activities that seem to fit together are indicated by the Xs. For example, in Figure 9-4, vocal imitation could be instructed during entry, activities of daily living, snack time, academics, and lunch. Similarly, the objective of reach and grasp can be taught during bathroom periods, activities of daily living, snack time, academics, and lunch. Highest priority skill targets should be scheduled for more frequent practice with a greater variety of materials and in as many locations as possible.

Knowing when and where a skill will be taught aids selection of cues and correction procedures, materials, and tasks.

There is not a "right" way to complete an ICS matrix. Its purpose is to point out which objectives can be taught during specified activities so that the teacher has a better idea of how to develop the specific training program for each objective. Knowing when and where an objective is to be taught helps her make decisions about cues and correction procedures,

A	B	C
Entry	Entry - health check	Entry - health check
Bathroom	Bathroom (toileting)	Bathroom
Activity of daily living	Self-help	Mobility to group area
Leisure	Snack	Music-group
Academics (at desk)	Group activity	Bathroom
Bathroom	Bathroom (toileting and	Snack
Lunch	washing)	Pre-academics (individual)
Pre-vocational (at long table)	Lunch	Mobility to lunch area
Gym	Rest	Vestibular stimulation
Academics	Pre-academics	Lunch
Bathroom/grooming	Music	Rest
Out - home/community	Bathroom (toileting)	Mobility to work area
	Exit home - dressing	Pre-academics (group)
		Bathroom
		Mobility to exit - home

FIGURE 9-5 Three sample schedules of daily activities for preschool or elementary level children

placement of materials, and the stimulus materials themselves. The next step is to construct the skill clusters, Step 4 of Figure 9-2.

Developing skill clusters Step 4 (Figure 9-2) uses information from the ICS Matrix to develop individualized skill clusters. These clusters are then listed on a data sheet (Figure 9-6). As noted at the beginning of the chapter, clusters are sequences of three to five responses (from different programs) organized in a functional or logical manner and repeated within and across activities. Which objectives to formulate into clusters should be apparent from the student's ICS matrix. In Figure 9-4 three objectives are repeated across four different daily activities. Vocal imitation, reach and grasp, and use of the communication board can be scheduled to occur during activities of daily living, snack time, academics, and lunch time. Since these objectives are logically related, they could form a useful cluster of responses for the student.

> Clusters are sequences of three to five responses organized in a functional or logical manner and repeated within and across daily activities.

Rolling could also be scheduled for each of these activities, but it does not fit logically and naturally with the other three responses. For this reason, rolling may be best taught as an isolated response. It could be scheduled once during the indicated activities (at entry/health check time, before snacks, and again before lunch), but should not be repeated any more often than this.

Note the organization of the data sheet shown in Figure 9-6 and the code letters. Portions of the data sheet are separated to indicate different activities. "t" before the behavior indicates that is is a teacher behavior, and "c" indicates a child's response. Trials with brackets form a skill cluster which is to be repeated as often as possible given the available time, student-teacher ratio, and stamina of the student. Figure 9-6 is a simple data sheet for one student. Other styles of data sheets which permit moni-

> On the ICS Data Sheet "t" indicates a teacher response and "c" indicates a child response; trials with brackets should be repeated as often as possible.

		ICS DATA SHEET (one option)	Student _____ Teacher _____ _____

		Date						
Entry/ **Health check**	c - roll into room							
	c - imitate "hi," "ah"							
	t - health check							
BR/ **Grooming**	t - point to BR on communication board							
	c - point to communication board							
	c - reach and grasp							
	c - imitate "ah"							
	t - indicate "wet" or "dry"							
Activity of **daily living/** **Dressing**	c - point to communication board							
	c - discriminate shoe/sock							
	c - reach and grasp							
	c - imitate "ah"							
	t - reinforce for watching other students							
Snack	c - roll to area							
	c - point to communication board							
	c - reach and grasp							
	c - imitate "ah"							
	c - drink from cup							

FIGURE 9-6 Sample data sheet showing training sequence for the first portion of a school day

toring of the interaction between students, easy graphic representation of the student's performance, or evaluation of larger sequences of activities are being developed.

Writing an instructional program The teacher can now develop instructional programs (Step 5, Figure 9-2) for each of the student's objectives. The ICS model does not specify how to write instructional programs since this topic has been well developed elsewhere (Williams, Brown, & Certo, 1975). A major concern should be developing programs applicable across settings, materials, and persons. The teacher can readily see the different settings and activities in which the program will be used by looking at the ICS Matrix and should get some ideas for naturally occurring cues, correction procedures, and reinforcers from the Data Sheet. For example, beginning snack preparation, or the verbalization "It's time for snack," could be the cue for the student to roll to the snack area. The naturally occurring consequence for arriving at the area is the opportunity to indicate a desired snack item. A natural cue for pointing to the communication board could be "What do you want?" (rather than the instructional cue of "Point to the juice/cookie"). The naturally occurring consequence for this nonverbal communication is offering the desired food, which becomes a cue for reach and grasp. The natural consequence of reaching and grasping is, of course, the snack item.

> The next step is deciding on cues, correction procedures, and reinforcers for the desired responses.

All sequences will not be as obviously related and inherently motivating as a snack time skill cluster. Instructional cues and corrections and more contrived reinforcers may be necessary when the student's performance requires additional assistance. The opportunity for utilizing the naturally occurring events of the environment is much greater, however, when the student's responses are sequenced in this manner.

Developing the classroom schedule Finally the teacher proceeds to Step 6 of Figure 9-2, the development of a classroom schedule. During this organizational activity the needs of all the students and data on the availability of personnel and materials are brought together. One of the teacher's functions, coordinating the individual sequences of all the students, is made more manageable by the fact that all the students follow the same schedule of daily activities.

> It is the teacher's responsibility to coordinate the individual sequences of all the students.

Concerns, common to all classrooms, include (a) the student/ teacher ratio required for different activities, (b) the time required for different activities, (c) the need to provide all teachers with the opportunity to observe others instructing the students, (d) collection of reliability data, and (e) program evaluation. A classroom schedule should be posted indicating the schedules of both the teachers and the students. In addition to providing structure to the day, this will help personnel see who is responsible for what.

Steps 7, 8 and 9 of Figure 9-2 reflect the transdisciplinary approach to be discussed in Chapter Eleven. Since all IEP objectives are incorporated into the student's ICS, all team members are involved in program implementation.

Revising sequence   Steps 11 through 13 of Figure 9-2 suggest which components of the student's ICS to evaluate if the student is not learning a skill. The model does not suggest specific procedures to investigate why the student is not acquiring a skill; some of the solutions, however, are directly related to the sequencing strategies.

If a particular skill is not being acquired, review the student's schedule first, then consider program or sequence revisions.

The teacher should first review the student's classroom schedule to determine if the program is actually being conducted, and if there are sufficient trials per day to optimize learning. The amount of time required for routine daily activities may have been underestimated in developing the ICS, so that in actual implementation, some skill clusters may not be repeated as often as planned because of lack of time. The classroom staff must be alert to the danger of not following the schedule and be willing to modify original sequences. Sometimes this can mean reducing the numbers of training trials per day of low priority or ancillary objectives to meet the target date for priority objectives.

Second, the teacher should analyze program data to see if any aspect of the instructional program needs revision. Possible targets for revision are the instructional cue, correction procedure, consequence, or level (step) of responses required. Haring, Liberty, and White (1980) have outlined the procedures for making program revision decisions. However, because these procedures assume a massed trials training strategy, they are only reasonable guidelines.

There is some evidence that the size of the skill cluster may affect acquisition.

Step 13 of Figure 9-2 suggests evaluating and revising the student's actual sequence. One factor to consider is the size of the skill clusters. There are some preliminary data indicating that acquisition of the skill may be negatively influenced if the skill clusters are too large (Holvoet, 1981). Four-response clusters appear to produce fewer errors during learning than clusters with two or five responses. The skill clusters Holvoet investigated were comprised of vocational and leisure skills for severely handicapped adolescents. Whether these findings generalize to all severely handicapped learners across all skill domains is an area for future investigation.

Finally, the teacher should determine whether the IEP goal is suitable. It may be necessary to proceed through the IEP process again, develop a new goal and/or objectives, and modify the ICS accordingly.

A sample case clarifies ICS procedures and provides some additional help in making decisions at the various steps. Figures 9-7 through 9-12 are the planning forms for this sample case.

SAMPLE CASE

Laura is a 2½-year-old with Down Syndrome. She scores below the 12-month level on the majority of items on the Callier-Azusa Scale (Stillman,

1977), and between the 6 and 8 month levels in language usage. Laura is a very playful, affectionate, and sociable little girl; she seems to enjoy being around adults. She can finger feed herself but needs total assistance in dressing and undressing. She has just begun to walk while holding onto furniture for support. Laura makes babbling sounds, especially when playing with dolls, but has no imitative skills. In terms of receptive language, Laura turns to look when her name is called and will come when called (by scooting along on the floor) but she does not follow other one-part commands such as pointing, giving named familiar items, or looking at familiar people. When she wants an item, she reaches for it rather than using a point or gesture response.

Laura lives at home with her natural parents. She is the youngest of six children and the only child still in the home. The other siblings have been removed to foster placements because of the parents' apparent inability to care for a large number of children. They seem to be doing very well with Laura, however; she attends school regularly, is well groomed, and appears to be happy.

Currently Laura attends a full day program for severely handicapped preschool children. She is in a class with four other children, one teacher, and one paraprofessional. The total class is structured using the ICS model for all the students. Figure 9-7 is a sample of Laura's IEP objectives, prioritized with target dates. Figure 9-8 is her ICS Activities Matrix. It is clear from this sequence of activities that the teacher's priorities were the motor and language areas.

From the ICS Activities Matrix, the teacher developed two types of data sheets for monitoring Laura's progress. Figure 9-9 is a sample data sheet for most of the morning activities. Both teacher and child behaviors are indicated; however, scoring is only done where a child action is indicated on the data sheet. The other items serve as cues to the teacher. The teacher scores the items as she proceeds through the data sheet. Skill clusters, as indicated by the brackets, are usually repeated three to four times within the sequence.

Figure 9-10 is the second type of data sheet developed by the teacher; it is a graphic representation of the student's acquisition of the entire lunch sequence. When using this form the teacher only records the first occurrence of the cluster, even though the cluster may actually be repeated five to ten times throughout the lunch period. In tabulating the data, the teacher has chosen to give Laura credit for prompted responses. A correct response is given the weight of a full point, a prompted response .5. For example, on day 11/5 Laura got one item in the sequence correct: "touches food/drink." She also was correct on two other items with prompting: walking and scooping/drinking without spilling. Her total percent correct out of the sequence for that day was 2/6 or 33%. Figures 9-11 and 9-12 are from the receptive language training program: the objective is to teach Laura to respond to the directions "Touch the _____." The ultimate goal of the program is to teach receptive labeling.

Individual Program Plan

Child's Name: Laura Birthdate: 11/10/81 IEP Date: 9/10/83

Priority	Objective	Definition of Success	Person Responsible	Target Date
1	Laura will cruise holding onto furniture	Distance of 4 feet, 3 times	Jan/Cozette	10/16/83
2	Laura will imitate "ba" for ball, when object is in front of her.	5 times per day for 3 days	Jan/Cozette	1/15/84
3	Laura will touch object when presented & given verbal cue "touch _____." (ball, baby)	5 times for each object per day for 3 days	Jan/Cozette	1/15/84
4	Laura will void in potty chair when placed on chair.	3 or less accidents/wk.	Jan/Cozette	1/15/84
5	Laura will drink out of glass, swallow liquid.	Will swallow 2 times consecutively for 3 days	Jan/Cozette	10/16/83
6	Laura will eat without assistance with spoon & fingers, entire meal.	Scoop food independently	Jan/Cozette	1/15/84
7	Laura will remove shoes & socks upon verbal cue "take off shoes & socks."	3 times per day for 3 days	Jan/Cozette	1/15/84
8	Laura will stack blocks on verbal cue.	Stacking 2 blocks 5 times per day for 3 days	Jan/Cozette	11/16/83
9	Laura will insert forms in form board on verbal cue.	Will insert 5 times per day for 3 days	Jan/Cozette	11/16/83

FIGURE 9-7 Laura's sample IEP objectives

ICS Activities Matrix
IEP Objectives in Order of Priority

Schedule	"Cruise" independent walking	Imitate "ba"	Follow direction "touch"	Toileting	Drink from glass	Eat w/ spoon	Take off shoes & socks	Stack blocks	Simple puzzle	Type of activity
Entry/ bathroom	X			X						Routine
Go to group area	X		X					X		Functional, hard
Story time		X	X							Age-appropriate, likes
Activity of daily living	X	X	X				X			Functional, hard
Snack	X	X			X	X				Functional, likes
Bathroom	X			X						Routine
Group/ leisure	X	X	X							Age-appropriate, hard
Lunch	X	X	X		X	X				Routine, functional
Total Trn. Opportun.	7	5	5	2	2	2	1	1	0	

FIGURE 9-8 Laura's completed activity matrix for morning activities

ICS Data Sheet

Student ____Laura____   Month/Year ____11-83____
Teacher(s) __Cozette/Jan__

	T-CUE/Behavior	C-ACTION	11-5	11-9	—	11-10	11-13	—
ENTRY	"Let's go potty"	walks	/	/		/	/	
	Toilet	W/D: void/BM	W	W		W	D	
	"let's go to class"	walks	1	1	1	1	1	O
	sit down in group							
GROUP	"touch block"	touches	1	1	1	1	1	O
	"stack block"	stacks						
	reward for waiting turn		3	2	4	3	3	2
	"Let's go to reading corner"	walks	1	1	1	O	1	O
	sit in group on floor							
STORY	touch picture/book	touches	1	1	1	1	O	4
	say "ba"	"ba"	O	O	O	O	O	O
	reward for waiting							
	"It's time to clean up"	walks	1	1	1	O	1	1
	sit before mirror							
	loosen shoes							
ACTIVITY OF DAILY LIVING	say "take off shoe/sock"	pulls off	O	O	1	1	1	2
	say "say ba"	"ba"	O	O	O	O	O	O
	play/range of motion							
	say "touch shoe/sock"	touches	1	1	1	O	O	O
	put on shoe/sock							
	"It's time for a snack"	walks	1	1	1	O	O	1
	sit at table							
SNACK	"touch food/drink"	touches	1	1	1	O	O	O
	drinks/eats	w/o spilling						
	say "say ba"	"ba"	O	O	O	O	O	O

Code: 4 - independent
3 - verbal direction
2 - model
1 - prompt
0 - refusal

FIGURE 9-9   Sample data sheet for Laura's early morning sequence

ICS DATA SHEET

TEACHER: Cozette   SEQUENCE: Lunch   YEAR: 1983

STUDENT: Laura

INSTRUCTION/COMMENTS: During drink, put one swallow in adapted cup for each opportunity to drink; shadow prompt scooping; correct walking in 5 steps.

CODE:
0 - correct   = 1 pt.
1 - correct with prompt = .5 pt.
x - error   = 0 pt.

Cues/Prompts	Student Actions	Correction Procedures
Place L. in standing		
"Let's go to lunch"	walks	hold hand
Point to chair		hold hand
Say "touch"	touches food/drink	put through sitting
Present food/drink	scoops/drinks w/o spilling	put through motions
Say "ba"	"ba"	prompt
Say "touch napkin"	touches	repeat
Say "Let's go potty"		put through motion
	L. walks	help L. stand
		hold hand

Data grid (columns: 11-5, 11-9, 11-10, 11-13, 11-16, 11-17, 11-19, 11-23, 11-24, 11-25, and % correct/prompt):

Step	11-5	11-9	11-10	11-13	11-16	11-17	11-19	11-23	11-24	11-25	% correct/prompt
10	10	10	10	10	10	10	10	10	10	10	
9	9	9	9	9	9	9	9	9	9	9	
8	8	8	8	8	8	8	8	8	8	8	70
7	7	7	7	7	7	7	7	7	7	7	
6	6	6	6	6	6	6	6	6	6	6	90
5	5	5	5	5	5	5	5	5	5	5	80
4	4	4	4	4	4	4	4	4	4	4	30
3	3	3	3	3	3	3	3	3	3	3	50
2	2	2	2	2	2	2	2	2	2	2	
1	1	1	1	1	1	1	1	1	1	1	45

FIGURE 9-10 Laura's lunch sequence on a self-graphing data sheet

Program Plan

STUDENT ___Laura___   DATE ___10-83___   LOCATION ___Preschool___

AUTHOR(S) ___Cozette___   PROGRAM NAME ___Receptive Language - "Touch the_____."___

Date of review	Objective/criterion terminal:	Antecedent/training natural & instructional	Correct response	Consequence	Scoring
10-83	L. will touch object with presentation of object array and direction "Touch ____."	Present two items ¾ arm's length in front of L; randomize location	Touches named object within 5 seconds	Correct: give item Incorrect: put through prompt using light guidance at the elbow	O - correct / - correct with prompt X - resists or refuses to respond
11-2-83	Intermediate: L. will touch single object with direction "Touch ____" and presentation of object.	Present one object at center, ¾ arm's length.		Correct: Incorrect:	

FIGURE 9-11 Page one of Laura's receptive language training program

Materials needed: block, book, shoe/sock, food/drink, blocks

Special positioning: place items in front of her, make sure she is supported and flexed at hips, feet, and back

How baseline differs from training: massed trials

Task analysis: N/A

Functional scheduling: Group activity, story time, ADL, snack, BR, leisure, lunch

Next program: Discrimination

Data graphed: (circle one)   rate latency duration frequency % correct # correct
other _____

FIGURE 9-12   Page two of Laura's receptive language training program

RESEARCH ON THE ICS MODEL

Mulligan, Lacy, and Guess (1982) conducted a general study of the effects of distributed trial sequencing with 11 severely handicapped students, ranging in age (5 to 20 years) and handicapping conditions. They compared the acquisition of cognitive and motor programs when distributed in a cluster containing four different programs. Results indicate that the mean level of responding in cognitive programs was positively affected by distributed trial training. The study, however, did not deal with the functionality of the items clustered together or the relationship of the training items to the variety of training persons, settings, and materials. Further investigation is needed on the effects of the curriculum structure and the sequencing of functional clusters.

Guess, Jones, and Lyon (1981) have summarized the effects of using the ICS model with 16 severely handicapped preschoolers. The data reflect substantial skill acquisition over a three year period. While there are no data on relative effectiveness of the ICS approach compared to other curriculum strategies, the evidence of skill acquisition by young and very severely impaired children is encouraging.

Two additional studies have investigated other effects of the distributed trials approach. Lacy (1982) questioned whether the distributed trials approach affected the student's spontaneous initiation of a response or response latency. A study by Brewer (1982) was concerned with how well vocational skills taught with the distributed model generalized across settings as compared to skills taught in a massed trial format. Both studies with severely handicapped adolescents demonstrated mild effects in favor of distributed trial training and the functional sequencing of training trials through the day.

Additional positive effects of distributed trial sequencing were identified in two tangentially related studies. Dunlap and Koegel (1980) have demonstrated that autistic children show an increase in "no responses" in massed trial training of typical cognitive programs. Distributed trial training decreased or removed "no responses." Dunlap and Koegel used the term "constant task presentation" instead of massed trial format and varied task presentation, rather than distributed trial format, but from all indications, their methods closely resembled those of the Kansas research group.

The intent is not to argue for eliminating massed trial training formats, but to suggest, based on past research (Dore & Hilgard, 1938; Ericksen, 1942; Kimble, 1949; Reynolds & Adams, 1953) and on the more recent data reported above, that some combination of the massed and distributed trial formats may produce the best learning and retention. Currently, the general assumption is that massed trials training would be most efficient during phases focusing on rapid acquisition. Generalization and the functional use of the skill would probably be learned most efficiently in the distributed trial format.

SUMMARY

1. The Individualized Curriculum Sequencing (ICS) model emphasizes (a) the teaching of skills in functional sets, called clusters, and (b) arrangement of clusters in natural and age-appropriate activities.

2. The ICS model emphasizes the importance of using natural cues, consequences, and materials whenever possible, and varying materials, trainers, and settings to enhance generalization.

3. The first step in the ICS process is prioritization of the student's objectives.

4. The second step in the ICS process is to complete an ICS Activities Worksheet which assists identification of relevant characteristics of the various classroom activities, and planning for time and staff scheduling.

5. The ICS Activities Matrix, Step 3, outlines the plan for when, where, and how to teach priority objectives.

6. Step 4 uses the skill sequences from the ICS Activities Matrix to develop a data collection format.

7. The next step is to develop instructional programs for each of the student's objectives.

8. The sixth step is developing a classroom schedule which considers the needs of all the students and the availability and utilization of personnel and materials.

9. Steps 7, 8, and 9 relate to the transdisciplinary team process. The schedule is submitted to the team for review and determination of staff training priorities and distribution of role functions.

10. The ICS model suggests three revision steps if a skill is not being acquired—schedule revision, program revision, and sequence revision.

11. Research investigating the effects of the ICS model indicates some superiority for distributed trials compared to massed trial training, and positive effects from using the ICS model with severely handicapped students. There are not, as yet, data comparing the effectiveness of the ICS model with that of other curriculum strategies.

REFERENCES

ADAMS, J.A. Warm-up decrement in performance on the pursuit rotor. *American Journal of Psychology,* 1952, *55,* 404–414.

BAYLEY, N. *The Bayley scales of infant development.* Atlanta: The Psychological Corporation, 1969.

BREWER, M. *The efficacy of distributed practice training on the facilitation of generalization skills of the severely retarded.* Unpublished manuscript. Lawrence, Kans.: Department of Special Education, University of Kansas, 1982.

BROWN, F., & ALDERSON, G. *Project LEARN curriculum manual.* Unpublished manuscript. Lawrence, Kans.: Department of Special Education, University of Kansas, 1978.

BROWN, F., HOLVOET, J., GUESS, D., & MULLIGAN, M. The individualized curriculum sequencing model (III): Small group instruction. *Journal of the Association for the Severely Handicapped,* 1980, *5,* 352–367.

BROWN, L., BRANSTON-McCLEAN, M.B., BAUMGART, D., VINCENT, L., FALVEY, M., & SCHROEDER, J. Using the characteristics of current and subsequent least restrictive environment as factors in the development of curricular content for severely handicapped students. *Journal of the Association for the Severely Handicapped,* 1979, *4,* 407–424.

BROWN, L., NIETUPSKI, J., & HAMRE-NIETUPSKI, S. The criterion of ultimate functioning. In M.A. Thomas (Ed.), *Hey, don't forget about me.* Reston, Va.: Council for Exceptional Children, 1976.

CHASEY, W.C. Distribution of practice, learning and retention. *Perceptual and Motor Skills,* 1976, *43,* 159–164.

DEESE, J. *The psychology of learning.* New York: McGraw-Hill, 1958.

DORE, L.R., & HILGARD, E.R. Spaced practice as a test of Snoddy's two processes in mental growth. *Journal of Experimental Psychology,* 1938, *23,* 359–374.

DUNCAN, C.P. The effect of unequal amounts of practice on motor learning before and after rest. *Journal of Experimental Psychology,* 1951, *42,* 257–264.

DUNLAP, G., & KOEGEL, R.L. Motivating autistic children through stimulus variation. *Journal of Applied Behavior Analysis,* 1980, *13,* 619–627.

ELMES, D.G., SANDERS, L.W., & DOVEL, J.C. Isolation of massed and distributed items. *Memory and Cognition,* 1973, *1,* 77–79.

ERICKSEN, S.C. Variability of attack in massed and distributed practice. *Journal of Experimental Psychology,* 1942, *31,* 339–345.

FRANKENBURG, W.K., & DODDS, J.B. *Denver developmental screening test.* Denver: University of Colorado Medical Center, 1969.

GUESS, D., HORNER, D., UTLEY, B., HOLVOET, J., MAXON, D., TUCKER, D., & WARREN, S. A functional curriculum sequencing model for teaching the severely handicapped. *AAESPH Review,* 1978, *3,* 202–215.

GUESS, D., JONES, C., & LYON, S. *Combining a transdisciplinary team approach with an individualized curriculum sequencing model for severely/multiply handicapped children.* Lawrence, Kans.: University of Kansas, 1981.

GUESS, D., KEOGH, W., & SAILOR, W. Generalization of speech and language behavior: Measurement and training tactics. In R.L. Schiefelbusch (Ed.), *Bases of language intervention.* Baltimore: University Park Press, 1978.

GUESS, D., RUES, J., WARREN, S., & LYON, S. *Quantitative assessment of motor and sensory/motor acquisition in handicapped and nonhandicapped infants and young children.* Volume I: Assessment procedures for selected developmental milestones. Lawrence, Kansas: Early Childhood Institute, University of Kansas, 1980. (ECI Document No. 135)

HALLE, J.W., BAER, D., & SPRADLIN, J.E. Teachers' generalized use of delay as a stimulus control procedure to increase language use in handicapped children. *Journal of Applied Behavior Analysis,* 1981, *14*(4), 389–411.

HARING, N. Infant identification. In M. Thomas (Ed.), *Hey, don't forget about me.* Reston, Va.: Council for Exceptional Children, 1976.

HARING, N., LIBERTY, K., & WHITE, O. Rules for data-based strategy decisions. In W. Sailor, B. Wilcox, & L. Brown (Eds.), *Methods of instruction for severely handicapped students.* Baltimore: Paul H. Brookes, 1980.

HOLVOET, J. *The effects of number and composition of interspersed trials on the learning of severely handicapped students.* Unpublished dissertation, Department of Human Development, University of Kansas, 1981.

HOLVOET, J., GUESS, D., MULLIGAN, M., & BROWN, F. The individualized curriculum sequencing model (II): A teaching strategy for severely handicapped students. *Journal of the Association for the Severely Handicapped,* 1980, *5,* 337–351.

KIENTZLE, M.J. Properties of learning curves under varied distributions of practice. *Journal of Experimental Psychology,* 1946, *36,* 187–211.

KIMBLE, G.A. An experimental test of a two-factor theory of inhibition. *Journal of Experimental Psychology,* 1949, *39,* 15–23.

KOEGEL, R., EGEL, A., & DUNLAP, G. Learning characteristics of autistic children. In W. Sailor, B. Wilcox, & L. Brown (Eds.), *Methods of instruction for severely handicapped students.* Baltimore: Paul H. Brookes, 1980.

LACY, L. *The effect of functional scheduling on the initiation and latency responses of severely handicapped students.* Unpublished master's thesis, Department of Special Education, The University of Kansas, 1982.

LENT, J.R., & McLEAN, B.M. The trainable retarded: The technology of teaching. In N.G. Haring & R.L. Schiefelbusch (Eds.), *Teaching special children.* New York: McGraw-Hill, 1976.

LYON, S., & LYON, G. Team functioning and staff development: A role release approach to providing integrated educational services for severely handicapped students. *Journal of the Association for the Severely Handicapped,* 1980, *5,* 250–263.

MITHAUG, D.E., & HAGEMEIER, L.D. The development of procedures to assess prevocational competencies of severely handicapped young adults. *AAESPH Review,* 1978, *3,* 94–115.

MULLIGAN, M., GUESS, D., HOLVOET, J., & BROWN, F. The individualized curriculum sequencing model (I): Implications from research on massed, distributed, or spaced trial learning. *Journal of the Association for the Severely Handicapped,* 1980, *5,* 325–336.

MULLIGAN, M., LACY, L., & GUESS, D. The effects of massed, distributed, and spaced trial sequencing on severely handicapped students' performance. *Journal of the Association for the Severely Handicapped,* 1982.

PREMACK, D. Reinforcement theory. *Nebraska Symposium on Motivation,* 123–128. Lincoln: University of Nebraska Press, 1969.

REYNOLDS, B., & ADAMS, J.A. Effect of distribution and shift in distribution within a single training session. *Journal of Experimental Psychology,* 1953, *46,* 137–145.

SAILOR, W., & GUESS, D. *Severely handicapped students: An instructional design.* Boston: Houghton Mifflin Co., 1983.

SNELL, M.E., & GAST, D.L. Applying time delay procedure to the instruction of the severely handicapped. *Journal of the Association for the Severely Handicapped,* 1981, *6*(3), 3–15.

SOMERTON, M.E., & TURNER, K.D. *Pennsylvania training model individual assessment guide.* Harrisburg, Pa.: Pennsylvania Department of Education, 1974.

STILLMAN, R. (Ed.). *Callier-Azusa scale.* Dallas, Tex.: Callier Center for Communication Disorders, 1978.

STOKES, T., & BAER, D. An implicit technology of generalization. *Journal of Applied Behavior Analysis,* 1977, *10,* 349–367.

UNDERWOOD, B.J., KAPELAK, S.M., & MALMI, R.A. The spacing effect: Additions to the theoretical and empirical puzzles. *Memory and Cognition,* 1976, *4,* 391–400.

VINCENT, L.J., SALISBURY, C., WALTER, G., BROWN, P., GRUENEWALD, L.J., & POWERS, M. Program evaluation and curriculum development in early childhood/special education: Criteria of the next environment. In Sailor, W., Wilcox, B., & Brown, L. (Eds.), *Methods of instruction for severely handicapped students.* Baltimore: Paul H. Brookes, 1980.

WILLIAMS, W., BROWN, L., & CERTO, N. Basic components of instructional program for severely handicapped students. *Theory into Practice,* 1975, *14*(2), 123–136.

CHAPTER TEN

AUGMENTATIVE COMMUNICATION

Linda McCormick and Howard Shane

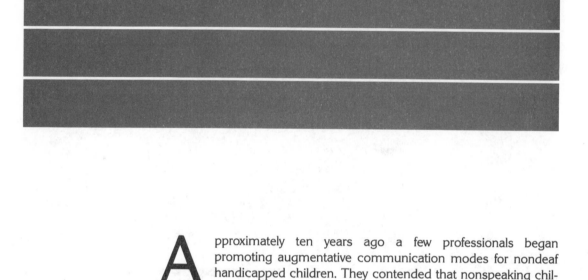

Approximately ten years ago a few professionals began promoting augmentative communication modes for nondeaf handicapped children. They contended that nonspeaking children could (and should) be provided with alternative modes—that these children have a right to the advantages of communication, even though speech may not be an attainable goal (Berger, 1972; Hodges & Deich, 1979; Kent, 1974; McLean (McCormick) & McLean, 1974). Denying the nonspeaking child an augmentative communication system, they argued, is tantamount to denying a physically handicapped child the use of braces, crutches, or a wheelchair. Certainly no one would say to a nonambulatory child, "If you will not or cannot learn to walk, you will be denied the advantages of mobility." However, this is a paraphrase of the argument against providing the nonspeaking child with an augmentative means of communication.

Acceptance of the value of augmentative communication systems for nondeaf handicapped children is now widespread. The most persuasive of the early arguments against the utilization of nonspeech communication methods (the possibility of interference with speech acquisition) has been countered by a number of investigators. Substantial data are available to document transfer from augmentative systems to speech (Carrier & Peak, 1975; Schaeffer, 1980; Silverman, 1980). There are even reports that "total communication" (sign language paired with oral language) instruction may facilitate speech acquisition and receptive language (Kohl, Karlan, & Heal, 1979).

A recent bibliography by Lloyd (1980) listing some 400 journal articles, chapters, and books directly concerned with implementing augmentative communication systems further substantiates the growing popularity of these approaches. Another source of information has been research with lower animals. In *Language Intervention from Ape to Child*, Schiefelbusch and Hollis (1979) summarize the accumulated efforts of researchers who have adapted and extrapolated from work with nonhuman primates to the development of nonspeech communication modes for handicapped children with these six points:

1. The analysis, planning, design, and implementation steps in primate research (technologically and experimentally) can be employed in developing language programs for handicapped children.

2. Functional language, including linguistic structures and functions, can be taught with various nonspeech symbol forms.

3. Both apes and children are able to produce generative forms and functions with nonspeech symbol repertoires.

4. Both apes and children demonstrate concept equivalence across stimulus modes.

5. The research with apes has a strong data orientation and provides explicit instructions for designing the operational maintenance.

6. The research with apes highlights both the similarities and the differences encountered in designing programs for the human child. The similarities are greatest in symbol mapping and in referential language exchanges. They differ in regard to the semantic range of, and pragmatic designs required for, a fully functional language (p. 362).

Research with nonhuman primates has contributed significantly to the knowledge base of augmentative communication.

Providing services to nonspeaking persons requires knowledge and training not, until recently, included in either Special Education or Speech-Language Pathology preservice curricula. In a recent position statement on nonspeech communication, the American Speech-Language-Hearing Association recommended that the following competencies be incorporated into preservice training programs for speech-language pathologists (ASHA, 1981). These skills are listed here because they are deemed equally important for special educators who are preparing to work with severely handicapped students. If both professionals (teacher and speech-language pathologist) bring these competencies to the task of assessing and programming for nonspeaking students, transdisciplinary communication, coordination, and subsequent intervention efforts will be enhanced significantly. The recommended competencies are:

1. Assessment procedures for determining augmentative communication system candidacy, and selection of system components

2. Assessment of prelinguistic communicative interaction strategies in nonspeaking persons

3. Knowledge of currently available aided and unaided techniques

4. Knowledge of available symbol systems

5. Knowledge of the nature of augmentative communication in interaction with speaking and nonspeaking persons

6. Development and evaluation of communication intervention program specifically designed to teach nonspeaking persons those skills needed in order to achieve communication competence via augmentative communication techniques

7. Knowledge of the effect of appropriate seating and positioning on the user's control of the speech mechanism and on a nonspeaker's communication techniques

8. Advocacy and funding procedures (ASHA, 1981)

Space limitation precludes thorough exposition of all of these competencies, but most will be touched upon. Our intent in this chapter is to provide an introduction to further study in the area. However, caregiver and family involvement are not specifically addressed because this subject is discussed at length in Chapter Eleven. Suggestions for further reading and more comprehensive resources are provided throughout the chapter. Studying this chapter should prepare you for that literature.

BASIC TERMS AND CONSTRUCTS

Mode refers to response method; *modality* refers to sensory channel.

The difference between the terms "mode" and "modality," as used in the augmentative communication literature, was briefly described in Chapter Five. *Mode* refers to response method. *Modality* refers to input channel. "Normal" speakers have a variety of possible response modes, including the oral mode (speech), manual-motor modes (pointing, gesture, signing, finger spelling, writing), and the ocular mode (directional eye movements). Physically handicapped persons have significantly fewer options. Decisions about which mode or modes will be most efficient and effective for the handicapped individual must be based on a case-by-case analysis of motor, cognitive, and linguistic capabilities, and on limitations and environmental considerations.

When the response mode requires external support, it is called aided communication; unaided communication relies solely on physical mechanisms.

A response mode may or may not require external physical support devices. If an external prop such as paper, writing implement, or communication board is required to enable the communicator to convey intended messages, the communication is said to be "aided." Communication boards range from simple poster-like charts with one or two pictures or symbols to sophisticated electronic devices costing thousands of dollars. They are categorized according to how the pictures or symbols are indicated: by direct selection, scanning or encoding.

Unaided response modes rely solely on physical mechanisms such as the vocal tract, face, upper limbs, and/or trunk. Gesture and mime are examples of natural unaided augmentative communication. Natural unaided communication can often be interpreted by a receiver without any special training. However, conventional unaided communication, which includes signing and oral language, cannot be decoded without training or a key.

Modality refers to the sensory channel (i.e., visual, auditory, tactile) through which information is received or transmitted. As discussed in Chapter Five, it is essential to identify a functional response mode before assessment of modalities. Until a functional and reliable response mode (means to indicate or answer) is identified or, if necessary, trained, there is no way to know the type and amount of sensory information the child is receiving. Sensory strengths and preferences affect the choice of methods to communicate with the child—the selection of means to *input* linguistic and nonlinguistic information. Motor control is the primary determinant of output modes.

The vocabulary and rules for combining signs and/or symbols to represent intentions and ideas about the world compose the *system*. As described below, systems may be aided or unaided. The term *device* is used to refer to the display (the hardware) for an aided system. The most common display device is the communication board or chart. Devices may be electronic or nonelectronic.

SYMBOL SYSTEMS

The best known *unaided symbol systems* are:

Unaided symbol systems do not require external equipment or devices.

1. **Signed English.** Signed English is a system of signing that parallels the English language. There is a sign for every word (including the copula and bound morphemes), and word order is identical to that in spoken or written English. Signed English has been taught to severely mentally retarded students (Browder, Morris, & Snell, 1981; Kohl, 1981) and autistic students (Carr, Binkoff, Kologinsky, & Eddy, 1978). A free guide to the system can be obtained by writing to the Gallaudet College Press, or see Bornstein, Hamilton, Kannapell, Roy and Saulnier (1973).

2. **American Sign Language.** Ameslan or ASL, as this system is called, is the language of the majority of deaf individuals in North America. ASL has its own morphology, semantics, and syntax. In some ways ASL is comparable to pictograph writing in that some of the symbols are quite arbitrary, while others are iconic. ASL has been used with autistic children (Cohen, 1981) and retarded students (Stremel-Campbell, Cantrell, & Halle, 1977). *A Dictionary of American Sign Language* (Stokoe, Casterline, & Croneberg, 1978) is a good resource for this system.

3. **Fingerspelling.** Fingerspelling is spelling words with the manual alphabet, which consists of 26 letters which have one-to-one correspondence with traditional orthography. In fingerspelling, one hand is held in front of the chest and words are spelled out letter by letter (Mayberry, 1978). It has been traced back to the work of Bonet in Spain in 1620 (Moores, 1978).

4. **Simultaneous (Total) Communication.** As the name implies, simultaneous communication refers to the simultaneous production of signs (usually one of the systems paralleling English) and speech and the teaching techniques associated with their production. It is theorized that the redundancy of information (visual plus auditory) facilitates learning (Kent, 1974).

Informal symbol systems include pantomime, natural gestures, and Amer-Ind.

There are also several informal systems that are not included in the above listing. Probably the most common are pantomime, natural gestures, and Amer-Ind. Natural, commonly understood gestures, which are used by most speaking persons (and the disabled) are limited in expressive capability compared to the standard systems, but they also have a number of advantages. The three major advantages of natural gestures are (Hamre-Nietupski, Stoll, Holtz, Fullerton, Ryan-Flottum, & Brown, 1977):

1. Easily understood by teachers, parents, and others without specialized training
2. Usually involve gross motor movements which are manageable for physically handicapped students
3. No aids or equipment are required

Hamre-Nietupski et al. (1977) provide an excellent resource for those considering the use of natural gesture. Their curriculum guide lists more than 160 generally understood gestures, plus strategies for teaching production and comprehension of these gestures.

As the name implies, Amer-Ind, or American Indian Hand Talk, derives from a gestural code used by Indian tribes (Skelly & Schinsky, 1979). Dr. Madge Skelly, who is herself a native American and was taught Hand Talk as a child by her Iroquois relatives, is credited with the modernization and adaptation of this code. The basic features of Amer-Ind—concreteness, flexibility and lack of grammatical structure—make it advantageous for individuals with minimal linguistic competence. Amer-Ind signs have been taught successfully to severely and profoundly retarded children (Daniloff & Shafer, 1981).

There are two types of aided symbol systems—alphabetic and nonalphabetic.

Aided systems are of two basic types: alphabetic and nonalphabetic. Nonalphabetic symbol systems include:

1. **Representational systems.** Rebus symbols and Blissymbolics are examples of representational systems. Although they use some abstract symbols and alphabetic characters, they rely primarily on pictures and line drawings. The most used Rebus system is the one presented in the *Peabody Rebus Reading Program* developed by Woodcock, Clark, and Davies (1969). Blissymbols are discrete symbols representing concepts. They were originally adapted for use with students with cerebral palsy. These students were capable of more sophisticated symboliza-

tion than pictures, but not yet ready to use the printed word for expressive communication (McNaughton & Kates, 1980).

2. **Abstract systems.**Symbol systems such as Non-SLIP, derived from Premack's (1970, 1971) work with chimpanzees, and the Yerkish lexigrams are examples of abstract systems. The symbols used in the Non-SLIP system (Carrier, 1976; Carrier & Peak, 1975) are plastic, color-coded shapes; each represents a word. Sentences are formed by placing them in the appropriate syntactic order on a form board. The Non-SLIP program was developed as a method of teaching language strategies. Use of the symbols for communication purposes was not the intent of the developer.

Yerkish lexigrams were developed for use in Project Lana at the Yerkes Primate Regional Research Center in Atlanta, Georgia (Rumbaugh, 1977, 1978). Each symbol, or lexigram, is a distinctive geometric figure that functions as a word. Each lexigram is composed of one or more of nine basic elements, such as a dot, a line, a diamond, and a circle. For Project Lana, they were depicted on a keyboard that was monitored by a computer.

3. **Direct reproductions.** Models (miniature objects), photographs and artist's drawings are also communication options. Theoretically objects, pictures, and drawings should not be included as symbol systems because they are fairly direct reproductions (as opposed to arbitrary representations) of their referents. However, particularly with young children and the more cognitively impaired, direct reproductions may be more appropriate than more sophisticated rule-bound systems.

Alphabetic symbol systems are the most common and therefore the most desirable for nonvocal communication. The codes represent the letters or sounds of a language. The only "listener" requirement is the ability to read, and even this requirement may be eliminated by Voice Output Communication Aids (VOCAS). The two primary alphabetic symbol system options are traditional orthography and the Initial Teaching Alphabet (i/t/a).

Alphabetic systems have the advantage of being easily interpretable.

1. **Traditional Orthography.** The child who is only moderately delayed in cognitive and receptive language skills, but experiencing severe expressive language problems, is the most logical candidate for traditional orthography. Traditional orthography has the advantage of being a "normal" system with the largest possible audience. Training involves teaching the child to produce (write, type, point to, etc.) words and sentences.

2. **Initial Teaching Alphabet.** The Initial Teaching Alphabet, developed by Sir Isaac Pitman, is the most popular of a number of phonemic alphabets. Phonemic alphabet systems provide a close sound-symbol relationship. Each sound in the language is represented by a single symbol, and each symbol represents only

one sound. These systems were originally designed as aids for teaching reading, but they are also well suited for use with an augmentative communication device. Shane and Melrose (1975) trained two persons (with severe quadriplegic involvement and functioning at or near age level on receptive language measures) to use i/t/a symbols displayed on a specially constructed electronic communication board. Both learned to use the set of trained symbols appropriately and demonstrated some generalization.

COMMUNICATION DEVICES

There are three basic communication board designs—direct selection, scanning and encoding.

The most common communication device or display is the communication board. Displays are of three basic types: direct selection displays, scanning displays, and encoding displays. In addition there are some devices that permit more than one indicating method.

Direct selection displays are designed for pointing, which is the easiest, fastest, and most normative method of indicating desired response elements. The child's motor capabilities determine the means of pointing (e.g., head pointing, fist, elbow, etc.), the size of the display, and the number of symbols on the display. The less reliable the child's motor

Communication boards often permit the use of several indicating techniques.

coordination, the larger the display must be to permit access to designated symbols (because the symbols must be farther apart). Eye pointing, or directed gaze as it is sometimes called, is the least desirable direct selection method because it places restrictions on the type of board that can be used. It also limits the number of symbols that can be placed on the board. A transparent board is usually best for selection by eye pointing. Then the message receiver can sit behind the display (opposite the communicator), so it will be easier to judge gaze direction.

Devices for direct selection range from basic communication boards fabricated by the teacher, communication specialist, or a local carpenter to adapted typewriters and other automated aids (i.e., the Canon Communicator, Auto-Com, Voice synthesis aids). Electronic devices allow for various types of input, such as a magnetized pointer, a keyboard, or switching mechanism. Voice output communication aids are among the more recent innovations in this area. One type uses prerecorded speech. The student selects words, phrases, or sentences from the prerecorded vocabulary.

Scanning displays may use techniques as simple as a "twenty questions" approach where only "yes" or "no" responses are required. The more complex direct scanning devices are designed so that the path to a desired vocabulary item may be controlled vertically, horizontally, angularly, or by a combination of the three. Message elements (e.g., pictures, words) or groups of elements are presented to the user one at a time so that the desired element can be indicated. In linear scanning, entries are pointed to (or highlighted in some way) one at a time until the desired entry is reached. In group-item (row-column) scanning, an entire group or row of entries is scanned until the child signals "stop." Then each entry in that row or group is scanned to isolate the desired element.

Scanning is more cumbersome than direct selection, but it may be necessary for the child with very restricted motion. Elements may be pointed to by the message receiver or illuminated by an electrical scanning device. The child may signal "stop" with a smile, nod, directional eye movement, or body movement. If the child has reliable motor control, he may use a switch to operate the indicator or stop the scanning light himself.

Encoding displays allow the child to indicate choices through a pattern or code. The code may be memorized or placed on a reference key. Figure 10-1 is an example of a simple pattern encoding display (Vanderheiden, 1976); a code display is more difficult. Letters of the alphabet are arranged in a matrix format on this display. The child would indicate "L" by pointing to 3 in the vertical column and 2 in the horizontal column. Because encoding requires a child to demonstrate cognitive and perceptual abilities at approximately the 4½-year level, this method has limited usefulness with severely retarded children (Crowder & Shane, 1981).

	1	2	3	4	5	6
1		A	B	C	D	E
2	F		G	H	I	J
3	K	L		M	N	O
4	P	Q	R		S	T
5	U	V	W	X		Y
6	Z	!	¿	?	Yes	

FIGURE 10-1 Example of an encoding display

The primary objective in designing or selecting an aided device is to maximize the child's communication potential; what is most desirable and appropriate for an individual child depends upon a number of considerations. The discussion that follows addresses the range of variables to consider in making this and other critical augmentative communication decisions. We will summarize the content of recent publications by Shane (1979, 1980, 1981), Vanderheiden and colleagues (1976, 1978), Sailor and colleagues (1980) and Reichle, Williams and Ryan (1981). Before you implement an augmentative communication program you should study one or more of these sources.

MAKING AUGMENTATIVE COMMUNICATION DECISIONS

Prior to selecting specific intervention strategies, the two major decisions are:

1. Is the child an appropriate candidate for an augmentative communication system?
2. What augmentative communication technique would be most appropriate for the child?

FACTORS RELATED TO CANDIDACY

You remember from Chapter Two that the normal infant begins cognitive and social learning at birth. Motor impairments have a profound and pervasive effect on these processes. The child's ability to explore, manipulate, and learn from the physical environment, as well as from play and social exchanges, depends heavily upon motor patterning and movement.

There is an urgent need for longitudinal research considering the effects of early introduction of augmentative communication on development in other domains.

To what extent the development of communication and social skills can be maximized and the deleterious effects of severe motor impairment minimized by introducing an augmentative communication system at a very early age is not known. One factor accounting for the lack of attention to this question is the difficulty in selecting and implementing appropriate augmentative systems with very young physically handicapped children. At the present time most systems require coordinated motor skills. However, as more sophisticated electronic and automated displays become available, this restriction may be overcome. A second factor hindering investigation of this question has been the contention that augmentative communication should not be considered unless there is incontrovertible evidence that speech is not a viable communication option. This position is beginning to attenuate.

Making predictions about a very young child's potential for developing speech is difficult but not impossible. Looking to the not-too-distant future, Shane (1980) forsees better assessment strategies to determine (a) those children who will not become oral communicators, (b) those children whose speech will improve as a function of learning an augmentative system, and (c) those children who will be served best if provided with several communication options to use as the situation requires.

Reliable predictive assessment of the type described above is not yet possible; however, there is rarely a good justification for delaying decisions about implementing augmentative communication systems with infants and young children. There is substantial evidence that augmentative communication skills neither prevent nor do they seem to delay oral language development. The opposite is true. Many reports describe *increased* speech following the implementation of an augmentative system (e.g., Duncan & Silverman, 1977; Rosenbek, Collins, & Wertz, 1976; Oxman, Webster, & Konstantaneas, 1978). (See Silverman, 1980, for a comprehensive look at this issue.) In addition to increasing productivity, augmentative systems appear to enhance intelligibility (Beukelman & Yorkston, 1977) and aid the child's organization of linguistic and semantic concepts (Chapman & Miller, 1980).

> There is reason to believe that an augmentative system should be introduced as early as possible.

These findings have relevance to decisions concerning the appropriateness of introducing an infant or very young child to an augmentative communication system. They suggest the reassuring conclusion that there is no possibility of undesirable consequences for false positives. (These are children thought to be incapable of speech who do, in fact, acquire it.) In other words, preparing an infant for and/or providing an augmentative system when such a system is unnecessary should not have any deleterious consequences for the child. There is more reason for concern if the error is in the other direction, that is, if the child is not provided with a communication option and does not develop speech as anticipated.

The problem reduces to determination of which infants are at-risk for speech. Careful consideration and analysis of the following factors will aid this determination. These factors are based on findings by Shane and Bashir (1980) and Shane (1981).

Medical history Medical information that suggests the possibility of mental retardation, autism, congenital dysarthia (a neuromuscular disturbance of oral motor functions caused by brain damage), or apraxia of speech (disturbance in oral motor planning ability) is one piece of data that contributes to making a decision about planning for an augmentative communication system. Not all children with neurological, physical, and/or social-emotional disability will fail to acquire intelligible speech. However, the presence of any one of these conditions suggests that the child is at-risk for speech.

Primitive oral reflexes With maturation of the central nervous system, the nonhandicapped infant's reflexes gradually become integrated or superseded by more mature responses controlled by higher centers of the brain. Table 10-1 shows the age span of reflexes important to feeding and eventually to speech. Difficulty with feeding and other evidence of the presence of primitive oral reflex patterns beyond ages 3 to 7 months are reason for concern about speech production.

TABLE 10-1 Primitive oral reflexes

Reflex	Typical age span	Description
Rooting	Birth to 3 months	Turns head in direction of facial stimulation and opens mouth (unless infant has just been fed)
Suckle-swallow	Birth to 6 months	Rhythmic sucking and swallowing pattern with lip closure
Bite	Birth to 7 months	Chewing movements during play or feeding when lips or gums are touched
Gag	Birth to 7 months (present throughout life but unusually strong during infancy)	Strong reaction (with tongue protrusion) to novel oral sensations

Source: Shane (1980).

Laryngeal functioning   The cessation of voice during vocal efforts, known as laryngeal block, is a characteristic laryngeal problem of children with cerebral palsy. In cases of laryngeal block or "abductor spasm," as this condition is termed by McDonald and Chance (1964), the vocal cords are held together with such force that the child cannot produce sounds, or blocking occurs during sound production and results in abrupt termination of voicing. Because the predictive value of laryngeal blocking relative to speech development has not, as yet, been established, this factor does not merit the same consideration as the two factors above. However, if there is reason to suspect laryngeal blocking, these data should figure in the augmentative communication decision.

Eating problems   Early problems with eating can be a risk factor because they suggest neuromotor involvement of the oral structures. According to Morris (1978), feeding assessment should consider:

1. jaw thrusting
2. tongue thrusting
3. tonic bite reflex
4. lip retraction
5. tongue retraction
6. nasal pharyngeal reflex

Problems in any of these areas are evidence that the coordination of the oral musculature necessary for speech is not developing properly.

Chronological age   The child's age will affect the relative weight assigned to the other decision factors. Morris (1975) suggests that 5 or 6 months of age is not too early to begin training indicating behaviors necessary for a communication board. The infant can be positioned and physically prompted to reach, point to, or look at named objects. Generally speaking, the older the nonspeaking child is (assuming appropriate intervention efforts), the greater the urgency to make a decision for and begin training an augmentative communication system.

Cognitive development   While there is some difference of opinion as to how much importance to assign to cognitive development, most feel that introduction of a *symbolic* (representational) system will not be maximally effective unless the child has, at the very least, attained sensorimotor Stage 5 (Chapman & Miller, 1980; Reichle & Yoder, 1979; Shane & Bashir, 1980; Yoder & Calculator, 1981). Shane (1979) suggests methods of assessing a child's ability to process representational information (models, photographs, pictures, line drawings) for communicative purposes. The objective of this assessment is to determine whether the child is able to associate (a) verbal labels with the objects, persons, or events they represent, or (b) line drawings, photographs, etc., with the objects they represent. If the child cannot deal with representational information, at least at a photograph level, he is probably not ready for an augmentative communication system. However, just because a child has not attained the level of representational ability considered prerequisite for use of an augmentative device or a symbolic communication system is not reason to delay attempts to foster effective communication and other readiness activities as described later in this chapter. Whatever communicative behaviors the child uses to indicate basic needs and affect should be shaped toward more acceptable and sophisticated communication forms.

Comprehension-production discrepancy   When a young child demonstrates a gap between comprehension and production skills, and if this gap appears to be continuously widening there is very good reason to consider an augmentative system. The wider the discrepancy, the greater the urgency to provide a functional expressive mode, particularly if appropriate oral language training has been tried and has been unsuccessful.

Imitation   Vocal imitation skills are highly predictive of success in oral language training. Keep in mind, however, that an initial reluctance (or inability) to imitate verbal models is not sufficient reason, in and of itself, to give up on the possibility of speech. Guess, Sailor and Baer (1978) report that 60 percent of the children who entered their program eventually learned to imitate. Some required as long as two years of training to acquire imitative skills, but the important point is that they were eventually acquired. Motor imitation ability should also be considered, because it seems to be predictive of the ability for vocal imitation.

Significant others   The importance of anticipating caregiver objections or resistance to augmentative communication cannot be overemphasized. There are two reasons why caregivers initially may reject the idea of their child being taught an augmentative communication system: they may interpret the recommendation for augmentative communication as meaning that the involved professionals have given up on the possibility of speech development, or they may view augmentative systems as hindering speech acquisition. These concerns should be anticipated and addressed even before they are explicitly stated by the caregivers.

Sometimes, even after the advantages of augmentative systems have been thoroughly explained and thoughtfully considered, caregivers continue to express some reservations about the recommendation to elect an augmentative system. One approach to deal with their misgivings is to arrange for them to see the positive effects of augmentative communication training and talk to other caregivers and system users. There is also the possibility that they may be open to a trial period of augmentative communication training. If neither of these strategies allays opposition to the proposal, there is no alternative but to put it aside. Even if the caregivers did not have the right, by law, to reject programming proposals, success of the intervention would be seriously threatened without their full cooperation.

SUMMARY OF CANDIDACY CONSIDERATION

Professionals with the responsibility of deciding whether or not to introduce augmentative communication training should consider the following factors:

1. Medical information—Is there evidence of a high risk disability?
2. Status of primitive oral reflexes—Are obligatory primitive oral reflex patterns present?
3. Laryngeal functioning—Is there evidence of laryngeal blocking prior to or during vocal efforts?
4. Eating problems—Is there evidence of problems with sucking, swallowing, or chewing (or coordination of these functions)?
5. Chronological age—Considering age weighed against other factors, how ready is the child for the introduction of a communication prosthesis?
6. Cognitive development—Is the child ready to deal with representational pictographic information?
7. Comprehension-production discrepancy—Is there a significant gap between comprehension and production functions?
8. Imitation—Is the child imitative?
9. Significant others—Are the caregivers and other significant adults in the child's environment receptive to the notion of an augmentative communication system?

The most powerful single indicator for an augmentative communication system is immature oral reflex behavior.

Some of these considerations are more important than others in the decision-making process. The strongest single indicator *for* augmentative communication seems to be immature oral reflex behavior. The strongest argument against augmentative communication is parental discomfort.

Plans for the introduction of an augmentative system should be held in abeyance if caregivers persistently object.

SELECTING AN APPROPRIATE TECHNIQUE

Once candidacy for an augmentative system has been determined, the next decision facing the service delivery team is whether to introduce an aided or an unaided system. Significant factors to be considered are (a) severity of neuromotor impairment, (b) imitative ability, (c) individual preferences, and (d) potential communication environments. In some cases, more than one system may be selected (one for the school and domestic settings and another for use in public environments).

Neuromotor impairment   Unaided systems require precise control of the arms and hands. Whether the child is capable of learning and using an unaided technique depends on his motor control deficits involving the upper extremities. Some children can execute gross functional signs such as "eat," which requires a cupped hand brought to the mouth with fingers pointed toward the face, but are not capable of forming more precise productions.

Imprecise productions may be adequate to communicate intentions *if* the child's repertoire includes no more than 10 to 20 signs and *if* teachers and caregivers are very familiar with the child's habits. However, as the child's expressive vocabulary increases, receiver comprehension decreases due to problems differentiating one imprecise sign from another. Whether any imprecise productions will be understood by audiences outside the immediate school and home environments is questionable.

The fact that there is little potential for development of a signing vocabulary in keeping with the child's cognitive abilities is reason to question exclusive reliance on signing, but it is not reason to reject manual communication altogether. Lack of fine motor coordination may preclude total dependence upon signing as a means of communication, but it does not preclude the use of gross functional signs and gestures as a means of signaling basic needs and desires to familiar adults. In cases like this the decision may be to teach two systems simultaneously, that is, gestures and gross functional signs for familiar environments and an aided technique that allows greater expression in more public environments.

Lack of fine motor coordination may preclude total reliance on signing, but some signs may still be used with familiar persons.

Motor imitation   With one notable exception—autistic children—motor imitation seems to be prerequisite for and predictive of success in learning manual communication. That nonimitative autistic children do learn to sign suggests that their imitation deficits may be more a reflection of atypical interpersonal behaviors than of inability to copy motor acts.

Reichle and Yoder (1979) suggest the use of sign approximations as stimuli from the beginning of motor imitation training, regardless of whether or not candidacy for augmentative communication has been established. If speech develops, there are no deleterious effects of having established imitative control with sign approximations rather than more tra-

Teaching signs in early imitation training is discussed in Chapter Six.

ditional (and nofnunctional) stimuli such as hand clapping. If, on the other hand, it becomes apparent that the child is not a good candidate for speech, then entry behaviors for unaided communication have already been developed.

Individual preferences Whether the child has a preference for pictorial or gestural communication should be considered. One method is to observe, record, and compute the rate of response to pictures versus gestures. If comparison is too time-consuming (or rejected for some other reason), other preference indicators may be considered. Just watch the child closely. Some children will demonstrate a definite attraction to pictorial stimuli of all kinds. Some may even begin to use pictures for items without instruction. Shane (1981) describes a child who would tear pictures from the Sears and Fisher-Price catalogues to communicate desired or misplaced items. He would pull out the family photograph album and point to the pictures of expected visitors or family members. Certainly, this behavior indicates a strong support for preference for pictorial stimuli and suggests selection of an aided communication technique using graphic content.

Other nonspeaking children demonstrate an equally strong preference for gestures. The use of gestures to compensate for lack of efficacy with oral language is a strong indicator for manual communication (provided there is adequate motor coordination).

Potential communication environments The extent to which an augmentative communication technique restricts or promotes culturally normative and independent transactions should be an important consideration in its selection. Nonspeaking individuals should be provided with techniques that will maximize productive interactions. In the final analysis, the greater the number of persons the child can communicate with, and the more community exposure a technique permits, the more desirable it is.

The greater the number of persons that can be communicated with, the better the technique.

Sign language is the third most used non-English language in the United States (O'Rourke, in Wilber, 1979) and the major communication mode for at least half a million deaf and hard-of-hearing persons. This does not mean that signing is necessarily the most desirable selection, however, even for the child who has sufficient coordination to acquire an extensive manual repertoire, because his communication partners are limited primarily to members of the deaf community.

SUMMARY OF TECHNIQUE CONSIDERATIONS

The desirability of an augmentative technique must be judged against the criteria specified above: (a) size of the potential audience and (b) likelihood of it contributing to independence. Because most people read and understand pictorial references, an augmentative technique using pictures or traditional orthography may best meet these criteria. Shane (1981) notes that, in many cases, professionals and parents request aided communication techniques—even for children who are effective manual communicators. The reason for requesting a second augmentative system is so the child can communicate with a larger and more varied audience than manual language often permits.

Another consideration related to achieving normality is appearance. Problems associated with the general reluctance of nonhandicapped persons to accept the individual who appears to be different cannot be overstated. There are at least three ways of dealing with these problems: (a) change the behavior judged as deviant to more closely conform to expectations of normality, (b) change the standards of the "normal" community so that the different behavior is no longer perceived and responded to as deviant, or (c) remove the individual to a setting where his behavior is not judged as deviant. The third option is unacceptable because it violates the rights of handicapped persons. This leaves two solutions for perceived deviancy: alter the child's behavior in the direction of normality and change society's standards and attitudes relative to deviancy. When applied to the selection of augmentative communication techniques, the solutions translate to two directives. First, consider providing the child with the technique that appears most normal. The child who goes into an ice cream shop and points first to the cones and then to the flavor of ice cream desired (or points to desired items on a menu) may appear more normal than the one who signs or uses a communication prosthesis. In some circumstances, signing has less stigma because the general public has had considerable exposure to the deaf and manual languages. In others (e.g., a department store), the use of pictures or printed words may be more appropriate. The ecology of the present and anticipated environments should dictate the selection of a communication mode or modes.

> Provide the child with a technique that conforms to expectations of normality while, at the same time, working to expand normality standards.

The second solution—changing the standards of the "normal" community so that the different behavior is no longer perceived as deviant —has become more important in recent years. As awareness of the importance of environmental factors and the consequent emphasis on changing the responding environment (an example is mainstreaming) increases, the parameters of "normality" should continue to expand. Augmentative communication techniques will become more common and, consequently, more accepted.

SELECTING AN APPROPRIATE SYSTEM

Once the child's appropriateness for augmentative communication has been established and a technique or techniques selected, the next task is to identify a symbol system. Again, the child's available input modalities and output modes will heavily influence this decision.

Unaided systems   Earlier in this chapter the four most common standard manual systems and some informal systems were discussed. Advantages and disadvantages of the various systems are delineated in Table 10-2. Deciding which system to introduce must be based on a thoughtful matching of the child's motor and sensory capabilities, the range of current and future expressive needs, and environmental support to system characteristics.

TABLE 10-2 Advantages and disadvantages of the most common manual systems

System	Advantages	Disadvantages
Signed English	Especially desirable for young and severely handicapped because of its focus on a limited vocabulary, paralleling of English word order, and use of a limited number (only 14) of inflection markers. Control of facial musculature less crucial than for ASL. Requires relatively little finger spelling.	Vocabulary is restricted to 2500 entries, compared to 5200 signs in ASL. Signs are generally not transparent (understandable from their form alone). Potential audience must have special training.
American Sign Language (ASL)	Broader audience as ASL is the language used by most deaf persons. The large number of users implies a larger number of trainers and better validated training strategies.	There is not a one-to-one correspondence between ASL signs and English words, which precludes direct translation from one to the other. Requires the simultaneous use of considerable facial expression of meaning. Most signs are not transparent. Potential audience must have training.
Finger spelling	May improve skills in written language, reading, and speech reading. Relatively easy to learn *if* child knows how to spell *and* has good fine motor coordination.	Not appropriate unless the child can spell. Requires greater manual dexterity than signs or gestures.
Simultaneous Communication	Designed to maximize the probability that a child will eventually produce spontaneous speech. Emphasizes word-sound associations.	Depending upon whether Signed English or ASL is the combined system (see above).
Pantomime and natural gesture	Gestures are easily understood without special training. The gross movements required may be easier for physicaly impaired students. Pantomime has greatest potential as an input system for the severely handicapped.	Severely limited expressive potential in comparison to standard manual systems. Pantomime requires at least Stage 5 cognitive development.

Aided systems Advantages and disadvantages of the different alphabetic and nonalphabetic symbol systems introduced earlier in the chapter are summarized in Table 10-3. In addition to weighing child and environmental characteristics as noted above, consider the following variables when selecting a communication system:

1. The system's potential for expansion or generalization to a more sophisticated system as the child's cognitive and motor skills increase
2. The needs and abilities of the child's audiences in critical present and future environments and their acceptance of the system
3. Available workers and time resources—an established ("ready made") system may be the best choice unless there is someone with the time to create symbols
4. The rate of communication the system permits; systems which rely on spelling are obviously much slower than those which permit expression of concepts

TABLE 10-3 Advantages and disadvantages of the most common aided symbol systems

System	Advantages	Disadvantages
NONALPHABETIC		
Representational systems (e.g., Rebus, Blissymbolics)	Production of syntax similar to English is possible. The pictographic nature of most of the symbols contributes to rapid learning. Blissymbols are particularly useful with physically handicapped students whose output is primarily restricted by physical limitations. The audience for Blissymbol and Rebus users includes all persons who can read English. Rebuses may also facilitate reading development.	Requires good visual discrimination skills. Blissymbols may require cognitive skills of *at least* a 2 year old. Decoding of the pictograhic symbols of the Rebus system may require sensorimotor Stage 5 cognitive development. The liberal use of traditional orthography in combined rebuses and the lack of a semantic base for many symbols may decrease learning rate.
Abstract systems (e.g., Non-SLIP, Yerkish)	Premack-type symbols (e.g., Non-SLIP symbols) can be identified by touch (as well as sight) so they can be used with the visually impaired. Premack-type symbols are not as visually similar as some other symbols so visual discriminations are somewhat easier. Can be designed to maintain English morphology, semantics, and syntax, which may facilitate speech and reading.	Require sensorimotor Stage 5 or 6 cognitive development. Non-SLIP was developed, and is used to *facilitate* language—its usefulness as a communicaion system, per se, has not been demonstrated. The Yerkish grammar is somewhat restricted compared to English. Because they are highly abstract, Yerkish symbols may be difficult for the severely handicapped to learn; also, they are relatively demanding on the child's visual discrimination skills. Not easily portable.
Direct reproduction (models, photographs and artists' drawings)	Models and photographs have a low level of abstraction—artists' drawings may be somewhat more abstract. Appropriate for children with very low cognitive levels. Only average visual discrimination skills required. Potential audience is unlimited. Models can be identified by sight as well as by touch. Good primary systems which can be faded when child is capable of dealing with a representational system or able to read.	Difficult to represent verbs and abstract concepts.
ALPHABETIC		
Traditional orthography	Can be used alone or in conjunction with other symbols—in the form of letters, syllables, or words. Considered to be a normative system with a very large audience of users. The potential vocabulary is unlimited if the child can spell.	Requires good visual discrimination skills, a high level of cognitive development (age 4 +), spelling skills (if child is to use letters), and some knowledge of the structure of language.
International teaching alphabet (i.t.a.)	Same as above.	Designed for use as a facilitator of reading—not as a communication system, so there is little research as to efficacy with handicapped children. Requires good visual discrimination skills and high level of cognitive development.

5. The degree of independence the system permits—the child should be able to initiate communications as well as respond.

SELECTING A DISPLAY DEVICE

There is one final technological decision before consideration of curricular content and procedures becomes paramount. If an aided technique is indicated, a suitable display device must be selected. There are as many display possibilities as there are students needing communication devices. These devices range from simple two or three picture communication boards to elaborate electronic displays, the content of which is limited only by the user's vocabulary, general language capabilities, and indicating skills. As a general rule, the simpler the board, the better, particularly with very young children. If an electronic device is being considered, Shane (1981) suggests considering the following factors:

With young children, the simpler the display device, the better.

1. *Indicating capabilities.* For some children the most efficient and precise means of indicating is an input switch. A variety of input switches are available. Some are activated by movements as subtle as wrist flexion or extension, also extension and neck flexion.
2. *Portability.* Vanderheiden (1978) differentiates devices weighing less than 25 pounds as portable and those weighing over 30 pounds as stationary. Because it is too heavy to go where the child goes, a stationary device cannot be available to the child in all environments. This limitation of many electronic displays is an important consideration when choosing between electronic and nonelectronic devices.
3. *Speed of message transmission.* A factor to consider is whether an electronic device will increase message transmission rate *enough* to outweigh the disadvantages, such as lack of portability and cost.
4. *Cost.* Purchase of an electronic communication device is not likely to be a one-time expense: the child should require a succession of more sophisticated devices or optional equipment purchases. While cost alone should not prevent purchase of an electronic display, it cannot be discounted. Unless there is reason to expect a more costly electronic device to have significant advantages, it may not be a wise purchase for a very young child.
5. *Benefit.* If the child is expected to do as well with a nonelectronic as with an electronic, more costly, and less portable one, the nonelectronic device is a better choice.

Selection of a board should be based on assessment of visual capacity, eye-head control, range of motion, and eye-hand control.

Again, we return to the importance of an accurate assessment of the child's physical and sensory capabilities. Visual capacity (acuity and range of eye movement) affects the precision of symbol discrimination and pointing. Eye-head control determines whether the child can use a head pointer (rod type or optical). Range of voluntary arm movements and eye-hand control influence the size and placement of entries on the display, board size, angle, and elevation.

Occupational and physical therapists should be consulted when determining the child's maximum voluntary arm extension, flexion, abduction, adduction, and which arm is preferred as a pointer and which is least likely to induce extraneous movement. All consistent and reliable motor movements should be assessed, as any one or all of these movements may be used in developing the child's interface with his communication aid.

Intended messages can be produced with a communication display by many response modes. Common indicating methods range from pointing with a finger, eye gaze, or stylus to activating a mechanical switch or lever. Any number of switches are available: push switches, paddle switches, sliding switches, moisture switches, eye controlled switches and tilt switches, to name but a few. Some can be activated by more than one body part, or a single movement can activate several switches. Information, descriptions and illustrations of commercially available switches may be found in Holt, Buelow, and Vanderheiden (1978), Silverman (1980), Silverman, McNaughton, and Kates (1978), and Vanderheiden and Grilley (1976).

TRAINING CONSIDERATIONS

The basic considerations in designing curricula for training an augmentative communication system are the same as those for oral language training: (a) entry skills, (b) what to teach, (c) how to teach, and (d) evaluation of child performance and progress. Even more so than in oral language training, each candidate for an augmentative communication system presents a unique programming challenge. These factors should be specifically addressed for each child. Only the basic purpose of intervention, to identify and develop functional exchanges, is the same for all children.

ENTRY SKILLS

As discussed earlier, the child's ability to deal with symbols, a sensorimotor Stage 5 attainment, influences the time when representational system and communication device should be introduced. If the child cannot yet deal with symbols, then initial programming should focus on (a) promoting interactions, (b) establishing the motivation for communication, and (c) developing functional response modes.

As discussed in several other chapters in this book, interaction is the starting point, basic activity, and primary goal of readiness training (Harris & Vanderheiden, 1980). The focus is on promoting and expanding forms of interaction through basic care and play activities. As the cognitive skills for symbolic representation begin to emerge, the child should be encouraged to substitute symbols for less sophisticated expressions of familiar functions (particularly the requesting function).

Begin interaction training by encouraging exchange rituals in all routine classroom activities, and teach caregivers how to identify and facilitate interaction possibilities in home routines. When necessary, adapt these routines to be compatible with the child's motoric abilities and arrange activities to maximize the child's control of the environment. Always imitate the child's vocalizations and gestures, no matter how subtle. Look at and talk about whatever the child focuses his gaze upon. Respond to all behaviors (crying, gaze, pointing) that indicate a request for objects or attention.

Promote both comprehension *and* production of signals.

Promote the understanding and use of pointing and iconic natural gestures (commonly understood signals such as a headshake to express affirmation and negation). The physically capable child can be prepared to point by such activities as giving and taking objects, touching objects when named, and poking a finger into wet sand or clay during play routines. You can facilitate acquisition of iconic natural gestures by encouraging imitation of functional object use and spontaneous functional object use behaviors, and use of gestures to communicate basic needs and desires.

In addition to focusing on increased interaction and establishing a desire to communicate, readiness programming should establish those motor skills the child will need to use an augmentative communication device. These can also be trained in the context of ongoing play and caregiving activities. If assessment of the child's motor capabilities suggests that he needs an input switch to gain access to a communication prosthesis, then develop play activities to teach switch activation. The idea is to develop mastery of the physical mechanism (electric or nonelectric) that will eventually be used as a means of communication.

Concentrate on teaching the motor skills the child will need to use an augmentative communication device.

Also keep in mind the perceptual and memory requirement of communication. Begin training visual discriminations, visual attention, tracking, matching, and short term memory. Perhaps most important is to begin pairing symbols from the vocabulary the child will eventually be taught with speech when communicating with the child (and with others while in the child's presence) (Harris & Vanderheiden, 1980). The child should have opportunities to see the signs or symbols used by others.

WHAT TO TEACH

Objectives for children functioning at sensorimotor Stage 5 or above should focus on (a) increasing already established interactions, and (b) using more sophisticated means to communicate basic intentions. Teach the child who is using such behaviors as gaze, pointing, crying, grunts, etc., that he can express basic intentions (requests, demands, comments) more efficiently and effectively through the use of symbols. The following recommendations can guide selection of initial content for augmentative communication training. Some are specific to one system, but most are applicable to any system.

If Blissymbolics is the system to be taught, Silverman et al. (1978) recommend selecting initial symbols that are:

1. Pictorial
2. Visually dissimilar
3. Related to concrete objects or persons in the immediate environment
4. Immediately functional

All of these suggestions are equally applicable to selection of initial Rebus symbols. The latter two are applicable to selections of any system for aided communication.

Holland (1975) emphasizes the importance of items that are functional—those that meet the child's needs for survival (e.g., "toilet," "drink"), sociability (e.g., "Hi," "My name is _____"), and expressing knowledge of the world (e.g., locative relationships, perceptual attributes). Additionally, the importance of items with "organicity" (items reflecting the child's unique preferences and current interests) is emphasized. Supplement school observations and data from reinforcer sampling probes with caregiver reports to identify these items. These are the items that the child is most likely to want to "talk" about. The important thing is to keep in mind what you know about the earliest productions of nonhandicapped children (see Chapter Two) and carefully study the child's unique communication needs and desires.

Substantially more variables need to be considered when selecting a system for unaided communication. Ease of production becomes as important a criterion as functional and motivational attributes when deciding which signs to teach first. After reviewing studies documenting the effectiveness of signing as an augmentative communication mode for severely handicapped students and their own clinical data, Reichle, Williams and Ryan (1981) suggest the following factors to consider when selecting an initial sign vocabulary:

> Ease of production is a primary consideration when selecting an initial sign vocabulary.

1. *Familiarity and representational level of the sign.* Iconic signs are acquired more readily than abstract ones. Two types of iconic signs can be differentiated: functional iconic signs that have a topography *identical* to the action being represented, and representative iconic signs that have a topography *similar,* but not identical, to the represented action. There is also evidence that signs for items or objects that are more familiar to the child are learned more readily.

2. *Functionality of the sign.* Signs that convey basic needs and desires will be acquired most easily. To determine if a sign has functional utility for the child, assess (a) frequency of use, (b) utility across different persons, places, and objects, and (c) association with reinforcing events and objects.

3. *Motor complexity.* Touch signs (where one hand comes into contact with the other hand or another part of the body) are learned more readily than signs that have no tactile component.

Signs performed with one hand are learned more rapidly than signs requiring the use of two hands. Signs where both hands perform the same action are easier to learn than signs requiring each hand to perform different actions.

Vocabulary expansion and, if an aided device is being use, board organization become major concerns once the child has the idea that the environment is responsive to symbolic communication. When the child has acquired a core requesting vocabulary, then new object and action symbols, symbols for places, prepositions, descriptors, question words, quantity, and time should be taught. The following questions will aid in ranking these second level training targets. Consider:

1. *Where* the child will want to "talk?"
2. What he will want and need to "talk" *about* in each of these settings?
3. Who he will want to "talk" *to* in these settings?

Use information about communication contexts, communication partners (prospective language teachers), and the child's specific interests and needs to generate a list of potential vocabulary additions. Relational and substantive functions that are first acquired and expressed by normal language learners can also be a reference for this list (See Table 2-5 in Chapter Two).

A communication board is always custom designed to its user's specifications.

Each communication board must be custom-designed to the user's specifications. A single-page display is the easiest to use but may have limited vocabulary space. Portability is also a concern. Unless the single-page display is small enough to wear around the neck or attach to a belt or wheelchair, its use may have to be limited to a single location.

Multi-page displays allow for the inclusion of more vocabulary about a particular topic or within a grammatical class. One way to organize these "book-like" displays is to place symbols about different settings on separate ("miniboard") pages (e.g., classroom page, lunchroom page, kitchen page, etc.). For a comprehensive presentation of board design and construction, see McDonald and Schultz (1973), Silverman (1980), and Vanderheiden (1977).

McDonald and Schultz (1973) and McDonald (1980) suggest arranging symbols in a "Fitzgerald Key" format. Columns represent the various parts of speech (the common word order in English). For example, from the left, the columns would be (a) subject (who, what, where), (b) verb, (c) modifiers, and (d) object.

In addition to teaching nonspeaking children the symbols to permit expression of ideas and intentions, programming should target skills to facilitate and maintain communicative interactions (Musselwhite & St. Louis, 1982). Not only do these communication skills contribute to the appearance of normality, but they also add information to the intended message.

1. *Eye contact.* Teach the child to establish eye contact with the message receiver prior to communication and between messages.

2. *Facial expressions.* Encourage the child to be as expressive as physically possible to emphasize the intent of a message.

3. *Appropriate head and body movements.* Body movements such as nodding the head and leaning forward slightly can add information to the message.

4. *Appropriate vocalization.* If the child is capable of some vocalization (particularly sounds that approximate "uh-uh") these vocalizations should be encouraged. Even minimal expressions of sound can support and maintain a dialogue and emphasize important points.

Keep in mind the extra linguistic behaviors that can aid "listeners" in interpreting intended messages.

HOW TO TEACH

The most common strategies for teaching manual signs are molding, shaping, and imitation (Mayberry, 1976). *Molding* is placing the child's hand(s) around the referent object, but it is only useful for teaching signs such as "cup" and "ball" that duplicate the shape of the object. *Shaping* is forming the child's hand(s) into the proper sign position. In *imitation* training a model of the sign is provided for the child to copy. Usually a combination of these strategies is used. Most important to remember is that *the verbal symbol is always paired with the sign.*

Use molding, shaping and imitation to teach manual signs.

Naturally occurring situations (as opposed to structured training sessions with massed trials) are the preferred training context (see Chapter Six). Situations to elicit the desired response can be contrived if there are not sufficient opportunities throughout the day to train a specific form or the structure. The idea is to arrange the environment to create the need to communicate as much as possible. Massed trials may be necessary at one time or another (e.g., when a new symbol is introduced), but this type of training format should be kept to a minimum (see Chapter Nine).

Ferrier and Shane (1980) suggest the following procedures to teach symbolic expression of early speech acts (requesting, labeling, commenting, describing, and questioning) with an aided device. Most training assumes what might be called a "parlor game format." To teach requesting:

1. Select three highly reinforcing objects and/or activities and represent them on the child's communication board. The complexity of the representations will depend on the child's cognitive level: size and placement are determined by his motor coordination.

2. Allow the child to sample (if food is one of the items) and/or manipulate the reinforcing objects. If an activity is included, allow the child to participate briefly in the activity.

3. Probe to see if the child can match the object or activity with its representation (e.g., "Point to juice," or "Show me swinging"). (If not, of course, symbol-referent correspondence must be taught.)

4. Point to each representation in turn and urge the child to indicate a choice by asking, "What do you want?"
5. Provide the appropriate object or activity immediately upon the indicating response.
6. Continue this "game" until the child indicates correct responses without prompting.
7. Generalize "requesting" to natural situations such as snack time, mealtimes, and toy play periods throughout the day.
8. Expand one-symbol requests to include an action symbol (e.g., want + object, blow + bubbles, eat + raisin).

These procedures can be used to teach a variety of requesting responses, depending upon the child's skill level. For example, if cookie is identified as a reinforcing item, the child might be taught to

☐ point to a Rebus symbol for cookie on a communication aid
☐ point to a picture of a cookie
☐ turn his head toward the cookie
☐ look at the cookie or picture of a cookie

Once basic needs and desires are being communicated, the child's repertoire can be expanded to include labeling, commenting, describing and questioning.

Once the child is communicating basic needs and desires (affecting the environment through representational means), the emphasis shifts to broadening his experiences and expanding intentional communication to include other speech acts such as labeling, commenting, describing, and questioning. Those objects and events in the environment that interest the child should be labeled repeatedly with the appropriate symbols always available on the communication device. Initially only objects and events that are immediately present will be appropriate vocabulary items. However, as cognitive skills increase, objects and events from the immediate past and anticipated activities should be represented. Further, attempts should be made to expand interactions beyond a single "round" to longer dialogues with two- and three-symbol comments and descriptions.

EVALUATION OF CHILD PERFORMANCE AND PROGRESS

Communicative behavior is usually only one of several constituent elements of a behavior cluster. As discussed in Chapters Six and Nine, reliable and continuous data collection is more of a challenge when instruction focuses on clusters, rather than on single behaviors, in the context of naturally occurring situations. Holvoet, Guess, Mulligan, and Brown (1980) recommend a format for recording the child's total performance in the skill cluster. Figure 10-2 depicts a sample data record for snack time interactions. A plus (+) indicates that the behavior was correctly performed; (p) indicates a prompt. When 10 distributed trials have been completed, the percentage of correct responses can be graphed separately for each behavior.

FIGURE 10-2   Example of a data sheet for snack time behavior cluster

SNACK TIME		DATES								
S^D	Child's R									
"It's time for snacks"	Moves to snack area in 5 sec. or less									
"Look what we have"	Raises head and looks at food items									
"What do you want?"	Indicates symbol for preferred food									
"Is this what you want?"	Nods "yes"									

Recording spontaneous, child-initiated communications poses a different problem. In some cases, tallies can be scored on an index card affixed to the child's wheelchair or the outside edge of his communication board. Another alternative is for the adults to carry or wear a type of event counter. If continuous daily recording becomes unmanageable, as can happen when initiations are at a high rate or when several children are being monitored at one time, probes may be the best solution. Set aside one day a week per child to record his spontaneous communication.

In conclusion, we want to stress the importance of maintaining a conditional attitude about decisions related to the selection and training of an augmentative communication mode. One of the measures of success of the program will be the extent to which it changes over time to accommodate the child's expanding communication needs and capabilities.

SUMMARY

1. The most persuasive argument against the use of augmentative communication systems—the possibility of inteference with speech acquisition—has been countered by research demonstrating transfer from nonspeech systems to speech and, in some cases, enhancement of speech acquisition.

2. A response mode which requires external support is said to be "aided"; those which rely solely on physical movements are called "unaided" modes.

3. The best known and most commonly used unaided symbol systems are Signed English, American Sign Language, Manual Alphabets, and Simultaneous Communication; informal systems include pantomime, natural gestures, and Amer-Ind.

4. Nonalphabetic symbol systems may use representational symbols such as Rebus symbols or Blissymbolics, abstract symbols such as Premack's plastic "chips," or direct reproductions such as models and pictures. Alphabetic systems usually rely on traditional orthography or the i/t/a.

5. Communication boards are of three basic types—direct selection displays, scanning displays, and encoding displays. Some boards permit use of several indicating methods.

6. Factors to consider when deciding if a child is an appropriate candidate for augmentative communication training include (a) medical history, (b)p rimitive oral reflexes, (c) laryngeal functioning, (d) eating problems, (e) chronological age, (f) cognitive development, (g) the comprehension-production discrepancy, (h) imitation skills, and (i) significant others.

7. Factors to consider when selecting an appropriate technique are (a) severity of neuromotor impairment, (b) imitative ability, (c) individual preferences, and (d) potential communication environments.

8. When selecting a display device, consider the child's indicating capabilities, portability of the device, speed of message transmission possible, and the cost of the device relative to its benefits.

9. If the child cannot deal with symbols, initial programming should focus upon (a) promoting interactions, (b) establishing motivation for communication and (c) developing functional response modes.

10. Objectives for children who demonstrate symbolic capabilities should focus on (a) increasing interactions and (b) use of more sophisticated means to communicate basic intentions.

11. When selecting initial signs to include in a manual signing program, consider their (a) familiarity and representational level, (b) functionality, and (c) motor complexity.

12. Teach manual signs in naturally occurring situations through molding, shaping and/or imitation.

REFERENCES

ASHA Committee Report. Position statement on nonspeech communication. *American Speech-Language-Hearing Association,* 1981.

BERGER, S.L. A clinical program for developing multimodal language responses with atypical deaf children. In J.E. McLean, D.E. Yoder, & R.L. Schiefelbusch (Eds.), *Language intervention with the retarded.* Baltimore, Maryland: University Park Press, 1972.

BEUKELMAN, D.R., & YORKSTON, K. A communication system for the severely dysarthric speaker with an intact language system. *Journal of Speech and Hearing Disorders,* 1977, *42,* 265–270.

BORNSTEIN, H., HAMILTON, B., KANNAPELL, B., ROY, H., & SAULNIER, K. *Basic preschool signed English dictionary.* Washington, D.C.: Gallaudet College, 1973.

BROWDER, D., MORRIS, W., & SNELL, M. Using time delay to teach manual signs to a severely retarded student. *Education and Training of the Mentally Retarded,* 1981, *16,* 252–258.

CARR, E., BINKOFF, J., KOLOZINSKY, E., & EDDY, M. Acquisition of sign language by autistic children. I: Expressive labeling. *Journal of Applied Behavior Analysis,* 1978, *11,* 489–501.

CARRIER, J.K., JR. Application of a nonspeech language system with the severely language handicapped. In L.L. Lloyd (Ed.), *Communication assessment and intervention strategies.* Baltimore, Maryland: University Park Press, 1976.

CARRIER, J.K., JR., & PEAK, T. *Non-speech language initiation program* (Non-SLIP). Lawrence, Kansas: H & H Enterprises, 1975.

CHAPMAN, R.S., & MILLER, J.R. Analyzing language and communication in the child. In R.L. Schiefelbusch (Ed.), *Nonspeech language and communication: Analysis and intervention.* Baltimore, Maryland: University Park Press, 1980.

CLARK, C.R., & WOODCOCK, R.W. Graphic systems of communication. In L.L. Lloyd (Ed.), *Communication assessment and intervention strategies.* Baltimore, Maryland: University Park Press, 1976.

COHEN, M. Development of language behavior in an autistic child using total communication. *Exceptional Children,* 1981, *47,* 374–379.

CROWDER, E., & SHANE, H.C. *Cognitive prerequisites necessary for matrix encoding.* Paper presented at ASHA, Los Angeles, 1981.

DANILOFF, J., & SHAFER, A. A gestural communication program for severely and profoundly handicapped children. *Language, Speech, and Hearing Services in Schools,* 1981, *12,* 258–267.

DUNCAN, J.L., & SILVERMAN, F.H. Impacts of learning American Sign Language on mentally retarded children: A preliminary report. *Perceptual and Motor Skills,* 1977, *44,* 11–38.

FERRIER, L., & SHANE, H.C. Communication skills. In J. Umbreit & P. Cardullias (Eds.), *Educating the severely handicapped: Curriculum adaptations,* (Vol. 4). Division of Physically Handicapped, CEC, 1980. Distributed by Special Press, Columbus, Ohio.

GUESS, D. Methods in communication instruction for severely handicapped persons. In W. Sailor, B. Wilcox, & L. Brown (Eds.), *Methods of instruction for severely handicapped students.* Baltimore, Maryland: Paul H. Brookes Publishing Co., Inc., 1980.

GUESS, D., SAILOR, W., & BAER, D. Children with limited language. In R.L. Schiefelbusch (Ed.), *Language intervention strategies.* Baltimore, Maryland: University Park Press, 1978.

HAMRE-NIETUPSKI, S., STOLL, A., HOLTZ, K., FULLERTON, P., RYAN-FLOTTUM, M., & BROWN, L. Curricular strategies for teaching selected nonverbal communication skills to nonverbal and verbal severely handicapped students. In L. Brown, J. Nietupski, S. Lyon, S. Hamre-Nietupski, T. Crowner, & L. Gruenewald (Eds.), *Curricular strategies for teaching functional object use, nonverbal communication, problem solving and meal-time skills to severely handicapped students* (Vol. 7, Part I). Madison, Wisconsin: Department of Specialized Educational Services, Madison Metropolitan School District, 1977.

HARRIS, D., & VANDERHEIDEN, G. Enhancing the development of communicative interaction. In R.L. Schiefelbusch (Ed.), *Nonspeech language and communication: Analysis and intervention*. Baltimore, Maryland: University Park Press, 1980.

HODGES, D., & DEICH, R.F. Language intervention strategies with manipulated symbols. In R.L. Schiefelbusch & J.H. Hollis (Eds.), *Language intervention from ape to child*. Baltimore, Maryland: University Park Press, 1979.

HOLLAND, A. Language therapy for children: Some thoughts on context and content. *Journal of Speech and Hearing Disorders*, 1975, *40*, 514–523.

HOLT, C.S., BUELOW, D., & VANDERHEIDEN, G. Interface switch profile and annotated list of commercial switches. In G.C. Vanderheiden (Ed.), *Non-vocal communication resource book*. Baltimore: University Park Press, 1978.

HOLVOET, J., GUESS, D., MULLIGAN, M., & BROWN, F. The individualized curriculum sequencing model (II): A teaching strategy for severely handicapped students. *JASH*, 1980, *5*(4), 352–367.

KENT, L.R. *Language acquisition program for the retarded and multiply impaired*. Champaign, Illinois: Research Press, 1974.

KOHL, F. Effects of motoric requirements on the acquisition of manual sign responses by severely handicapped students. *American Journal of Mental Deficiency*, 1981, *85*, 396–403.

KOHL, F., KARLAN, G., & HEAL, L. Effects of pairing manual signs with verbal cues upon the acquisition of instruction following behaviors and generalization to expressive language with severely handicapped students. *AAESPH Review*, 1979, *4*, 291–300.

LLOYD, L.L. Unaided nonspeech communication for severely handicapped individuals: An extensive bibliography. *Education and Training of the Mentally Retarded*, 1980, *15*(1), 15–34.

MAYBERRY, R. If a chimp can learn sign language surely my nonverbal client can too. *ASHA*, 1976, *18*, 223–228.

MAYBERRY, R. Manual communication. In H. Davis & S. Silverman (Eds.), *Hearing and deafness* (4th ed.). New York: Holt, Rinehart and Winston, 1978.

McDONALD, E.T. Early identification and treatment of child at risk for speech development. In R.L. Schiefelbusch (Ed.), *Nonspeech language and communication: Analysis and intervention*. Baltimore, Maryland: University Park Press, 1980.

McDONALD, E.T., & CHANCE, B. *Cerebral palsy*. Englewood Cliffs, New Jersey: Prentice-Hall, Inc., 1964.

McDONALD, E.T., & SCHULTZ, A. Communication boards for cerebral palsied children. *Journal of Speech and Hearing Disorders*, 1973, *38*, 73–88.

McLEAN (McCORMICK), L., & McLEAN, J. A language training program for nonverbal autistic children. *Journal of Speech and Hearing Research*, 1974, *35*, 186–193.

McNAUGHTON, S., & KATES, S. The application of Blissymbolics. In R.L. Schiefelbusch (Ed.), *Nonspeech language and communication: Analysis and intervention*. Baltimore, Maryland: University Park Press, 1980.

MILLER, A., & MILLER, E. Cognitive developmental training with elevated boards and sign language. *Journal of Autism and Childhood Schizophrenia*, 1973, *3*, 65–85.

MOORES, D.F. *Educating the deaf: Psychology, principles, and practice*. Boston: Houghton Mifflin Co., 1978.

MORRIS, S.E. A neurodevelopmental approach to communication boards. In S.E. Morris (Ed.), *Pre-speech and language programming for the young child with cerebral palsy: A workshop training manual.* Workshop Training Manual, Evanston, Illinois, 1975.

MORRIS, S.E. Oral-motor development: Normal and abnormal. In J. Wilson (Ed.), *Oral motor function and dysfunction in children.* Division of Physical Therapy, Chapel Hill, N.C., 1978.

MUSSELWHITE, C.R., & ST. LOUIS, K.W. *Communication programming for the severely handicapped: Vocal and nonvocal strategies.* Houston, Texas: College-Hill Press, 1982.

O'ROURKE, T.J. *A basic course in manual communication.* Silver Spring, Maryland: National Association of the Deaf, 1973.

OXMAN, J., WEBSTER, C.D., & KONSTANTANEAS, M.M. The perception and processing of information by severely dysfunctional nonverbal children: A rationale for the use of manual communication. *Sign Language Studies,* 1978, *21,* 89–316.

PREMACK, D. A functional analysis of language. *Journal of Experimental Analysis of Behavior,* 1970, *14,* 107–125.

PREMACK, D. Language in chimpanzees? *Science,* 1971, *172,* 808–822.

REICHLE, J., WILLIAMS, W., & RYAN, S. Selecting signs for the formulation of an augmentative communicative modality. *Journal of the Association for the Severely Handicapped,* Spring, 1981, *6*(1), 48–55.

REICHLE, J.E., & YODER, D.E. Assessment and early stimulation of communication in the severely and profoundly mentally retarded. In R.L. York & E. Edgar (Eds.), *Teaching the severely handicapped (Vol. 4).* Columbus, Ohio: Special Press, 1979.

ROSENBEK, J.C., COLLINS, M.J., & WERTZ, R.T. Intersystemic reorganization for apraxia of speech. In R.H. Brookshire (Ed.), *Clinical aphasiology: Conference proceedings.* Minneapolis: BRK Publishers, 1976.

RUMBAUGH, D.M. (Ed.). *Language learning by a chimpanzee: The Lana project.* New York: Academic Press, 1977.

RUMBAUGH, D.M. LANA Project helps retarded children learn language. *Yerkes Newsletter,* 1978, *15,* 20–23.

SAILOR, W., GUESS, D., GOETZ, L., SCHULER, A., UTLEY, B., & BALDWIN, M. Language and severely handicapped persons: Deciding what to teach to whom. In W. Sailor, B. Wilson, & L. Brown (Eds.), *Methods of instruction for severely handicapped students.* Baltimore, Maryland: Paul H. Brookes Publishing Co., Inc., 1980.

SCHAEFFER, B. Spontaneous language through signed speech. In R.L. Schiefelbusch (Ed.), *Nonspeech language and communication.* Baltimore: University Park Press, 1980.

SCHIEFELBUSCH, R.L., & HOLLIS, J.H. (Eds.). *Language intervention from ape to child.* Baltimore: University Park Press, 1979.

SHANE, H.C. Approaches to communication training with the severely handicapped. In R.L. York & E. Edgar (Eds.), *Teaching the severely handicapped* (Vol. 4). Columbus, Ohio: Special Press, 1979.

SHANE, H.C. Approaches to assessing the communication of non-oral persons. In R.L. Schiefelbusch (Ed.), *Nonspeech language and communication: Analysis and intervention.* Baltimore, Maryland: University Park Press, 1980.

SHANE, H.C. Decision making in early augmentative communication system use. In R.L. Schiefelbusch & D. Bricker (Eds.), *Early language intervention.* Baltimore, Maryland: University Park Press, 1981.

SHANE, H.C., & BASHIR, A.S. Election criteria for the adoption of an augmentative communication system: Preliminary considerations. *Journal of Speech and Hearing Disorders,* 1980, *45,* 408–414.

SHANE, H.C., & MELROSE, J. An electronic conversation board and an accompanying training program for aphonic expressive communication. A paper presented at the American Speech and Hearing Association Convention, Washington, D.C., 1975.

SILVERMAN, F. *Communication for the speechless.* Englewood Cliffs, New Jersey: Prentice-Hall, Inc., 1980.

SILVERMAN, H., McNAUGHTON, S., & KATES, B. *Handbook of Blissymbolics for instructors, users, parents and administrators.* Toronto, Ontario: Blissymbolics Communication Institute, 1978.

SKELLY, M., & SCHINSKY, L. *Amer-Ind gestural code based on universal American Indian Hand Talk.* New York: Elsevier North Holland, Inc., 1979.

STOKOE, W., JR., CASTERLINE, D.C., & CRONEBERG, C.G. *Dictionary of American Sign Language,* (revised edition) Silver Spring, Md.: Linstock Press, 1978.

STREMEL-CAMPBELL, K., CANTRELL, D., & HALLE, J. Manual signing as a language system and as a speech initiator for the nonverbal severely handicapped student. In E. Sontag, J. Smith, & N. Certo (Eds.), *Educational programming for the severely and profoundly handicapped.* Reston, Va.: Council for Exceptional Children, 1977.

VANDERHEIDEN, G.C. Providing the child with a means to indicate. In G. Vanderheiden & K. Grilley (Eds.), *Non-vocal communication technique and aids for the severely physically handicapped.* Baltimore, Maryland: University Park Press, 1976.

VANDERHEIDEN, G.C. Design and construction of a laptray: Preliminary notes. Madison, Wisconsin: The Trace Research and Development Center, 1977.

VANDERHEIDEN, G.C. (Ed.). *Non-vocal communication resource book.* Baltimore, Maryland: University Park Press, 1978.

VANDERHEIDEN, G.C., & HARRIS-VANDERHEIDEN, D. Communication techniques and aids for the non-vocal, severely handicapped. In L.L. Lloyd (Ed.), *Communication assessment and intervention strategies.* Baltimore, Maryland: University Park Press, 1976.

WILBER, R.B. *American sign language and sign systems.* Baltimore: University Park Press, 1979.

WOODCOCK, R.W., CLARK, C.R., & DAVIES, C.O. *The Peabody Rebus Reading Program.* Circle Pines, Minnesota: American Guidance Service, 1969.

YODER, D.E., & CALCULATOR, S. Some perspectives on intervention strategies for persons with developmental disorders. *Journal of Autism and Developmental Disorders,* 1981, *2*(1), 107–121.

CHAPTER ELEVEN

EXTRACURRICULAR ROLES AND RELATIONSHIPS

Linda McCormick

No one person or profession has an adequate knowledge base and sufficient expertise to make unilateral decisions and perform all functions associated with the provision of educational services for handicapped students. Professionals, paraprofessionals, parents, and volunteers must learn to communicate with one another, to make joint decisions, and most importantly, to coordinate their service delivery efforts, if they are to achieve maximum behavior change goals. In schools, the machinery for making decisions, solving problems, and taking action on a wide range of problems is clearly defined and described by law. How well the system works, of course, depends upon the people involved. Recognition of the importance of understanding group behavior, particularly the dynamics of work teams, is relatively new in the human service fields, but it is an area that will undoubtedly receive considerably more attention in the eighties than ever before.

This chapter on extracurricular role functions begins with a brief introduction to the various teams mandated by P.L. 94-142 and their respective functions in the assessment, planning, and intervention processes. It then describes three approaches to team organization at the service delivery level. Strategies and procedures for one of these approaches, the transdisciplinary team model, are presented. The remainder of the chapter focuses on school-home partnerships—specifically, parent involvement.

P.L. 94-142 MANDATED COMMITTEES

P.L. 94-142 mandates four work groups at the school level; each has different goals, composition, and responsibilities.

This law provides for involvement of four groups, each with somewhat different composition and responsibilities in the educational intervention process. This process begins when a child is first referred as possibly needing special services and ends when those services are no longer deemed necessary. The goals, composition, and responsibilities of each of these teams are outlined in Table 11-1.

TABLE 11-1 Goals, composition, and responsibilities of teams in the intervention process

Team	Goals	Composition	Responsibilities
Special education committee	*Coordination of all procedures* from referral to IEP review *Monitoring* IEP development and implementation	Permanent members — LEA special education personnel and principals Changing members — relevant professionals concerned with a particular child	Organize services Appoint evaluation and IEP teams Assure P.L. 94-142 compliance Review referrals Assure that parental rights protected Authorize evaluation Monitor programming
Evaluation team	*Nondiscriminatory evaluation* for eligibility determination and program planning	Membership depends on severity and complexity of suspected disability Team must include at least one teacher or other specialist with expertise in the area of child's disability All members must have certification and/or license appropriate to their area of expertise	Select and administer appropriate formal and informal assessments Collect and review data from other sources Document any potentially biasing factors Interpret and report evaluation data Serve on IEP team if requested

TABLE 11-1 (continued)

Team	Goals	Composition	Responsibilities
IEP committee	*Development of the IEP*	Child's teacher (special and/or regular) Special education supervisory personnel Child's parents Child (if appropriate) Member of the evaluation team (or person able to interpret the evaluation data) Other relevant professionals (as appropriate)	Review evaluation data and other information Develop a total service plan (IEP) which includes: 1. statement of present performance levels 2. annual goals and short-term objectives 3. statement of special education and related service needs 4. projected date for initiation and termination of services 5. appropriate objective evaluation criteria and evaluation schedule 6. statement of the extent to which child will participate in regular education Approve IEP revisions (if required)
Service delivery team	*Implementation of IEP goals and objectives*	Teacher (special and/or regular) Representative of each related service required to assist child to benefit from special education. Examples: speech pathology and audiology psychological services physical therapy occupational therapy counseling and guidance medical diagnosis social work parents paraprofessionals	Comprehensively plan and coordinate services Provide instructional, management and therapy programs Monitor instruction, management and therapy programs Train and coordinate parents and paraprofessionals Mobilize community resources Plan and program transition to less restrictive environments

The school special education committee (sometimes called the special services committee) is a coordinating and monitoring group to assure that all special services are provided as mandated by P.L. 94-142. Turnbull, Strickland, and Brantley (1978) describe this committee as "the hub of the wheel for the coordination of all procedures related to the identification, evaluation, and placement of handicapped students" (p. 32).

Upon receipt of a written referral and the signed parental permission form, the special education committee identifies appropriate professionals to comprise an assessment team. This second group, called the multidisciplinary assessment team (because its members come from different disiplines) is responsible for preplacement (pre-IEP) assessment as described in Chapter Four.

The IEP committee (except the parents) is also appointed by the special education committee. The composition and responsibilities of this planning group are discussed at length in Chapter Five. The fourth group is responsible for IEP implementation (the functions outlined in Chapters Five and Six). At the very least, this team includes the teacher and a professional representing each of the related services designated in the child's IEP.

There is not a specific legal requirement for parents, paraprofessionals, and professionals (other than those providing specialized educational services) to be members of this work team; however, their participation is highly desirable. The team may also include representatives from medical and dental professions, nutrition, and social services.

SERVICE DELIVERY TEAM MODELS

Service delivery teams may adhere to multidisciplinary, interdisciplinary, or transdisciplinary tenets. (Note that in this context the term "multidisciplinary" denotes an approach to organizing and apportioning service delivery functions, rather than simply "a group of professionals from different disciplines"). Members of the service delivery team are responsible for postplacement assessments to verify and/or expand IEP goals and objectives, for planning of teaching strategies, for service delivery functions, and for evaluation. As team leader, the special education teacher organizes and coordinates the group's efforts so they function as a cohesive unit.

The three approaches to service delivery team organization are termed multidisciplinary, interdisciplinary, and transdisciplinary.

The variables that most clearly differentiate multidisciplinary, interdisciplinary and transdisciplinary approaches are coordination, collaboration, and communication. In a *multidisciplinary* approach, which is most commonly associated with the medical model, professionals maintain their respective discipline boundaries with only minimal, if any coordination, collaboration, or communication. Each assesses and, in some settings, attempts to remediate that aspect of the child's problem that is considered her particular specialty. The limitations of this approach are most apparent after the assessment stage where, as Hart (1978) states, "The chance of opposing recommendations is great. There is potential that important data will be overlooked because the person receiving it may not recognize the implications of some of the recommendations" (p. 392). In this approach the student is dissected into problem domains and never properly reassembled as a "whole child."

The *interdisciplinary* team approach was a response to dissatisfaction with the multidisciplinary model. However, it has not turned out to be a particularly good response because of the persistence of team communication problems. Assessment procedures are much the same as in the multidisciplinary approach and therapy conforms to the same isolation tenets (described in the next section). Where problems become apparent is in linking programming to assessment. Too often, the programming recommendations provided to the teacher are more ideal than manageable. The teacher may not have the skills to implement the recommended programs, nor the authority to arrange for their provision (Hart, 1978).

Despite an *avowed* commitment to coordination, collaboration, and communication, in practice the interdisciplinary approach does not assign an equal role to teachers in the decision-making process. While there may be some exchange of information prior to intervention, it generally ends at that point. Recommendations and information flow only one way—to the teacher—so they are rarely subjected to any reliability or validity criteria. If the teacher has sufficient skills and resources to implement a recommendation, and subsequent program evaluation results suggest a need for revision, there is no mechanism for communicating this information to the professional who provided the programming recommendations. It is not altogether clear who is accountable for what in this model—whether it is the teacher or the professional(s) who have recommended particular programming objectives and procedures.

The *transdisciplinary* model addresses the majority of these problems. Originally conceived by Hutchison (1974), this model suggests specific procedures for sharing information and skills among professionals and across discipline boundaries. It is unique in advocating (a) joint functioning (team members performing assessment, planning, and service delivery functions together), (b) continuous staff development (expansion of each team member's competencies) and (c) role release (sharing functions across discipline boundaries) (Lyon & Lyon, 1980). Whenever possible, assessments are implemented in the classroom so that teaching staff, other professionals, and parents can observe and provide input. Planning is a group effort integrating all of the assessment information.

Transdisciplinary team members are accountable for seeing that the best practices of their respective disciplines are implemented; however, their responsibility does not stop there. They are also responsible for monitoring program implementation, training others if necessary, and revising programs when evaluation data indicate that the procedures are not working. With the teacher as coordinator and manager of all program elements, there is no duplication of efforts or splintering of services.

TRANSDISCIPLINARY TEAM STRATEGIES

There is no single activity that we can point to as *defining* the transdisciplinary approach. However, there are two interaction strategies—integrated therapy and consultation—which have come to be closely identified with it and which distinguish it from the other two approaches.

Integrated therapy In the multidisciplinary and interdisciplinary approaches, language assessment and training (and other specialized therapy services) are generally provided in a segregated environment (usually a clinic or therapy room). In the transdisciplinary approach they are provided in the classroom and in other natural environments. This has been termed "integrated therapy" (Nietupski, Schutz, & Ockwood, 1980; Sternat, Nietupski, Messina, Lyon, & Brown, 1977).

> "Integrated therapy" can be defined as training in environments where the skill is to be performed.

Nietupski et al. have discussed some of the problems associated with providing services in a segregated environment, called the "isolated therapy model." One problem is the episodic nature of the intervention. In an isolated therapy model, language training sessions are usually provided only two or three times a week, for perhaps 30 minutes per session. This type of brief spaced intervention is rarely effective with severely handicapped students. Similarly, because the conditions of isolated therapy differ so drastically from normal language learning circumstances, this approach is not well suited to the language intervention needs of young language-delayed children. Certainly the language instruction of young nonhandicapped children is not restricted to brief intervals spaced throughout the week; it is, in fact, limited only by their waking hours.

A second problem with isolated therapy conditions has to do with sharing information and skills among therapists and teaching staff. When therapy is provided in a location removed from the classroom, communication specialists often find it difficult to keep teachers abreast of programming procedures and child progress. It is difficult to overemphasize the importance of communication specialist-teacher exchanges, and the expansion of teacher skills; neither is as likely to occur unless language instruction techniques are demonstrated in the classroom.

A third problem with isolated therapy conditions is the potential to impede rather than enhance generalization. Because they rarely demonstrate skill generalization or transfer, it is highly unlikely that severely handicapped students will perform new skills in other than the training environment (Harris, 1975; Stokes & Baer, 1977). This means that many of these students, if trained in a separate therapy room, will not learn to communicate in other environments. Similarly, generalization is a primary concern with young children (Bricker & Carlson, 1980; Mahoney & Weller, 1980); training should be provided in all of the child's potential communication environments and include as many "significant others" as possible.

A fourth related and equally compelling issue has to do with the nature of the language-learning experience. When language training is provided under isolated therapy conditions, the instructional content and procedures are constrained by the limited physical and social context. Verbal exchanges are often unidimensional, with the child in the role of passive respondent rather than active initiator (Mahoney & Weller, 1980), and too often, language instruction centers on objects and pictures from kits that have little or no intrinsic appeal to the child. You remember from Chapters Two and Six that normal communicative exchanges center around familiar activities, objects the child finds especially interesting, caregiving routines, turntaking games, and social rituals. It is difficult to manufacture these "real world" conditions in a therapy room and, as Nietupski et al. (1980) have argued, "a legitimate question can be raised about why it is necessary to create 'real-life' situations in the therapy room, when these situations already exist in the classroom and in the home" (p. 16).

There is a variety of theoretical and practical considerations (e.g., the importance of longitudinal intervention in natural environments, the reality of limited resources and personnel) which suggest the superiority of integrated therapy conditions in most school situations. It must be stressed, however, that the effectiveness of integrated therapy will depend on the professionals involved—specifically, the willingness of communication specialists, teachers, and ancillary personnel to alter traditional beliefs and practices and negotiate new role functions. If there is a commitment to making the integrated therapy model work, there is every reason to believe that the results will be gratifying to all of those involved.

The integrated therapy approach requires some redefinition of traditional role functions.

Nietupski et al. (1980) suggest the following long-range goals for communication specialists and teachers in shifting to an integrated therapy model. For communication specialists, the first task is to consolidate time allocated to individual therapy sessions into several weekly time blocks for each classroom being served. Communication specialist role functions would include:

1. *Consulting* the language and communication needs of all children in the class
2. *Demonstrating/modeling* for the teaching staff to enhance their ability to teach the needed language and communication skills
3. *Assessing* (and possibly providing some direct instruction) to continuously monitor child progress and program effectiveness
4. *Making decisions* related to program development and modifications

Role functions of the teacher would include:

1. *Sharing information* about all aspects of each child's programming
2. *Soliciting suggestions* for incorporation of language and communication objectives into classroom routines and parent training activities
3. *Implementing* language and communication recommendations

4. *Documenting* acquisition, mastery, and generalization

5. *Revising* curricula in line with the communication specialists' suggestions

Such a redefinition of role functions requires teachers, parents, and related services personnel to discard the notion that only therapists can provide therapy. (This is analogous to insisting that only teachers can teach.) There are, of course, some role functions specific to each discipline: for example, assessment and articulation therapy responsibilities will undoubtedly be retained by communication specialists. However, these will be a relatively small subset of the many competencies the specialist brings to the intervention arena. A proportionately greater number of skills can and should be shared with parents and other professionals, paraprofessionals and volunteers. The transdisciplinary team approach provides both a vehicle and a context for this type of sharing.

Consultation   Caplan (1970) describes consultation as ":.. a process of interaction between two professional persons—the consultant and the consultee, who invokes the consultant's help in regard to a current work problem with which he is having some difficulty and which he has decided is within the other's area of specialized competence" (p. 19). What this definition and others fail to mention, and what preservice preparation curricula have failed to target, are the skills required by such a process. Teachers and therapists alike need instruction and practical experiences focused on the dynamics of effective consultative interactions (as well as other forms of professional communication).

Consultation is one means of promoting and initiating workable solutions to the problems of handicapped children; however, it requires specialized skills that many professionals have not had the opportunity to develop.

Professional preservice training programs are beginning to develop consultation competency modules to prepare students for sharing in a mutually supporting atmosphere. Prospective teachers and therapists need background and experiences in areas of human relations such as building trust and taking risks, seeking and providing feedback, listening and communicating, confronting limits and expectations, and negotiating. Leaving acquisition of these skills to chance is unconscionable, because a large part of the job of a professional in human services areas is maintaining good relations with other adults.

There are basically two approaches to consultation: the directive model and the process model (Schein, 1969). The major difference between these two approaches relates to the source of information and how much emphasis is placed on joint problem diagnosis. Directive consultation relies on data collected by the consultant, while the process model focuses on data provided by the consultee. An optimal consultation model would integrate the strengths of both approaches, matching consultation strategies to the problem. The consultant should progress through these steps:

An optimal consultation model would *integrate* directive and process models.

1. Help the consultee precisely define the problem
2. Clarify the level and type of consultant involvement desired

3. Suggest and assist data collection procedures to assess the problem

4. Discuss intervention and evaluation options

5. Seek consensus as to the specific role functions for those involved

6. Assist and monitor implementation and evaluation of the selected strategies

There is no question that productive consultant-consultee exchanges are most difficult when the professionals involved represent different disciplines. It is ironic that the very conditions which constitute the strength of a team of professionals from different disciplines—their diverse backgrounds and skills—are also the major cause of their problems (McCormick, 1982). The potential for role conflicts resulting from arbitrary jurisdictional boundaries and differing emphases is obvious. Communications across disciplines are complicated because the different disciplines usually (McCormick, 1982) (a) hold differing views as to etiology, prognosis, and treatment; (b) use special professional terminology (jargon) to express discipline-specific concepts; and (c) assign different intervention priorities. To compound the problem further, many professionals become defensive when they perceive some threat to their discipline's beliefs and practices.

The intent of this discussion is not to inject a pessimistic outlook, but rather to provide an objective appraisal of some of the factors responsible for counterproductive attitudes and professional conflicts. These problems can be overcome or prevented. For professionals who are willing to invest some time and effort in developing effective reciprocal relationships, the transdisciplinary team approach provides a viable framework for sharing and professional growth. However, it requires (a) attention to team organization procedures; (b) concern for developing and documenting team accountability; (c) commitment to keeping open communication channels; and (d) receptiveness to new and/or different approaches (McCormick, 1982).

TEAM ORGANIZATION AND MANAGEMENT PROCEDURES

A shortcoming of most of the literature on team functioning has been the concentration on describing unique discipline functions, rather than on *team* functions, *team* accountability, and consensus procedures. Another problem, alluded to earlier, is the assumption that participating professionals understand group dynamics and know how to apply group decision-making strategies, role negotiation procedures, and conflict management techniques. This is not usually the case; teachers are not prepared for their seemingly incompatible roles as team leaders, adult trainers, and consultees, and ancillary personnel are not adequately prepared for their roles as team members, adult trainers and consultants. Generally speaking, neither group has been prepared to address the specific requirements of organizing and managing effective work teams as outlined below.

Team composition, tasks, and objectives vary from one team to another; however, it is possible to outline some specific organizational activities and accountability procedures. Table 11-2 presents the three transdisciplinary processes proposed by Lyon and Lyon (1980) and possible outcomes to evaluate whether the processes are actually occurring.

If the three transdisciplinary team processes—joint functioning, continuous staff development, and role release—are occurring, there will be observable outcomes such as those suggested in Table 11-2. These are not the only possible data sources, of course. These are simply examples. There will be other evidence that these processes are occurring—in children's folders, teacher records, and routine reports/logs maintained by ancillary personnel.

The first order of business for any group of individuals who aspire to team status is organization (McCormick, 1982). There are at least three processes that should be undertaken *before* tackling such child-related issues as assessment, curriculum planning, service delivery, and program evaluation. The core group (teaching staff and related services personnel) must reach some consensus on (a) team goals and objectives, (b) functional roles and responsibilities of individual team members, and (c) oper-

> The service delivery team needs to undertake three tasks—goal specification, role negotiation, and definition of ground rules—prior to student-specific problem solving.

TABLE 11-2 Transdisciplinary team processes and outcomes

Process	Measurable Outcomes of These Processes
1. **Joint functioning**—team members perform required service delivery functions together whenever possible	a. Skill cluster approach[1] to *all* programming b. Data in each child's folder (evaluating training and generalization) collected by teachers *and* ancillary personnel c. Documentation of parent contacts and training in teacher *and* ancillary personnel records d. Therapy services, when required, provided in the classroom
2. **Continuous staff development**—team members train and receive training from one another	a. Records of ongoing training needs, assessment, and inservice training by and for all team members b. Teacher notebook/log with questions/concerns addressed to, and answered by, ancillary personnel c. *All* team members competent to provide most services d. Therapy services, when required, provided in the classroom
3. **Role release**—team members share information and functions	a. Skill clusters (in each child's programs) demonstrating input from ancillary personnel b. Changes/adaptations on programs demonstrating input from ancillary staff c. Teacher notebook/log (#2 above) indicating sharing of information d. Other evidence (in daily schedules) that professionals are providing services not traditionally associated with their discipline e. All team members current on each child's programming progress

[1]Note: See Chapters Six and Nine.

ating ground rules (McCormick, 1982). When these issues have been resolved, the core group will be well on the way to becoming a working team.

Initial negotiations should generate two documents, an informal contract specifying the *team's* goals and objectives, and a list of role functions for all participating professionals (Table 11-3). When consensus has been reached on these issues, the team is ready for more specific discussions and the apportioning of responsibilities related to assessment, program development, service delivery, and program evaluation for specific children. Parents, paraprofessionals and volunteers may be included in team meetings at this point.

Table 11-3 is an example of a Team Functioning Agreement developed by one transdisciplinary team. Using the procedures manual *Combining a Transdisciplinary Team Approach with an Individualized Curriculum Sequencing Model for Severely/Multiply Handicapped Children* by Guess, Jones, and Lyon (1981), and the article "Service Delivery Teams: Content and Process Issues" by McCormick (1982) as guides, the team formulated (a) team organization and service delivery objectives, (b) activities to operationalize the team objectives, and (c) possible sources of data to verify that these objectives were being met. The data sources specified on this contract (child, teacher, and ancillary personnel records) are already being routinely maintained, so there is no requirement for additional record keeping.

> It is simply a matter of identifying appropriate sources of data to establish that the team is meeting its goals and objectives.

The team accountability document presented in Table 11-3 could be a model for other service delivery groups. Service delivery objectives and opportioning of responsibilities will, of course, vary from one team to another, depending on a range of variables (e.g., professional representation, severity of student handicapping conditions). At the same time, there will be elements in common across teams.

The next section considers parent involvement, another of the significant and meaningful "extracurricular" responsibilities of teachers and communication specialists. In a way, school-home interactions are similar to interactions among professionals; they have the potential to significantly affect the success of intervention efforts.

SCHOOL-HOME PARTNERSHIPS

> During the past decades there has been a marked increase in attention to the importance of involving families, particularly primary caregivers, in the educational intervention process.

The need for professional-parent interactions to be mandated is regrettable when there are so many logical and ethical reasons for involving parents with the educational process. Beyond simple compliance with legal requirements, there is a considerable rationale, deriving from substantive data generated by normal development research and early intervention programs, for including family members in all assessment, planning, and service delivery activities.

TABLE 11-3 Sample transdisciplinary team functioning agreement

Objectives	Activities	Evaluation Data Sources
A. Team Organization		
1. Reach consensus on team goals	1.1 Formal clarification of team goals—general statements of core missions, e.g., chronological age-appropriate curricula, functional skills development, preparatory curriculum activities, individualized educational programs, arrangements for interactions with nonhandicapped peers and other persons, opportunities for partial participation, curricula which do not rely on instructional inference, home/school interactions, maximum use of instructional time, efficient measurement procedures, and effective teaching techniques	Team contract specifying goals and measurable performance objectives
2. Identify and reach consensus on objectives	2.1 Reach consensus on specific team objectives 2.2 Formulate measurable team functioning objectives for team's responsibility domains—assessment, program development, service delivery, evaluation 2.3 Prioritize objectives in each responsibility domain 2.4 Assign responsibilities for evaluation of objectives	
3. Negotiate role functions	3.1 Participate in role negotiation process (possibly using the "role message" approach) 3.2 Reach agreement on each team member's functions (clarification of each member's contributions in the four responsibility domains)	List of negotiated role functions
4. Identify and reach consensus on team operating procedures	4.1 Discuss importance of an open communication system/information sharing 4.2 Discuss interfering self-oriented behaviors 4.3 Agree on discussion-making procedures—whether unanimous vote or consensus procedures will be used and how subsequent actions will be treated	Notes from organizational meetings delineating team operating procedures

TABLE 11-3 (continued)

Objectives	Activities	Evaluation Data Sources
	4.4 Define group "norms"—attitudes and behaviors that constitute being a "good" versus a "bad" team member	
	4.5 Decide on meeting times and scheduling of other interactions	
B. Service Delivery		
1. Collaborate on assessment efforts	1.1 Teaching staff will conduct general assessments and schedule ancillary staff assessments	Assessment schedule for general and specific assessments
	1.2 Teaching staff will explain to parents and other staff what is being assessed, arrange for them to assist and observe when possible, and interpret results for them	
	1.3 Ancillary staff will conduct in-depth assessments in their respective areas	Record of each student's present level of performance across skill domains
	1.4 Ancillary staff will explain to parents and other staff what is being assessed, arrange for them to assist and observe when possible, and interpret results for them	
2. Collaborate in program development efforts	2.1 Teacher will assume responsibility for development of IEPs—explain the process to parents and instruct them on involvement, collect/share assessment information, schedule/coordinate IEP conferences, write final IEPs	IEPs
	2.2 Teacher will develop instructional clustered skill activity plans with input and feedback from other team members and develop student and classroom schedules	Evidence of ancillary staff input to clustered skill activity plans and schedule
	2.3 Ancillary staff will contribute to IEP development in areas related to their expertise, including the provision of procedures to measure progress in their recommended skill targets	Evidence of ancillary staff input to IEP objectives

TABLE 11-3 (continued)

Objectives	Activities	Evaluation Data Sources
	2.4 Ancillary staff will assist in allocating instructional time, prioritizing objectives, and specifying caregiving procedures	
	2.5 Ancillary staff will assist in developing clustered skill activities and scheduling	
	2.6 Ancillary staff will determine the training that teaching staff need to perform specific functions related to their respective disciplines or areas of expertise	Needs assessment by ancillary staff of teaching staff's training needs
3. Collaborate in service delivery efforts	3.1 Teacher will assure that programs, activities, and caregiving procedures are implemented and evaluated as planned	Ongoing programs, activities, and caregiving procedures related to IEPs and activity schedules;
	3.2 Teacher will assure that the physical environment is arranged to facilitate learning and assign routine "housekeeping" tasks	Schedule for routine "housekeeping" tasks
	3.3 Teacher will maintain communications with and among parents and provide instruction to parents and paraprofessionals	Home-school communications in diaries
	3.4 Teacher will decide when to change/modify programs and activities with input from ancillary staff and parents	Evidence of joint decision making re: change/modification of student programs/activities;
	3.5 Ancillary staff will train the teaching staff and parents to perform specific functions related to their respective disciplines or areas of expertise	Evidence of training teaching staff
	3.6 Ancillary staff will continuously monitor and provide assistance with programming strategies, materials, and equipment and caregiving procedures related to their respective disciplines or areas of expertise	Evidence of ancillary staff response to observed programming, equipment and caregiving inadequacies and teaching staff questions/concerns
	3.7 Ancillary staff will respond to questions and concerns of teaching staff and parents as these concerns relate to their respective disciplines	

TABLE 11-3 (continued)

Objectives	Activities	Evaluation Data Sources
	3.8 Ancillary staff will continuously monitor and evaluate the performance of functions related to their respective areas of expertise to identify training and development needs	Ongoing training needs assessment
4. Collaborate in program evaluative efforts	4.1 Teacher will assure data collection, analyses, and feedback of data for decision making	Current data on all student program/activities and program modification where indicated
	4.2 Teacher will assure full implementation of evaluation procedures as specified on IEPs	
	4.3 Teacher will train and assist other team members and parents in the collection of data and monitoring of health-related information as needed	Current health-related data where required
	4.4 Teacher will design, construct and maintain graphs and other reporting devices with assistance from other team members	Current graphs for ongoing programs/activities (student records)
	4.5 Teacher will interpret evaluation data to other team members to assist team decision making and make necessary program changes as necessary	Evidence of data justification and ancillary staff input into program/activity changes
	4.6 Ancillary staff will provide input and assistance for data collection and program changes	
	4.7 Ancillary staff will participate in IEP reviews, updating, and revisions	Evidence of ancillary staff participation in IEP reviews/updating/revisions when appropriate
	4.8 Ancillary staff will assist development of forms for and monitoring of health-related records	Appropriate forms for health-related data

NORMAL DEVELOPMENT RATIONALE

As discussed in Chapter Two, one of the more interesting developments in the study of language/communication acquisition has been the parent-child interaction data. It is difficult to justify exclusion of parents from the intervention process when, in fact, the family is the natural teaching/learning context. Caregivers are ideally suited to be their children's teachers and/or consultants to the professionals who share concerns for their children. Their participation can make the difference between adequate and inadequate programming.

EARLY INTERVENTION RESEARCH RATIONALE

The most successful early intervention programs in the past decade have been those supporting caregivers as primary teachers and working to strengthen parent-child and family relationships (Bronfenbrenner, 1974; Gray, 1971; Lazar, 1977; Schaefer, 1972). Research and experience have demonstrated that parents are natural reinforcing agents and generalization facilitators (Hayden, 1976; Lillie, 1975; Shearer & Shearer,1977), and that intervention with parents benefits siblings as well as the target child (Goodson & Hess, 1975). Parent involvement takes many forms in early intervention programs; however, the one feature that successful programs share is commitment to the concept of parent-professional partnership, meeting the needs of the family, as well as of the child.

LEGAL RATIONALE

There are also legislative and legal bases for current parent involvement practices. P.L. 94-142 mandates involvement of parents in the processes of identification, diagnosis, placement, and programming for every child receiving special educational services. A parent participation philosophy also permeates the Head Start legislation (O'Keefe, 1979).

TYPES OF PARENT INVOLVEMENT

The concept of parent involvement is broadening and, at the same time, becoming more flexible. There is general acknowledgment of changing life styles and modified family patterns and a new sensitivity to family needs. As Foster, Berger, and McLean (1981) state, there is no longer any basis for the assumption that "mothers are the primary caretakers for their children, that caring for children is the major or sole employment of most mothers, that children are raised by their two biological parents, and that fathers show their concern for their children through participation in organizational efforts such as fund raising, meeting with legislators, and so forth" (p. 57). The demise of traditional households, with the mother at home and the father employed, does not mean that there is less desire on the part of parents to be involved in their children's education and development; however, it does point out the need to be more flexible in parent involvement activities.

Parent involvement no longer implies particular types of activities.

Most parents enter into a cooperative relationship easily if they feel they are contributing members of a team trying to do what is best for their child.

A review of the literature by Welsh and Odum (1981) found five prevalent forms of parent involvement:

1. Parents receive social and emotional support from program staff and other parents (including aid in obtaining needed economic help and social services)

2. Parents participate in program planning, policy making, evaluation, dissemination of program information, and promotion of legislative action

3. Parents provide child data to facilitate reliable assessment and valid programming

4. Parents learn to work with their own child at school and at home (following demonstrations of appropriate interactions and teaching techniques)

5. Parents serve as observers, aides, and volunteers in the classroom

It is less important how parents participate than that they are involved—that whatever roles they want to play in their child's education, and whatever activities they want to participate in, are available to them and valued by professionals.

GUIDELINES FOR PROFESSIONAL-PARENT INTERACTIONS

Parents should (and, according to the law, *must*) have the opportunity to become involved at all stages of the intervention process. Begin with the assumption that parents want what is best for their child and assume responsibility for establishing an open, supportive, and accepting atmosphere. The vast majority of parents will chose to involve themselves at some level in their children's education. Professionals must realize that the extent of this involvement depends on many factors, such as the needs of other family members, economic pressures, and the amount of child-related stress the family is experiencing. The important thing is to give parents an opportunity to be involved at the following stages.

AT THE ASSESSMENT STAGE

Parents are primary informants and "validators" of information from other sources.

The purposes of professional-parent interactions at the assessment stage are (a) consolidation of data pertinent to development of a valid and comprehensive IEP, and (b) establishment of ongoing information-sharing practices. Swick and Hobson (1978) suggest that professionals can maximize the potential for productive and positive interactions by being:

1. *Approachable:* ready to listen to parents' ideas and generally open to both verbal and nonverbal communications

2. *Flexible:* willing to make necessary adjustments to accommodate to parents' schedules

3. *Sensitive:* responsive and sympathetic to parents' pressures and
unique coping styles

4. *Dependable:* reliably and consistently supportive of parent perspectives

To supplement language/communication information from formal
assessment procedures, history profiles, and parent interviews, communication specialists and teachers may schedule opportunities to observe the
child's interactions with various family members in naturalistic settings
(see Chapter Four). These observations can be of considerable value.
They can provide important perspectives on the quality of caregiver-child
interactions and sibling-target child relationships.

P.L. 94-142 sets forth procedural guidelines that bring the parents
into the assessment process. Parent consent must be obtained before
preplacement evaluation, and parents must be informed of their right to
examine all relevant records and reports concerning their child and obtain
an independent evaluation if so desired. To comply with regulations and
assure full understanding on the part of parents, it is often desirable to set
up a preassessment conference and review the procedural safeguards of
the legislation. Keep in mind that there is a difference between obtaining a
signature giving approval for testing and informed consent as defined in
P.L. 94-142.

AT THE PLANNING STAGE

Membership on the IEP committee is intended to provide parents with the
opportunity to (a) specify the services they want for their child, (b) share information they consider relevant to their child's education, (c) participate
in the placement decision, and (d) indicate to what extent they are willing
and able to become directly involved in the intervention process (Turnbull,
1978). In practice, unless parents have been prepared for this level of participation (their role in the IEP process and the reasons for the IEP conference), they may not fully appreciate and use this opportunity to affect the
planning process.

*Unless professionals pre-
pare parents for their role
on the IEP committee, they
may not fully appreciate
and take advantage of this
opportunity to influence
programming directions.*

Turnbull (1978) suggests providing parents with a list of questions to
be thinking about before the IEP conference, such as:

1. What specific skills would you like your child to learn?
2. Do you have specific concerns about your child's home behavior
which school programming could address?
3. What do you see as your child's strengths and weaknesses?
4. What objects and events would you consider to be rewarding for
your child?
5. How do you feel about your child having opportunities to interact
with nonhandicapped children?

Additional questions specifically addressing communication skills might include:

6. How would you feel about your child being provided with an augmentative communication system (manual signing or a communication board), if such strategies were considered by professionals to be appropriate?
7. When, where, and with whom does your child interact most often?
8. What specific communication skills would you view as most useful to your child?

If parents enter the IEP planning process knowing what to expect, their contributions will be more useful and the resulting document will be more meaningful and appropriate. The key to creating a conference atmosphere where everyone is comfortable and communicative is advance planning and preparation.

AT THE SERVICE DELIVERY STAGE

Under ideal circumstances each school would provide a parent involvement specialist to coordinate home-school activities and assume major responsibility for parent counseling and training. In practice, because of limited resources, this is rarely the case. This means that teachers and ancillary personnel must consider parent interactions as a part of their responsibilities.

If adequately prepared for and encouraged to contribute at the assessment and planning stages, most parents will also participate, at some level, in programming. Professional-parent interactions at the service delivery stage may be characterized in somewhat the same way as interactions among professionals in the transdisciplinary team process. Parents and professionals should perform required programming functions together whenever possible, and parents should receive training to maximize their skills and effectiveness in teaching and managing their children and facilitating generalization. Reciprocally, parents should share relevant information with professionals and teach professionals any special techniques found to positively influence the behavior of their children at home and in other nonschool environments.

It is most important to assess and respond to parents' expressed needs and interests, rather than attempting to coax and/or coerce involvement in activities that are presumed to be beneficial. In a recent study, Winton and Turnbull (1981) surveyed parents regarding their actual desires to be involved in various program aspects (as opposed to what others have assumed to be their participation choices). Information was collected on a sample of 31 mothers' attitudes toward the following eight activities: (a) volunteer outside the class, (b) volunteer inside the class, (c) serve on policy board, (d) parent training opportunities, (e) parent coun-

There are many parallels between professional interactions in the transdisciplinary model and parent-professional interactions.

seling opportunities, (f) informal contact with teachers, (g) opportunities to help others understand child, (h) no role, if desired.

Almost a fifth of the parents, 19 percent, indicated that they liked having the choice of not participating (no role). These parents said that they did not necessarily dislike the other activities; it was simply that they appreciated the option of *not* being involved sometimes when noninvolvement seemed to be in their own and their families' best interests. The parents' need not to be involved is not evidence of lack of concern or involvement with their child. It is certainly a legitimate parent prerogative, and one which should be treated with respect. Informal involvement options, such as home-school notebooks, and telephone contacts are alternatives to direct involvement.

> Professionals should not assume that all parents want or need to participate in all activities or at all times.

Another finding of interest from the Winton and Turnbull study was that the activity most preferred by the greatest number of mothers was informal contacts with their child's teachers. In describing these contacts, the mothers emphasized (a) that they liked them to be frequent (e.g., at drop-off and pick-up time), and (b) that they liked informal *sharing* of information.

Most parents will choose to allocate some time, energy, and resources for active participation in programming. Vincent, Dodd, and Henner (1978) have provided a comprehensive outline for planning and implementing a program for these families. Though originally developed in a program for severely and profoundly handicapped students, these guidelines apply equally well to developing services for families of young handicapped children. This outline could very easily be made into a planning checklist.

> When parents express interest in a formal parent program with regular meetings and planned activities, one should be provided.

I. Plan program goals
   A. Seek input from parents
   B. Formulate tentative goals and objectives
   C. Outline possible activities to attain the goals
   D. Involve supervisors and obtain preliminary support and cooperation
   E. Set a time line for program review by appropriate administrators

II. Identify potential referral/assistance resources
   A. Compile a list of community agencies concerned with handicapped children and their families
   B. Contact the agencies and find out
      1. eligibility
      2. cost
      3. time between referral and service delivery
      4. information requested at referral
      5. relative emphasis on episodic versus longitudinal intervention
   C. Record and file the information so that it is easily retrievable

III. Prepare for the first meeting
   A. Set a time and invite the parents
   B. Determine parents needing transportation and arrange to provide it
   C. Arrange for child care during the meeting (for students and siblings)
   D. Arrange for physical space—if possible, set aside a specific parent room
   E. Send reminder home (after the initial invitation) with clearly stated purpose of the meeting

IV. Conduct the first meeting
   A. Give parents reason for hope and optimism and some idea of the work that will be needed to help their children
   B. Introduce the parents-as-partners construct and discuss the natural teaching-learning relationship between parent and child
   C. Discuss the learning and practice of new techniques to improve the *quality* of the time they spend with their children
   D. Present a prospective agenda for the next meeting and solicit suggestions
   E. Specifically ask parents if they will return for a second meeting

Eventually, the parents themselves may assume responsibility for planning and conducting the meetings. However, this management shift should occur gradually over time as the parents become more competent and independent, not all at once. The most important concern initially must be to establish trust and provide parents with support, knowledge, and access to resources.

There are numerous commercially available language training programs that are specifically designed for parent implementation.

Parent involvement in language/communication programming   In addition to generally supporting and consulting to parents, and keeping them informed about their child's educational progress and trends in the field, teachers and ancillary personnel may assume direct parent training responsibilities. There is a particularly strong justification for involving parents in their child's language programming. In fact, some commercially available language training programs are specifically designed for parent implementation. For example:

1. "Managing behavior 8, Behavior modification: Teaching speech to a nonverbal child"
Developed by: S.L. Harris
Published by: H and H Enterprises, Inc., Lawrence, Kansas
This book presents a four stage program: I. Teaching Attention, II. Teaching Nonverbal Skills, III. Teaching Verbal Imitation, IV. Teaching Functional Speech. Though designed primarily for use with autistic children, the procedures are easily adapted and appropriate for other nonverbal children.

2. "Ready, set, go: Talk to me"
Developed by: D. Horstmeier and J. MacDonald
Published by: Charles E. Merrill Publishing Co., Columbus, Ohio
This program is designed for use by parents or teachers, with consultation from a communication specialist. It is a noncategorical program intended for young children who have not learned prelanguage and initial verbal communication skills. A diagnostic screening test is provided to assist selection of specific targets. The program includes prescriptive packets for (a) preliminary skills, (b) functional play, (c) motor imitation, (d) receptive procedures—objects, (e) receptive procedures—actions, (f) following directions, (g) sound imitation, (h) single word production, and (i) beginning social conversation.

Many parents welcome the opportunity to work toward specific language and communication targets. Presumably they have already been given the opportunity to contribute to development of their child's goals and objectives at the planning stage. With encouragement and support, they can also contribute to selection of teaching strategies and reinforcers and, particularly with very young children, assume a primary language/communication training role.

Among the programs to help parents become the primary language intervention agents for their children, Hart's (in press) milieu therapy model is worthy of special consideration. This model is based on the premise that handicapped children do not acquire language in naturally occurring situations because they are deficient in the social and cognitive learning strategies required to benefit from typical caregiver-child interaction contexts. The broad goal of the training program, called "Incidental Language Teaching," is to arrange the caregiver-child interactions to facilitate the child's development of interactional strategies and generalized use of new skills. There are five teaching strategies (as outlined below), along with some guidelines to follow in training parents to use these strategies with their children. Each technique should be thoroughly explained to parents and then demonstrated. Application should be monitored continuously. The parents' training may take place in the classroom, at home, or in some other convenient location.

Hart has provided some guidelines for parents to use in facilitating their child's communication strategies.

1. Arranging the environment   There are three steps in this technique, which is designed to encourage child verbal initiations and responses. The first step is to identify a set of materials that the child finds interesting and desirable. These reinforcing materials should be placed within view, but out of the child's reach, so that requesting (either assistance or the stimuli) becomes obligatory. Once the child is consistently requesting assistance or materials, the third step is to improve the quality of the request. The parent makes assistance and/or the desired objects contingent upon more intelligible, complex, or semantically correct request forms (depending upon the child's level).

2. Child-directed modeling The technique of child-directed modeling has five primary goals: (a) establishing joint attention as a cue for verbalization, (b) teaching turn-taking skills, (c) training generalized imitation skills, (d) developing and expanding vocabulary, and (e) teaching generalized conversational skills. The first step is to establish joint attention on an object or event the child is interested in (or something the parent has selected as an appropriate discussion topic). Then, while manipulating the object, the parent models a word (or words) to be imitated. An imitation (or approximation) is reinforced by expanding the child's utterance and offering the object. If the child does not respond, or responds with an unintelligible, incorrect, or unrelated response, the procedure is repeated. If the second trial is not successful in eliciting an appropriate imitation, the parent provides corrective feedback (the desired response), provides the object, and repeats the three-trial process.

3. Manding and modeling When the child is consistently imitating the parents' models and has at least a limited spontaneous vocabulary, the third technique, called "manding," is begun. Manding is a behavioral term (Skinner, 1957), used in this context to refer to an instruction to verbalize or imitate. Parents may ask for old information (information that the child has demonstrated sometime in the past) or new information. In the latter case, the parent asks a question and then provides a model of the correct response for the child to imitate.

The first step in this procedure, as in child-directed modeling, is to establish joint attention. Then the parent mands for a verbalization about the target stimulus (e.g., "Tell me what that is," or "Tell me what you're doing.") A correct response is praised and expanded, and the child is given access to the stimulus object. If the child does not respond or responds incorrectly, the parent may provide either a corrective mand or a corrective model for the desired response. If a corrective model is presented and the child again responds incorrectly, the parent should present a second corrective model.

4. Time delay The purpose of a time delay procedure is to teach the child to initiate interactions. Rather than telling the child what to say (modeling) or asking her what she wants (manding), in the arranged environment the parent takes a position near to the child and looks at her to indicate a willingness to listen. The parent should delay at least five seconds. If the child initiates a request, comment, or question, the parent praises, expands the utterance, and provides the stimulus object. The parent may delay a second time or shift to modeling or manding for an incorrect response.

Chapter Seven provides additional suggestions for parent-implemented communication training.

5. Incidental teaching Incidental teaching procedures are also applied to prompt more elaborate and complex utterances and improve conversational skills. In the arranged environment (a setting with preferred, high interest stimuli), the parent applies one or all of the techniques (modeling, manding, or time-delay) to elicit more sophisticated responses and additional information about the stimulus object(s).

By the time parents have reached this last technique, the child has learned to respond appropriately to and initiate requests, turn-taking skills, and more complex structures. The parents have learned a technology for, and demonstrated their competencies in, teaching social-communication skills.

When intervention involves an augmentative communication system, parent involvement is no longer optional: as many family members as possible *must* be trained if the system is to be truly functional for the child. Chapter Ten suggests reasons for, and ways of dealing with, caregivers' resistance to introduction of an augmentative system. Most important to keep in mind is that, as stated earlier, even if the caregivers did not have the right, by law, to reject programming proposals, success of the intervention is seriously threatened without their full cooperation. If the parents feel they cannot commit the time and effort augmentative communication requires, then it should not be attempted. The symbols and procedures learned at school must be functional for the child in other environments, or school programming time is virtually wasted.

When parents approve introduction of an augmentative system, their preparation for successful interactions with a nonverbal child may be approached through one (or all) of the following formats (Musselwhite & St. Louis, 1982):

1. Lecture-discussion sessions
2. Hands-on demonstrations and modeling
3. Role-playing

The skills parents and other family members will need to be appropriate "listeners" for a nonverbal child will vary according to the type of augmentative technique and device adopted (Harris, 1982). Some types of simple communication boards require the "listener" to assume an active role in message formulation and expression. More sophisticated devices, such as electronic prosthesis with printouts, require less participation by the "listener." Though this may seem to be an advantage, most consider it a disadvantage of many of the more sophisticated devices: they take the social element out of interactions. The "listener" may not even be present when the message is composed (Harris, 1982).

Shane and Cohen (1981) have described some of the nonproductive communicative interaction patterns that can occur between augmentative communication users and communicative partners. It is important for parents and other potential "listeners" to be aware of these phenomena, since they have the potential to undermine programming efforts. (Interestingly enough, these same phenomena can be observed when naive communicators interact with foreign language speakers.) Those who interact with nonverbal children should guard against these unproductive behaviors:

Family involvement is imperative when an augmentative communication system is involved.

Through training and practice, parents and other communication partners can learn appropriate interpretive and "listening" skills.

1. using unnecessarily simple structures and vocabulary
2. feigning comprehension
3. anticipating answers and speaking *for* the nonspeaking persons
4. speaking louder than necessary

Finally, you should emphasize these critical points with parents, whether their children are learning vocal or nonvocal communication systems. First, unless children are placed in the position of having to understand and use language, language growth will be minimal. Second, how consistently they stimulate and respond to their children's communicative efforts will significantly affect the learning process. Third, whether language and communication skills trained at school generalize to the home and other environments will depend largely upon the parents' ability to make the skills functional for the child in those settings.

Appropriate use of the combined knowledge and expertise of parents, ancillary personnel, and teaching staff can add up to a quality program. However, there is more to it than being consistently available and prepared to talk with one another; there must be a sensitivity to one another's needs, exchange of ideas and sharing of functions to maximize programming efforts. In the final analysis, the only factor sufficiently powerful to dissolve professional-parent partnerships in special education should be their success. When the child is no longer in need of special services, the partnership can be dissolved—it has successfully accomplished all of its goals.

SUMMARY

1. P.L. 94-142 provides for four types of working teams: one to coordinate and monitor all mandated procedures, a second to assess and formulate eligibility procedures, a third to plan and write the IEP, and a fourth to deliver services.

2. Service delivery teams may organize according to multidisciplinary, interdisciplinary, or transdisciplinary models; the transdisciplinary approach is characterized by joint functioning, continuous staff development, and role release.

3. Disadvantages of the isolated therapy model include episodic intervention, logistical barriers to sharing information and skills, lack of generalization, and the artificial nature of the training conditions.

4. An optimal consultation approach is one that uses both directive and process procedures, depending upon the nature of the problem.

5. The team should reach consensus on team goals and objectives, functional roles and responsibilities, and operating rules before tackling child related issues such as assessment, planning, service delivery, and program evaluation.

6. There are at least three very good reasons for involving parents in the education of handicapped children—normal development data, the findings of early intervention research, and legislative and legal requirements.

7. Parents should have the opportunity to become involved at all levels of the intervention process—assessment, planning, and service delivery. They should have the option of not being involved.

8. The "Incidental Language Teaching" program provides specific guidelines to aid parents in facilitating their child's development of interactional strategies and generalized use of new skills.

9. As many family members as possible *must* be involved in implementing an augmentative communication system, or programming will not be generally effective.

10. Parents and professionals alike must guard against nonproductive and atypical listener behaviors with nonspeaking persons.

11. Two related themes are stressed as central to parent involvement: (a) the importance of taking into account the needs, skills, *and* desires of the parents, and (b) the importance of professional-parent reciprocity.

REFERENCES

ALLEN, K.E., HOLM, V.A., & SCHIEFELBUSCH, R.L. *Early intervention—A team approach.* Baltimore: University Park Press, 1978.

BRICKER, D., & CARLSON, L. An intervention approach for communicatively handicapped infants and young children. *New directions for exceptional children.* San Francisco: Jossey-Bass, Inc., 1980, *2,* 33–48.

BRONFENBRENNER, U. Is early intervention effective? *Teachers College Record,* 1974, *76*(2), 279–303.

CAPLAN, G. *The theory and practice of mental health consultation.* New York: Basic Books, 1970.

FENTON, K.S., YOSHIDA, R.K., MAXWELL, J.B., & KAUFFMAN, M.J. Recognition of team goals: An essential step toward rational decision making. *Exceptional Children,* 1979, *45,* 638–644.

FOSTER, M., BERGER, M., & McLEAN, M. Rethinking a good idea: A reassessment of parent involvement. *Topics in Early Childhood Special Education,* 1981, *1*(3), 55–65.

GOODSON, B.D., & HESS, R.D. *Parents as teachers of young children: An evaluative review of some contemporary concepts and programs.* Washington, D.C.: Bureau of Educational Personnel Development, DHEW/OE, 1975. (ERIC Document Reproduction Service No. ED 136 967)

GRAY, S.W. The child's first teacher. *Childhood Education,* 1971, *48*(3), 127–129.

GUESS, D., JONES, C., & LYON, S. *Combining a transdisciplinary team approach with an individualized curriculum sequencing model of severely/ multiply handicapped children: A procedures manual.* Lawrence, Kans.: University of Kansas, 1981.

HARRIS, D. Communicative interaction processes involving nonvocal physically handicapped children. *Topics in Language Disorders,* 1982, *2*(2), 21–37.

HARRIS, S.L. Teaching language to nonverbal children—with emphasis on problems of generalization. *Psychological Bulletin,* 1975, *82,* 565–580.

HART, B., Incidental strategies. In R.L. Schiefelbusch (Ed.), *Communicative Competence: Assessment and Intervention.* Baltimore: University Park Press, in press.

HAYDEN, A.H. A center-based parent-training model. In D.L. Lillie, P.L. Trohanis, & K.W. Goin (Eds.), *Teaching parents to teach.* New York: Walker, 1976.

HUTCHISON, D. A model for transdisciplinary staff development (A nationally organized collaborative project to provide comprehensive services for atypical infants and their families). A monograph: *Technical Report 8, 1974.*

LAZAR, I. *The persistence of preschool effects: A long-term follow-up of fourteen infant and preschool experiments. Final report.* Washington, D.C.: Administration for Children, Youth and Families (DHEW), 1977. (ERIC Document Reproduction Service No. ED 148 470)

LILLIE, D.L. The parent in early childhood education. *Journal of Research and Development in Education,* 1975, *8*(2), 7–12.

LYON, S., & LYON, G. Team functioning and staff development: A role release approach to providing integrated educational services for severely handicapped students. *JASH,* 1980, *5*(3), 250–263.

MAHONEY, G., & WELLER, E. An ecological approach to language intervention. *New Directions for Exceptional Children,* 1980, *2,* 17–32.

McCORMICK, L. Service delivery teams: Content and process issues. In N. Haring & M. Noel (Eds.), *Progress or change: Issues in educating the emotionally disturbed* (Vol. 2: Service Delivery). Seattle: University of Washington, 1982.

McCORMICK, L., & GOLDMAN, R. The transdisciplinary model: Implications for service delivery and personnel preparation for the severely and profoundly handicapped. *AAESPH Review,* 1979, *4*(2), 152–161.

MUSSELWHITE, C.R., & ST. LOUIS, K.W. *Communication programming for the severely handicapped: Vocal and non-vocal strategies.* Houston, Tex.: College-Hill Press, 1982.

NIETUPSKI, J., SCHEUTZ, G., & OCKWOOD, L. The delivery of communication therapy services to severely handicapped students: A plan for change. *Journal of the Association for the Severely Handicapped,* 1980, *5*(1), 13–23.

O'KEEFE, A. What head start means to families? (Department of Health, Education, and Welfare, Pub. No. OHDS 79-31129). Washington, D.C.: Government Printing Office, 1979.

SCHAEFER, E.S. Parents as educators: Evidence from cross-sectional, longitudinal, and intervention research. In W.W. Hartup (Ed.), *The young child: Review of research* (Vol. 2). Washington, D.C.: National Association for the Education of Young Children, 1972.

SCHEIN, E.H. *Process consultation: Its role in organization development.* Reading, Mass.: Addison-Wesley, 1969.

SEARS, C.J. The transdisciplinary approach: A process for compliance with Public Law 94-142. *Journal of the Association for the Severely Handicapped,* 1981, *6*(1), 22–29.

SHANE, H.C., & COHEN, C.G. A discussion of communicative strategies and patterns by nonspeaking persons. *Language, Speech, and Hearing Services in Schools,* 1981, *12*(4), 205–210.

SHEARER, M.S., & SHEARER, D.E. Parent involvement. In J.B. Jordan, A.H. Hayden, M.B. Karnes, & M.M. Wood (Eds.), *Early childhood education for exceptional children: A handbook of ideas and exemplary practices.* Reston, Va.: The Council for Exceptional Children, 1977.

SKINNER, B.F. *Verbal behavior.* New York: Appleton-Century-Crofts, 1957.

STERNAT, J., MESSINA, R., NIETUPSKI, J., LYON, S., & BROWN, L. Occupational and physical therapy services for severely handicapped students: Toward a naturalized public school service delivery mode. In E. Sontag, J.J. Smith, & N. Certo (Eds.), *Educational programming for the severely and profoundly handicapped.* Reston, Va.: Council for Exceptional Children, 1977.

STOKES, T.F., & BAER, D.M. An implicit technology of generalization. *Journal of Applied Behavior Analysis,* 1977, *10,* 349–367.

SWICK, K.J., & HOBSON, C.F. Working relationships: Parents and teachers. Champaign, Ill.: Stipes Publishing Co., 1978.

TURNBULL, A.P. Parent-professional interactions. In M.E. Snell (Ed.), *Systematic instruction of the moderately and severely handicapped.* Columbus: Charles E. Merrill, 1978.

TURNBULL, A.P., STRICKLAND, B., & BRANTLEY, J. *Developing and implementing individualized education programs.* Columbus: Charles E. Merrill, 1978.

VINCENT, L.J., DODD, N., & HENNER, P.J. Planning and implementing a program of parent involvement. *Teaching the Severely Handicapped,* 1978, *3,* 282–297.

WELSH, M.M., & ODUM, C.S.H. Parent involvement in the education of the handicapped child: A review of the literature. *Journal of the Division for Early Childhood,* 1981, *3,* 15–25.

WINTON, P.J., & TURNBULL, A.P. Parent involvement as viewed by parents of preschool handicapped children. *Topics in Early Childhood Special Education,* 1981, *1*(3), 11–19.

YOSHIDA, R.K., FENTON, J.S., MAXWELL, J.P., & KAUFFMAN, M.J. Group decision making in the planning team process: Myth or reality? *Journal of School Psychology,* 1978, *16,* 237–244.

CONCLUSION

ADAPTING AN IDEAL TO THE CONSTRAINTS OF THE REAL WORLD

Richard L. Schiefelbusch and Linda McCormick

M ost published language intervention programs have been carefully planned, implemented, and validated to assure that they do what they were designed to do—teach language. They both contribute to and draw from research technology and theory, as well as our knowledge of language. The problem facing teachers and communication specialists is analysis and synthesis of these programs to answer "real world" questions such as who, when, where, and how to develop effective and efficient language intervention services. There is no simple solution or formula for translating research information into guidelines, but this summary chapter provides suggestions for organizing the available information. We will also briefly review the programming suggestions in Chapter Seven (infant intervention), Chapter Eight (preschool intervention for language delayed children), and Chapter Nine (intervention with the severely handicapped).

A DESIGN

There is no such thing as one program to meet the intervention needs of all language delayed/deficient children. Some need communication training, others need speech training, and still others need training in the basic semantic functions and vocabulary. In the face of this diversity, what we need is an organizational design flexible enough to incorporate individual programs for each child.

A design is defined (in this context) as a system with three basic subsystems: (a) the program *environment*, (b) program *strategies*, and (c) program *operations* (Schiefelbusch, 1983). Its purpose is to do the things necessary to produce important and desired outcomes. Its source is the theoretical and applied research literatures.

PROGRAM ENVIRONMENTS

In Chapter Six the instructional environment was defined as essentially a context to enhance and support learning. Program environments should be flexible, age-appropriate and functional—a context for generalization as well as for acquisition and practice. Alone, or in combination, they include the classroom, playground, clinic (in some instances), home, grocery store, etc. Because the purposes of language intervention vary, the environments must also vary.

A preschool classroom arranged to optimize communicative interactions is an example of a program environment.

The cues, consequences, and materials of most natural environments are maximal for language learning for most children, including many who are language-impaired. For others, there may be a need to arrange prosthetic environments. These contexts should include features to compensate for the child's learning problems and prepare him for functioning in natural contexts. Cues, consequences, and materials in these artificial environments should simulate as nearly as possible those in natural environments.

The environments described in Chapters Seven, Eight, and Nine meet these important criteria. The environment for the infant program described in Chapter Seven is an early childhood demonstration center, but every effort is made to simulate the conditions of normal language learning. Caregivers are taught to arrange their interactions in the home (mostly caregiving and play activities) to profit from what we know about infant language learning.

The language programs described in this book use multiple environments.

The primary program environment for the language impaired children described in Chapter Eight is the preschool classroom. However, parents are also taught how to arrange instruction in the home. In this preschool environment, all activities (e.g., free play, arts and crafts, snack time) are arranged and used for instructional purposes.

Chapter Nine emphasizes the use of natural contexts and routine activities for the language instruction of severely handicapped students. The unique aspect of the ICS model described in that chapter is its integration of divergent theoretical approaches, and the teaching of skill clusters across developmental domains. Rather than dividing the curriculum and the school day into traditional development areas (e.g., social, motor, language), the ICS approach focuses on the activity parameters and natural skill sequences inherent in routine activities.

PROGRAM STRATEGIES

Program strategy decisions have to do with what to teach and how to teach it. Both types of decisions require substantial information about the strengths and capabilities of the child and the purposes of intervention. The purpose of designing strategy is to adapt the language program to fit the child, rather than requiring the impaired child to learn a standard program in a standard way.

Program strategies reflect prevailing research and theory: they include early intervention (described in Chapters Seven and Eight), nonspeech intervention (described in Chapter Ten), milieu or incidental teaching (described in Chapter Eleven), developmental intervention (also described in Chapters Seven and Eight), and remedial intervention (described in Chapter Nine). Each of these broad strategies includes a variety of unique teaching procedures—arrangements to increase the probability of achieving important and desired outcomes.

PROGRAM OPERATIONS

Program operations denote the purposeful system for teaching language to a child. The system can be broken down into five functional categories: planning, development, maintenance, evaluation, and generalization. These operations are common across all intervention programs regardless of goals, design and strategies.

Program planning   Program planning is usually based on initial assessments of the child's language functioning and other related case information relevant to the child's language learning.

Planning is based upon initial assessment.

Chapters Four and Five discuss assessment and planning. Attention is focused on the IEP process, procedures for asking instructionally relevant questions, and atypical learning strategies.

Each of the programs described in Chapters Seven, Eight, Nine, and Ten provides an initial assessments plan for children individually. The tactics vary among and within programs to accommodate differences among the children.

Program development   Program development refers to the systematic plan followed in teaching language to any child. Chapter Eight discusses the language program under the heading of "Curriculum Design." It includes fine- and gross-motor skills, personal social skills, listening and attending skills, language and perceptual skills, and preacademic skills.

Chapter Nine describes a language curriculum for severely handicapped children. This curriculum features functional communication skills that would occur naturally in the child's environment.

Program maintenance refers to effective continuing management of the training activities.

Program maintenance   Since language training programs may extend over a substantial period of time, the teacher or clinician may need to give careful attention to motivation strategies (Schiefelbush, 1976; 1981). *Maintenance* includes the implicit interest that the training activities provide, as well as the contingencies that are applied to increase functional responding. (In Chapter Eight, maintenance features are discussed under the heading, How to Structure Training.)

Clinical hunches may be useful to guide preliminary choices of procedure, but they cannot substitute for direct, objective information about the effects of instruction.

Program evaluation   Program evaluation might also be called continuing assessment. The importance of such assessments is developed in Chapter Four.

Program generalization   Each of the language programs in this book (Chapters Seven, Eight and Nine) gives careful attention to generalization issues. In Chapter Seven caregivers are active participants in a range of natural activities and functions. In Chapter Eight the teachers and parents share in extending the contextual language activities to other settings. In Chapter Nine they use an individualized curriculum sequencing model to teach for generalization. The important issue common to each of these programs is the generalization to new circumstances that require a broad range of language uses.

CHANGING IDEALS

Language intervention environments, strategies, and operations change over the years to reflect the information generated by basic and applied research. In the past decade, ideals have generally shifted from formal, artificial, and contrived arrangements to informal, natural intervention designs. There has been considerable growth in our knowledge *about* language, and about how, when and where to teach it. A major shift in primary training agents has also occurred. Verbal behavior is no longer the exclusive province of speech pathologists; training responsibilities are now shared by teachers, parents, and other significant adults in the child's life.

The role of the speech pathologist has changed from that of an itinerant clinician working directly and individually with a large number of children to that of a specialist with responsibilities for (a) consultation, (b) demonstration/modeling, (c) assessment, and (d) program decision making (Nietupski, Scheutz, & Ockwood, 1980). The specialist also may provide inservice training in areas related to language and communication.

> The specialist is responsible for assessment, demonstration, and monitoring functions.

We are tentative in our description of language/communication specialist roles because functions vary according to the size and organizational philosophy of the school system, and the level of language training of teachers and other team members. In general, however, the professional skills of the language/communication specialist should extend across the full range of activities discussed in Chapter Four (assessment), Five (planning), Six (design), and Eleven (integration). In working with teachers and parents within the framework of the transdisciplinary team, the specialist must recognize that precise professional operation alone will not assure optimal language intervention procedures. The language/communication specialist is also responsible for designing program evaluation and data gathering procedures to refine and improve the services.

The teacher, as discussed in Chapter Eleven, has a number of critical role functions that include (a) sharing information; (b) soliciting suggestions for routine daily activity; (c) implementing recommendations; (d) documentating progress; and (e) revising curricula. These activities posit the teacher as the one who actualizes the help of the specialist in teaching the children. The teacher is also usually the primary interface with the home, sharing information with parents, and devising home programs.

> The teacher is the actualizer who teaches the children, shares with parents, and combines activities.

These suggestions place the teacher in the center of the transdisciplinary process as the person responsible for integrating language and communication activities with overall curriculum.

The teacher's efforts to directly instruct language can be enhanced by these reminders (Mattick, 1977): (a) the language of all children can be improved; (b) language can be enhanced by provision of naturally occurring experiences in an encouraging classroom environment; (c) frequent verbal transactions are essential to learning language; (d) encourage both comprehension and production skills; (e) if important topics are creatively arranged, they are likely to be prolonged; (f) both the quality and the quantity of communicative experience is important to language development; (g) frequent peer experiences enhance interaction skills in children of all ability levels; and (h) the most important language teaching strategy is to listen with interest to the child's communications, regardless of their quality.

Parents should participate according to their motivation. Minimally, they should share information and extend the activities of teachers and specialists.

The obvious trend toward parental involvement is supported by documented results showing home-based or home-supported programs to be generally effective. Hawkins and Hawkins (1981), however, urge professional planning in accordance with parental motivations. The best plan may be to suggest a small number of teaching tasks each day. The tasks should have the following characteristics: (a) they should be brief, requiring no more than three or four minutes each; (b) their ultimate value should be obvious to the parents; (c) they should fit into daily home routine rather than require special training sessions; (d) they should be tasks that cannot be accomplished if training is limited to the classroom environment.

In conclusion, the complexities of language and the needs of special learners have influenced, and will continue to influence, the nature and directions of language intervention. Increased production of practical, reliable, and validated programs will depend on whether consumers (teachers, communication specialist, and parents) continue to demand more effective and efficient designs. The future of language acquisition research and language intervention techniques is as much your responsibility as a consumer as it is the responsibility of researchers.

REFERENCES

HAWKINS, R.P., & HAWKINS, K.K. Parental observations on the education of severely retarded children: Can it be done in the classroom? *Analysis and Intervention in Developmental Disabilities,* 1981, *1*(1), 13–22.

MATTICK, I. The teacher's role in helping young children develop language competence. In C.B. Cazden (Ed.), *Language in Early Childhood Education.* Washington, D.C.: National Association for the Education of Young Children, 1977.

NIETUPSKI, J., SCHEUTZ, G., & OCKWOOD, L. The delivery of communication therapy services to severely handicapped students: A plan for change. *Journal of the Association for the Severely Handicapped,* 1980 *5*(11), 13–23.

SCHIEFELBUSCH, R.L. Language training strategies for retarded children. In D.V. Sankar (Ed.), *Mental Health in Children,* Vol. III. Westbury, N.Y.: PJD Publications LTD, 1976.

SCHIEFELBUSCH, R.L. A philosophy of intervention. *Analysis and Intervention in Developmental Disabilities,* 1981, *1,* 373–388.

SCHIEFELBUSCH, R.L. Language intervention: What is it? In D. Yoder, J. Miller, & R.L. Schiefelbusch (Eds.) *Language Intervention.* Rockville, Md.: American Speech-Language-Hearing Association, 1983.

NAME INDEX

SUBJECT INDEX

Contributors

Linda McCormick is an Associate Professor of Special Education at the University of Hawaii and Coordinator of the Early Childhood Handicapped Graduate Teacher Preparation Program. She received her Ph.D. from George Peabody College of Vanderbilt University in 1973. In addition to primary professional commitments to early language acquisition and infant and preschool intervention, she has published numerous articles on, and consults to, application of the transdisciplinary service delivery model. Prior to joining the faculty of the University of Hawaii, Dr. McCormick was a member of the graduate faculty at the University of Alabama in Birmingham and was associated there with the Center for Developmental and Learning Disorders. She is currently a consultant to numerous public and private agencies in Hawaii, providing workshops and teaching courses for various universities in the South Pacific, an active member of several professional organizations, and reviewer for numerous journals.

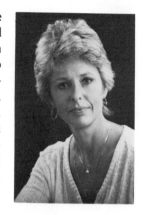

Richard Schiefelbusch is a University Distinguished Professor of Speech-Language-Hearing and Director of the Bureau of Child Research and the Kansas Center for Mental Retardation and Human Development at the University of Kansas. He received his Ph.D. from Northwestern University in 1951. He has directed a series of funded research projects and programs focused on language and communication disorders of retarded, culturally deprived, perceptually impaired, learning disabled, and language-deviant children. He has also directed research training and clinical training projects in these areas. He has edited a series of books on procedures and strategies for language intervention. Concurrently, he has prepared articles, chapters and monographs on language and communication topics and has lectured widely in the United States, Latin America, Japan, Israel, Great Britain, France, and the Netherlands. He has received the honors of the American Speech-Language-Hearing Association and the Special Award of the American Association on Mental Deficiency. He is listed in *Who's Who, Leaders in Education, The World Who's Who of Au-*

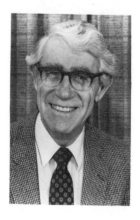

413

thors, American Men and Women of Science, and *The Directory of American Scholars.* Currently he is on the editorial board of six scholarly journals.

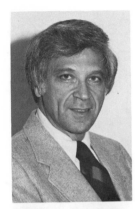

Ronald Goldman, who received his Ph.D. from the University of Pittsburgh, is Professor of Biocommunications at the University of Alabama in Birmingham and Director of Training at the Center for Developmental and Learning Disorders in Birmingham. He is a member of numerous professional and scholarly organizations, and the recipient of many awards and honors. He is a member of the editorial boards of several publications in the field of language disorders.

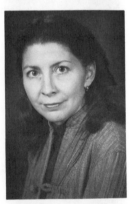

Diane Bricker received her doctorate from George Peabody College. Currently, Dr. Bricker is Professor of Special Education and Director of the Early Intervention Program at the Center on Human Development at the University of Oregon in Eugene. Her list of publications indicates many of her research interests: the high-risk infant; language intervention for communicatively handicapped infants and young children; personnel training; and intervention and integration of handicapped preschool children into curriculum settings.

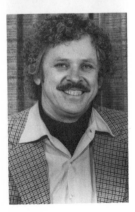

Kenneth F. Ruder, who received his Ph.D. in communication sciences from the University of Florida, is presently a research associate in the Bureau of Child Research, an associate professor of linguistics, and an associate professor of speech-language and hearing at the University of Kansas. Dr. Ruder has published widely on language training and language acquisition and has produced three films: *Where to Start with Non-Verbal Children, Perspectives on Language Training,* and *Comprehension and Production: A Study of the Acquisition of Color Terms.* His current major scientific interest is psycholinguistics and language intervention.

Betty Hazard Bunce has been a kindergarten teacher, a research assistant for the Bureau of Child Research at the University of Kansas, a co-coordinator of the Varsity House Language Preschool, a clinical supervisor and a speech-language pathologist. She is presently working on her doctorate in speech-language pathology at the University of Kansas. She has presented several workshops on language training and published several papers. Her present professional interests include articulation training and research, language training and research, and reading research.

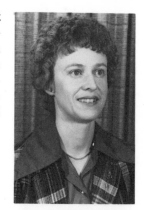

Charlotte Collins Ruder received an M.S. in Speech and Hearing from the University of Wisconsin in 1964. She was employed as a pediatric audiologist at Eye and Ear Hospital at the University of Pittsburgh and as a clinical supervisor and instructor in the Department of Speech and Hearing at the University of Florida. For the past ten years she has been employed as a research assistant at the Bureau of Child Research in the area of language training and as a coordinator of a language training research preschool for language delayed children. Currently she is a teacher of the hearing impaired for the Lawrence, Kansas school district.

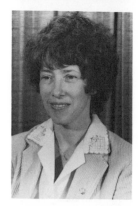

Marilyn Mulligan is Project Coordinator-Curriculum Development for the Project for Deaf-Blind Youth and Courtesy Assistant Professor in the Department of Special Education at the University of Kansas, where she also earned her Ph.D. She has published articles, chapters, and monographs, given workshops and presentations, and is a member of many organizations devoted to the language problems of the handicapped. She serves on the board of editors of the *Journal of the Association for the Severely Handicapped.*

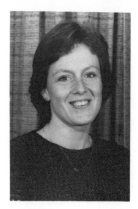

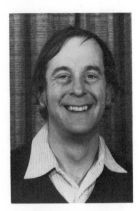

Phillip Douglas Guess is a professor in the Department of Special Education at the University of Kansas, where he received his Ed.D. He has published books, papers, articles and chapters on the communication problems of the handicapped, and, from 1981 to 1983, he was the editor of the *Journal of the Association for the Severely Handicapped.*

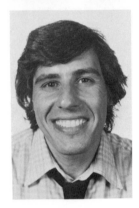

Howard Shane is Director of Speech Pathology and Audiology, Developmental Evaluation Clinic, of Children's Hospital Medical Center in Boston. He is also Associate in Pediatrics at the Harvard Medical School and an associate professor at Emerson College in Boston. In his work on communication methods, Dr. Shane has given seminars and workshops all over the country, published numerous articles and papers, and served as a consultant to many organizations. He received his doctorate in speech pathology from Syracuse University.

Glossary

Accommodation   The mental process through which an organism's existing cognitive repertoire changes and modifies in accordance with new and different information.

Aphasia   Acquired language disorder caused by brain damage, resulting in partial or complete impairment of language comprehension, formulation, and use for communication.

Assimilation   The process, complementary to accommodation, through which new information and new experiences are incorporated into an organism's existing cognitive repertoire.

Association   A strategy for increasing long-term memory; new event or events to be remembered are deliberately linked to similar and easily recalled categories of events.

Augmentative communication   Nonspeech communication which may be either aided or unaided depending upon the individual's congitive and motor abilities.

Autism   A syndrome of developmental disabilities involving multiple perceptual, cognitive, and language disturbances, extreme social isolation and such behavioral excesses as self-stimulation.

Categorical knowing   Knowing the different categories a word can belong to, based on its semantic, perceptual, or functional attributes.

Cerebral palsy   The term applied to a general category of motor deficits resulting from brain damage prior to age 6.

Chaining   A procedure to teach complex behaviors by linking together a series of responses already in the child's repertoire; as each step is mastered, reinforcement is shifted to the next step of the series.

Chunking   A strategy for grouping related bits of information for easier retrieval from short- or long-term memory.

Cognitive knowledge   The mental organization of sensory impressions into perceptually and/or functionally equivalent categories or concepts.

Communication   The encoding of a message to stimulate meaning in the mind of another and the accurate decoding of the intended meaning of others; entails an *exchange* of ideas and intentions.

Content   The semantic or meaning aspect of language—mental representations of objects, events, and relations linked to and expressed through language.

Communicative readiness   Refers to behaviors such as gazing at the adult, head orientation, leaning toward the adult while vocalizing or gazing, pausing in activities upon hearing an adult voice, etc., which are evidence that the child is prepared to participate in a communicative exchange.

Comprehension   Understanding what a word or series of words means; the association of sound sequences with appropriate concepts.

Concept formation   Mental activity of interpreting, transforming, organizing and comparing selected sensory information into nonlinguistic and linguistic categories; the process of mental representation.

Context   The social, linguistic and/or physical circumstances surrounding a particular event.

Design   A specification of environments, strategies, and operations to affect desired intervention outcomes.

Discrimination   Differential responding controlled by the relevant features and properties of environmental stimuli or events.

Duration recording   A behavioral assessment procedure used to measure the length of time a target behavior occurs; data may be reported in seconds, minutes, or percentages.

Extended knowing   Knowing something about the range of objects and events that a particular word can refer to.

Fading   The gradual removal of instructional supports and assistance—called prompts, cues, or correctional procedures—so that the desired behavior is performed independently (with only naturally occurring supports).

Features   A set of constituent elements or attributes that accounts for what the child knows about the meaning of a word.

Form   The "how" element of language—includes phonology, morphology, syntax, and the means for linking sounds with meaning.

Function   In speech act theory, function refers to the purpose or desired effect of an utterance—the act which an utterance is intended to perform.

Generalization   Stimulus generalization is the carryover or extension of trained behaviors (e.g., words, signs, gestures) to new situations (with different persons, in different settings with different stimuli and removed in time from training.) Response generalization is the use of newly acquired skills to expand existing repertoires.

Grammar   (1) A theory, or hypothesis, about the organization of language in the mind of speakers of that language—the underlying knowledge which permits understanding and production of language. (2) Language usage relative to some standard of linguistic etiquette.

Holophrastic utterance   Single word used by a child to convey what an adult would say with a sentence.

Iconic symbol   A word, gesture, sign, or picture which closely resembles that which it refers to or represents.

Imagery   A strategy for storing information in long-term memory which involves visualizing (imagining a picture of) either the event or events to be remembered or something that symbolizes the event(s).

Integrated therapy   Instruction provided in the classroom and/or other natural environments where the target behaviors are ultimately to be performed—facilitates generalization and teacher-therapist exchange of information and skills.

Interval recording   A behavioral assessment procedure in which the observation period is divided into equal time intervals; it permits relatively precise measurement of low and medium rates of responding.

Language   "Knowledge of a code for representing ideas about the world through a conventional system of arbitrary signals for communication."[1]

Language Acquisition Device (LAD)   Chomsky's explanation or theory of the origins of language; characterized as a set of rules or underlying principles for forming sentences, and procedures for discovering how these principles apply to the particular language to which the child is exposed.

Latency recording   A behavioral assessment procedure in which the time that elapses between stimulus and response initiation is recorded.

Learning disabilities   "A disorder in one or more of the basic psychological processes involved in understanding or in using language, spoken or written, which may manifest itself in an imperfect ability to listen, think, speak, read, spell..." (Section 5(b)(4) of P.L. 94–142).

Learning strategies   Activities undertaken by an individual to cope with the requirements of a task or to solve a problem—cognitive responses intermediary between sensory input and language.

Lexicon   A speaker's mental dictionary which includes words and information about their meanings, pronunciation, and associations.

Linguistics   The scientific study of language to describe its elements and the way it works.

Mand   A functional class of verbal behavior such as demanding, commanding, requesting, and asking which usually is acted on by the hearer.

Mean Length of Utterance (MLU)   A method for quantifying language development—most reliable as an index of linguistic competence when children produce sentences with fewer than four words.

Metalinguistic knowing   Knowing about a word—that it is composed of sounds, inflections, etc.

Mode   Refers to the particular method of communication, i.e, oral mode (speech), manual-motor mode (pointing, gesture, signing, finger spelling, writing), ocular mode (directional eye movements).

Modality   Refers to the particular sensory channel (i.e., visual, auditory, tactile) through which information is received or transmitted.

Modeling   An instructional procedure wherein a demonstration of the desired response (motor or verbal) is provided by the teacher.

Morphology   The study of words and their meaningful units, i.e., roots, prefixes, suffixes, etc., and the rules for forming words out of morphemes.

Narrative recording   A behavioral observation method which entails continuous and precise description of relevant behaviors and setting events as they occur.

Object permanence   The understanding that objects continue to exist even when not immediately perceptible.

Overextension   The overgeneralization of a word to inappropriate objects, events, or contexts.

Paralanguage   Refers to suprasegmental phenomena such as laughter, crying, sighs, and whining which are used to signal emotional and attitudinal aspects of communication.

Phoneme   The smallest sound unit in a language that signals a meaningful difference; phonemes are divided generally into consonants and vowels.

Phonology   The study of the system of speech sounds employed by native speakers of a language.

Pragmatics   Study of the rules governing how language is used in social contexts.

Program environment   The teaching context designed to support instructional operations and strategies.

Program operations   The procedures and technology used in planning, maintaining, and evaluating an instructional program.

Program strategies   Program and procedural responses which derive from consideration of the child's strengths and capabilities.

Prompt (or Cue)   These two terms are often used interchangeably to denote stimuli which function to assist or "prime" a desired response; a prompt is not effective unless it occasions the desired response and eventually can be removed without weakening the desired response.

Prosodic features   Those tonal/rhythmic characteristics of language that are used to signal word and sentence differences.

Psycholinguistics   The scientific study of language acquisition, general language behavior and psychological mechanisms, especially how language influences and is influenced by memory, attention, and perception.

Reciprocal actions   A jointly or mutually regulated system in which each member adapts behavior to dovetail with the other.

Referent   The person, action, or event to which a word refers and for which it serves as a symbol.

Referential knowing   Knowing the object or event to which a word refers, and also the range of objects or events to which it can be extended.

Rehearsal   A memory strategy involving the covert practice of units to be remembered.

Reinforcement   Any event that immediately follows a response and has the effect of increasing the probability that the response will be repeated.

Relational knowing   Knowing the meanings a word assumes when used with other words.

Representational systems   Nonalphabetic symbol systems that rely primarily on pictures and line drawings.

Semantics   Study of language meaning and how it is acquired; the semantic component of language includes meanings and rules for linking meaning with words and with word sequences (phrases and sentences).

Semantic knowledge   That subset of cognitive knowledge or those mental representations which have become properly linked to words or sequences of words.

Shaping   The process of reinforcing closer and closer approximations to a desired terminal response.

Skill cluster   A group of trials (tasks) sequenced in a logical relationship to each other and useful across a variety of environments.

Sociolinguistics   The study of how language varies in relation to social situations and cultures.

Speech   The phonatory-articulatory language mode: one media/means of realizing or expressing language.

Speech act   The basic unit of analysis in pragmatics—an intentional verbally encoded social gesture directed by one person to another.[2]

Suprasegmental features   The tonal/rhythmic characteristics of language such as intonation contour (where stress is placed on a word, phrase, or sentence), pitch, and rhythm or pause time.

Syntax   Sentence structure, i.e., word order, inflections, and relationships between words; syntactic rules specify which strings of words are acceptable and which are not.

Telegrahic speech   Term used to describe early sentences which tend to resemble telegrams—articles, prepositions, and conjunctions are frequently omitted while nouns and verbs are overrepresented.

Time sampling   A behavioral observation method where data are scored at the end of equally spaced intervals rather than during the intervals.

Transformations   Operation for generating an infinite variety of sentences from five basic deep structure sentence patterns.

Use   The "why," "when," and "where" of language—its pragmatic or social exchange dimension.

---

[1]Bloom, L., & Lahey, M. *Language development and language disorders.* New York: John Wiley & Sons, 1978. p. 4

[2]Garvey, C. *Play.* Cambridge, Mass.: Harvard University Press, 1977.